Chronic RELIEF

A Guide to Cannabis for the Terminally and Chronically Ill

By Nishi Whiteley

Disclaimer

The contents of this book, all text, graphics, images, tables, and studies are for informational purposes only. The content is not meant to be a substitute for professional medical advice, diagnosis, or treatment.

This book is written as an introductory guide to cannabis. You are urged to read all the referenced studies, books, websites, and videos to deepen your understanding of cannabis.

This information is not meant to prevent, alleviate, or cure any disease or disorder. Always seek the advice of a physician, doctor or chiropractor, or other qualified health provider with any questions you may have regarding a medical condition.

This information is not intended to promote the misuse of cannabis or any other drug. If you suspect you are abusing drugs, we urge you to seek professional medical help.

Neither the publisher nor the author shall be liable or responsible for any loss or damage allegedly arising from any information or suggestion within this book or on our website.

Chronic Relief: A Guide to Cannabis for the Terminally and Chronically Ill
Author: Nishi Whiteley
Foreword: Ethan Russo, M.D.
Editors: Kurt Wilson and Anne Tara Szostek
Index: Theresa Raymond
Cover & Interior Design: Jeanette Dickens
Cover Photo: Mojave Richmond, Enhancements by Drew Rice

ISBN: 978-0-9971491-0-4
PCN/LCCN: 2016947106
Publisher: Alivio, LLC
Austin, Texas

Website: *http://mychronicrelief.com*

This book is dedicated to my parents,
James and Nadine Whiteley, for their
remarkable example of true love
in sickness and in health.

Contents

Foreword xi

Disclaimer xv

Prologue xvii
    Intention xvii
    Why Chronic Relief xviii
    Coming Full Circle xviii
    I Wish I Were a Fairy Godmother xix
    Why Does This Book Matter? xx
    How to Use This Book xxi

Chapter One: NADINE: 1
    Moving Nadine Forward 4

Chapter Two: Cannabis Introduction:
Is It Snake Oil or Real Medicine? 7
    The Difference between Medical Marijuana and Hemp 12
    An Abbreviated History of Cannabis 15
    Cannabis Prohibition: Rooted in Fear,
        Greed, and Misinformation 17
    The Cannabis Revolution 23
    Pioneers of the Cannabis Movement 25
    Legality 27
    The DEA Ignores Their Own Advisors 29

Chapter Three: The Science of Cannabis 33
    The Endocannabinoid System – The Reason Cannabis Works 37
        The Cannabinoid Receptors 39
        Agonist and Antagonist 41
        Endocannabinoids: AEA and 2AG 42
    Introducing the Cannabinoids 43
        Therapeutic Effects of Various Cannabinoids 50
    Decarboxylation – How to Activate Cannabis 52
    Terpenes 53
        Therapeutic Effects of Select Terpenes 56
    Fingerprinting 59

Chapter Four: Your Body's Control Center **61**
The ECS: Our Internal Harm Reduction System 61
The Nervous System. 62
    Feed Your ECS with Essential Fatty Acids 65
The Brain: The Master Organ 65
    Neurotransmitters 66
    Keeping the Brain Healthy 67
    Aging in the Brain and Body 69
    Protecting the Brain as You Age. 71
Cognition. 72

Chapter Five: The Common Denominators of Illness **75**
Oxidation. 75
Inflammation 77
    Monitoring Inflammation through Blood Testing 79
    Inflammation Related Disease 80
    How Cannabis Reduces Inflammation 82
Pain. 84
    My Story: Using Cannabis to Manage Pain 85
    Relieving Chronic Pain 87
    The American Pain Epidemic. 95

Chapter Six: Diseases and Symptoms
Benefited by Cannabis. **99**
Cancer 99
Anxiety and Depression 101
Neurodegenerative Disorders. 103
ALS. 103
Elder Care and Alzheimer's. 104
Post-Traumatic Stress Disorder (PTSD) 107
Other Conditions Cannabis Can Help 109
Why Is Cannabis So Safe? 113
The Research Conundrum 114
Why It's Harder to Research Cannabis than LSD. 116
Chasing the Research Rabbits. 119

Chapter Seven: The Benefits of Whole Plant Cannabis vs.
Currently Legal Medicines and Intoxicants **123**
Cannabis vs. Prescription Pharmaceutical Medications 123
Cannabis vs. Alcohol 126
Cannabis vs. Tobacco. 129
    Cannabis and the Lungs 132

Chapter Eight: Cannabis Guide **137**
What Is Your Health Strategy? 137
    Checklist for Better Living 141

Prevention Plan 143
Recovery Plan. 144
Maintenance and Management Plan. 145
Disease Curing Plan 147
Palliative Care Plan 148
Risks, Side Effects, and How You Might Feel – What to Expect . . . 149
Risks and Harm Reduction. 149
Possible Positive Effects. 154
Contraindications and Cautions –
Who Should NOT Use Cannabis?. 160
Before You Inhale or Ingest. 166
Don't Let Perfect Be the Enemy of Good 169
Using the Whole Plant: Making the Most of Your Medicine 170
Cannabis Plant Uses 171
Varieties: Indica vs. Sativa 172
Potency and Quality. 174
What to Buy?. 176
What to Ask For 177
Weights and Pricing. 178
Mold, Bacteria, and Other Biologicals. 178
Storage 179
Antidotes 180
Intake Methods. 180
Ingestion for Lasting Relief. 194
Raw Cannabis 195
Cannabis Oil 196
Is Hemp Oil the Same as Concentrated Cannabis Oil? 197
How Is Concentrated Cannabis Oil Made? 197
How to Use Cannabis Oil 199
The Rise of Concentrated Cannabis Oil –
The Rick Simpson Story 201
Is Concentrated Cannabis Oil Right for Me?. 202
Tinctures and Extractions 204
Ethanolic Extraction Recipe. 206
Dosing with Tinctures. 207
Cannabis Tea Recipe 209
Cannabis Gel Caps. 209
Suppositories. 211
Dosing and Titration Best Practices 214
Finding the Ideal Therapeutic Dose Range 216
Making Sense of Dosing with Dried Buds 217
Dosing with Edibles. 220
Dosing with Dispensary Edibles 221
Dosing Homemade Edibles 222
Tolerance 223
Sensitizing and Re-Sensitizing the Endocannabinoid System. . 223

Re-sensitizing the Endocannabinoid System. 224
Cannabis Analysis 225
Know Your Testing Lab 228

Chapter Nine: Onward **231**
The American War on People Who Use Drugs 231
Your Voice Counts 234
Three Simple Ways to Use Your Voice. 235
Tips for Talking about Cannabis with Friends and Family 236
Dispelling Cannabis Propaganda. 238
Conclusion. 240

Acknowledgements **245**

Cookbook Extra **249**
Nutrition Is Key! Tips for Healing the Body with Food 249
Kitchen Must Haves for Patients and Caregivers. 254
How to Make Basics. 256
  Butter. 256
  Vegetable Glycerin Tincture Recipe 258
  Cannabis Cooking Tips!. 259
Drinks 260
  Green Drink. 260
  Happy Apple Seed 260
  The Kiwi 261
  Peppermint or Lavender Fizz. 261
  Lemonade 262
  Snickerdoodle Smoothie 262
  The Smooth Tropical. 263
Breakfast 264
  Hot Oatmeal. 264
  Cold Oatmeal. 264
  Quiche. 265
  Two Minute Egg Tower. 266
  Sautéed Apples 267
Condiments. 268
  Pesto. 268
  Lemon Edamame Spread 268
  Croutons 269
Dressings 270
  Garlic Lemon Dressing. 270
  Dijon Dressing. 270
  Blueberry Balsamic 271
Appetizers and Basics. 272
  Cheese Bread 272
  Soda Bread (Gluten Free) 272

Hummus 273
Soups 275
   Sweet Potato Soup with Cilantro Cream 275
   Beef and Barley Soup. 275
   Lentil Soup 276
   Ecuadorean Quinoa Stew 276
Main Dishes. 278
   Cilantro Beef. 278
   Chicken Pot Pie 278
   Veggie Beef Turnovers. 280
   Tuna Noodle Casserole 280
   Green Chicken Enchiladas 281
   Sautéed Cabbage and Sausage 283
   Parmesan and Herb Pasta 283
   Herb Spring Rolls. 284
   Black Gold Chili. 284
Sides and Salads 286
   Squash Ribbon Salad. 286
   Quinoa Tabouli 286
   Broccoli Slaw. 287
   Herbed Rice 287
   Stir Fried Rice. 287
   Robin Hood Corn 288
   Baked Broccoli with Lemon Garlic Sauce. 288
   Spaghetti Squash 289
   Fiery Mashed Sweet Potato. 289
   Sautéed Kale with Balsamic Reduction. 290
Dessert 291
   Elaine's Pastry Crust 291
   Apple Crumble Pie. 292
   Oatmeal Chocolate Cookies. 292
   Foster Styled Bananas 293
   Mexican Chocolate Sauce 311
   Chocolate Torte 294
   Gluten Free Brownie 295

Appendix. 297
   Email to Friends - Moving Nadine Forward. 297

Bibliography 301

Index 317

Foreword
by Ethan B. Russo, MD

Cannabis has been documented as a medicinal plant for four thousand years or more, and between 1840 and 1940, enjoyed a century as a mainstream pharmaceutical throughout the civilized world. Its modern prohibition in the USA in the last 75 years is a historical aberration, a political decision despite the expressed testimony of the American Medical Association that it should remain in the pharmacopoeia. That ban was ruled unconstitutional by the US Supreme Court in 1969, only to be instituted once again in the following years despite the expressed scientific enquiry of the Shafer Commission that recommended its decriminalization and availability for medicinal use. Cannabis was last reviewed scientifically by the World Health Organization in 1965, just one year after the discovery of its primary psychoactive component, tetrahydrocannabinol, THC, with no subsequent follow-up despite the availability of decades of additional data. Although this plant is easily grown and provides a versatile fabric and extraordinarily nutritious seed, it has still been forbidden to cultivate or possess in most nations. It is often falsely claimed that there is no proof of medical benefit for cannabis. In truth, a 2011 assessment by the International Association for Cannabinoid Medicines yielded 34 pages of clinical trial study data and reports attesting to its efficacy and safety with no attributable major toxicity or mortality *(http://www.cannabis-med.org/english/studies.pdf)*. The pejorative view of this plant has so poisoned political opinion that it has almost completely suppressed knowledge of the endocannabinoid system (ECS), a fundamental physiological system. That prejudice has ensured that the ECS is rarely covered in medical school curricula ostensibly merely because its name is based upon that very plant. Thus, another generation of physicians remains ignorant of a critical topic that portends to provide relief from medicine's many recalcitrant disorders that beg for improved therapy. Patients around the world have decried denial of the availability of cannabis-based medicines as a violation of their most basic human rights to access its ability to provide palliation of their pain and suffering.

The discovery of the endocannabinoid system in the last decade of the 20th century has provided the rational basis for understanding the therapeutic value of cannabis and its components. The role of the ECS in modulating virtually every aspect of human physiology to maintain homeostatic balance explains the myriad claims that patients around the world have made in relation to cannabis as an analgesic, sleep-aid, anti-inflammatory agent, anti-nausea drug, anticonvulsant, gastrointestinal remedy, autoimmune disease palliative, anti-spasticity drug, primary chemotherapeutic agent in cancer, antidepressant, anti-anxiety and even antipsychotic. While the primary psychoactive chemical of cannabis, tetrahydro-cannabinol (THC) is often vilified, fear of its adverse effects has been constantly exaggerated in perpetuation of a global political agenda based on an extremely shaky foundation anchored solely on ideology and a political agenda, rather than on science. Worse, it has impeded necessary research into cannabis therapeutics, especially regarding another key cannabinoid, the non-intoxicating cannabidiol (CBD), whose analgesic and anti-inflammatory activity complement those of THC, but which also counteracts many THC side effects such as anxiety and tachycardia.

Longer life spans and toxic exposures have both contributed to an epidemic of cancer in humans and our companion animals. The usual and customary approach to chemotherapy involves use of cytotoxic agents in the hope that they will kill all the cancer but not the patient nor their other critical organs and function. While therapeutic advances are clear with this approach, it remains a terrible ordeal for the affected patient, and one sometimes worse than the disease itself. Current research supports the promise of cannabinoids in treating cancer much more selectively, as these drugs are capable of targeting malignant cells, and diminishing their blood supply without corresponding damage to the surrounding normal tissues. To date, research on the cannabinoids has been slow to take hold in oncology because of intellectual property issues coupled with an irrational fear of the psychoactivity of THC and the plant from whence it came.

The prohibition of a fabulously therapeutic plant has denied a palliative and potentially curative healing agent to millions of people around the globe, and simultaneously criminalized and alienated countless people who deign to employ it for whatever reason. In doing so, it has also removed the hempen shirt from their back and nourishing hempseed from their mouths. The attempts to eradicate this prolific plant in a continuing culture war have poisoned the landscape, eliminated livelihoods, and pitted neighbor against neighbor. The costs to society have been astronomical, with no demonstrable gain. Instead a major crime against humanity and crime against nature have been perpetrated and perpetuated.

Contemporaneously, Sativex° (USAN: nabiximols), an oromucosal whole cannabis-based medicine containing roughly equal proportions of THC and CBD as well as terpenoids is approved for treatment of spasticity in multiple sclerosis in 27 countries around the world, and is also approved for pain in MS and cancer pain unresponsive to optimized opioid treatment in Canada. Additionally, Epidiolex°, a purified cannabidiol extract is currently in Phase III clinical trials in the intractable pediatric epilepsies, Dravet and Lennox-Gastaut syndromes, with a notable benefit. These medicines prove that properly constituted cannabis-based medicines can fulfil all the necessary requirements for safety, quality, consistency and efficacy required of any pharmaceutical. In so doing, they underscore that the prohibitions placed on cannabis are fatally flawed and deleterious to public health around the globe.

It is the proper time for the international community to recognize its error, and end the prohibition of cannabis so that it can meets its potential as food, fiber, and pharmaceutical. It is only in this manner that cannabis can be legally regulated and fundamental human rights for medical treatment of personal choice can be restored.

The book that you hold in your hands provides testament to these principles. There are countless volumes on the topic of cannabis, written with widely disparate points of view and emphases. Nishi Whiteley has provided a great service in delivering a clear and refreshing voice and orientation to the subject of cannabis, born of necessity, and answering the critical questions: If I or my loved one suffer from an illness that "conventional medicine" has failed to treat adequately, might cannabis help, and if so, how would I go about using it properly? In addressing these questions, she has accurately portrayed the scientific literature on cannabis and "brought it down to Earth" in a very heartfelt and personal account that will be accessible to a much wider audience beyond the academic world. My hope is that it will be widely read, not only by patients and their families, but by thought leaders and politicians that may take its message to heart and positively change direction on cannabis policy in this country and around the world.

Disclaimer

I am not a medical or legal professional. **The information in this book does NOT constitute nor replace sound medical or legal advice.** I've taken every precaution to ensure the information I share is rooted in science and, when that is not possible, in sound anecdotal evidence. Although this book has been reviewed by expert cannabis physicians/researchers, reading the book does not replace medical advice. If you are ill or experiencing pain, seek the counsel of a licensed medical professional. If you are unhappy with the first physician you see, keep looking until you find the right one. Trust your instincts!

Cannabis is classified in the U.S. as a Schedule I illegal drug according to the U.S. Controlled Substances Act (CSA). At the time of publication, twenty-five states and the District of Columbia have some sort of medical cannabis law, yet the U.S. government is steadfast in its persecution (yes, I mean that) of cannabis users regardless of state laws. **If you choose to use cannabis, you do so at your own risk—regardless of what your state law says.** I encourage you to understand your rights and the penalties for breaking the law. Visit the *Americans for Safe Access* website for state specific legal information.

While this book is written to educate the public about the therapeutic merits of cannabis and advocate for its therapeutic use, it is important to keep in mind that cannabis is neither a cure-all nor the answer to every ill. Cannabis use does come with risks outlined later in this book.

Prologue

Intention

The purpose of this book is to support the sick and suffering (and their caregivers) in finding relief. This information is not intended to promote the misuse of cannabis (also known as marijuana, sinsemilla, sensi, dank, kind bud, weed, pot, chronic, ganja) or any other drug.

My desire is that this book:

- Provide a starting point for first-time cannabis users.
- Provide evidence about the therapeutic importance of cannabis in order to broaden people's perspectives.
- Bring science to the forefront of the cannabis conversation.
- Reduce fear of cannabis and increase understanding of how it works in the body and why it is a safe and effective medicine.

The U.S. Federal Government's prohibition on cannabis is based on fear, misinformation, and the blatant dismissal of repeated strong scientific evidence showing its therapeutic benefits. This failed policy contributes to the unnecessary suffering of people who could benefit from the medicinal effects of cannabis, makes it more dangerous to acquire, gives power to drug cartels and gangs, and removes a large amount of taxable cash from our legal economy.

Some of the information in this book is readily available by visiting people at dispensaries in states where medical cannabis is legal. However, the level of knowledge varies at every dispensary. For the suffering souls who don't live in those states, it's more difficult to get access to good information. Many mainstream Americans don't have a clue where to start. Instead, they suffer in silence and fear. Does this describe you? If so, this book is for you!

What if we lived in a world where no one had to take legal and personal risks to get needed healthcare and relief? What if we lived in a world where people could afford healthcare? What if the patient's knowledge of their body and what works for them were considered an important part of healthcare and wellness? And what if we lived in a nation where the best and safest medicine was prescribed as the first line of treatment? I hope this book helps us move closer to these possibilities.

Why Chronic Relief

The term "chronic" is generally associated with something negative, ongoing, and habitual. In the context of illness, it refers to the ongoing symptoms of disease and the layer of ongoing negative effects many pharmaceutical medicines can create.

The word "chronic" is also a street term for the highest quality cannabis. In this book, I use the term "chronic relief" in alignment with what I want for all who are suffering: the best possible ongoing, high quality, loving, compassionate, divine, and natural relief —a deliverance from the prison of suffering. I hope "chronic relief" will take on a holistic and symbolic meaning for you as it has for me.

Coming Full Circle

My mother's death from lung cancer in 2010 inspired me to educate others with chronic illnesses about the medical benefits of cannabis. When I first started this project, I was very secretive about it. Before long it became clear that this project is more than a labor of love or passion; it is my duty to use my unique perspective, teaching skills, interest in medicine and integrated therapy, knowledge of health, nutrition, agriculture, and professional marketing background to help educate people about the merits of cannabis.

At the beginning of my writing journey, an unlikely teacher emerged. I call him Sensei, the Japanese word for teacher. The timing of when he came into my family's life was curious—my sister Shana, a restaurant owner, desperately needed help to execute an extended catering contract. Mom had been gone only a year. We were awkwardly trying to find our new normal. This catering job was a great distraction for us because it was so big that we all had to pitch in either at the restaurant or with child care for my nephew. It happened that another local restaurant was closing that day, so my sister called to see if any of their employees needed work. The manager recommended only one person: Sensei.

At the end of the catering project, I served as the designated driver for the catering crew's night out on the town. As Sensei and I came to know one another, we realized each of us had knowledge the other needed. A true friendship was born.

I cannot help wondering if this was the work of Heaven's new angel, my mom Nadine. Sensei has shared so much knowledge with me about cannabis and wholeheartedly encourages me at every turn. Without him I am not sure this book would have been written. He has picked up the phone and responded to emails and texts at all hours. He has answered thousands of questions, told me the truth when others were blowing smoke up my skirt, sniffed out the bull-shitters trying to ride on my coattails, and taught me what goes on in the street, in grow rooms, and inside the criminal justice system as a result of our failed war on drugs.

One of the rabbit trails that characterized our conversations led us down the path of the often taboo topic of religion. I was surprised to discover that Sensei believes in God rather vigorously (maybe more than he wants to admit). He once said, "I am not religious, but spiritual. There is no way one can understand the cannabis plant and still deny that God exists." This statement has stuck with me and in many ways driven my dual path of scientific discovery and my own personal spiritual journey during the four years of writing this book.

I liken writing this book to jumping from a cliff without being able to see what is at the bottom. I've had to trust that I will either grow wings and learn to fly or there will be water at the bottom to break my fall.

Luckily, I have been surrounded by family and close friends who have been supportive, talked me off many a ledge, and politely listened as I rambled on ad nauseam about what I have learned. People have crawled out of the woodwork to share personal stories of pain and suffering and how cannabis gave their lives back. Each story reminds me how fragile life is and how vulnerable we are.

I am grateful to all who supported this project financially, made critical introductions for me at the right time, said yes to my request for interviews, shared recipes and techniques, let me into their grow rooms and homes, answered questions, allowed me to cite their work, and provided legal advice. This book is proof that none of us make great things happen alone.

The irony is not lost on me that Sensei and others showed up in my life at the exact time I needed to learn what they had to teach and when I most needed their support or encouragement. This brings me full circle. Maybe Sensei is right about the divine nature of the cannabis plant and life itself. Through learning how this plant works in the human body, I now find it hard to deny a higher power exists. I am happy to share what I have learned with you.

In many ways this book is the beginning of me: a coming out party for who I am and what I believe with no apologies. So here is a piece of my heart and soul I hope will help others get the relief we all desire, deserve, and need. Every word is written with profound love. It is my hope this work is a ripple in the wave of society's understanding of the therapeutic merits of cannabis resulting in a shift towards sustainable national laws that are good for people, the economy, and most importantly, reducing suffering.

I Wish I Were a Fairy Godmother

Life is about living even when you are dying! And we are all dying. It's about how to live our best lives with dignity, how to live in comfort, and how to savor the sweet miracles of those moments when we are confronted with our mortality and that of those we love, and we find the courage to be completely present, connected, and fearless. I love this well-known quote by an unknown author, which becomes especially poignant when tomorrow becomes an uncertainty: "It's not how many breaths you take but how many moments take your breath away."

Suffering is the singular thing that most disturbs me about the human experience. I've always wanted to be the one who could fix what ails my family and friends—a fairy godmother of sorts. It doesn't work that way. People suffer physical, mental, emotional, and spiritual pain for different reasons. Sometimes I can help. Sometimes I cannot. There was a time I took on the suffering of others as if it were my own, but I have learned that each of us has a different path, and I can only walk my own and support others, when asked, in walking theirs. As I wrestled with my empathy for others, I discovered it is through objectivity about suffering that I can be of greatest service (way easier said than done). When feeling someone else's pain too personally, we are without the full force of our own wellness and thus less able to help them.

Caregivers take note: Energy is like water —a precious resource. Not caring for your loved one from an overflowing cup eventually depletes your resources leaving little for yourself and nothing to share. Then you both go thirsty. Whom does that serve? Remember that your self-care is critical to the person you are supporting. Martyrdom serves no one.

It is through my own suffering, and that of loved ones, that I have found courage to offer this book. While I cannot take away your suffering, and writing this book doesn't heal my heart from the loss of my sweet momma, it is comforting to think this book may help you move beyond pain to a joyful, peaceful place. Oftentimes it is through suffering that we have our greatest opportunities for physical, spiritual, religious, or personal expansion. Suffering is in contrast to the comfort and pleasure we all desire, yet it is often the vehicle that opens the heart to healing and happiness.

I ask you to consider the following:

- How is your current situation leading you to expand your thinking and open your heart?
- How does it expand what you desire?
- How might following your heart's desire and your inner knowing improve your life?

Why Does This Book Matter?

This book matters because too many people suffer severely and unnecessarily from a variety of ailments that are treatable with cannabis. Yet cannabis is misunderstood, wrongly demonized, and undervalued as a medicinal plant. Many legal medicines are ineffective and cause horrible side effects—even death. Cannabis is one of the safest, if not the safest, known medicine. People deserve to know the truth so they can make their own decisions about whether or not to use it for their wellness and their highest good.

The vast majority of people who go into the medical field do so because they want to be healers, yet the healthcare system, which might be more appropriately named the "sickness care system," is not generally designed to support, encourage, or benefit doctors who work to heal their patients—especially when it comes to chronic illness. Let me also point out that pharmaceutical companies make money when their customers are sick; they stop making money when they get well.

Rather than being taught how to heal dis-ease, doctors spend most of their time in medical school learning to manage symptoms. For example, most medical schools teach only three to six hours of nutrition, and they do not teach students about the body's endocannabinoid system (your innate harm reduction system that mimics chemicals in the cannabis plant—more about this later) or cannabis as medicine. In fact, most doctors are taught that cannabis is a dangerous, illicit drug with no medical value.

The point is that you alone are responsible for your health and life. You have the most to gain or lose by being well or getting sick. Do not give this power to your doctor, caregiver, or anyone. Instead, tune in to your body; learn about your ailment—not just what it is doing to you but how it came about. How do mindset, genetics, lifestyle, and environment contribute to where you are? How do you utilize your doctor as a resource and an important part of your wellness team? Recognize that you may need more than one person on your team including physicians, cannabis experts, nutritionists, acupuncturists, counselors, spiritual guides, etc., to achieve the healing you desire. When you are willing to fight for your wellness and actively and carefully choose your medical team, you will attract doctors, nurses, and other healers who will go the extra mile.

How to Use This Book

Chronic Relief is one part research paper, one part personal narrative, and one part guidebook. You can read it from cover to cover or flip around to topics that are most important to you. The book is peppered with my personal stories as well as a few from others who have generously allowed me to share them.

The book begins by explaining how this project came about and my personal evolution on transitioning from a business and marketing consultant to a cannabis educator and author. The "Introduction to Cannabis" chapter is intended to give a comprehensive overview of all that we will explore. In this section you will also find an "Abbreviated Cannabis History" as well as a quick look at "Legality."

My voice changes substantially in the "Science" section. There I am trying to stick to the science but present it in a way that gives everyone a basic context for how and why cannabis works in the body. I hope it will give a foundation for understanding how cannabis can support health and healing. For my fellow cannabis science geeks, hopefully the references will help you down whichever rabbit trail most intrigues you.

What you will not find in this book is a comprehensive explanation of how cannabis can be used for specific ailments. While that is covered in part throughout the book, developments in science are happening too quickly to provide comprehensive coverage of every ailment that could benefit from cannabis. Instead, the book looks at the "Common Denominators of Illness" and how cannabis addresses them.

Cannabis use is commonly compared to using tobacco, alcohol, and prescription drugs. In "The Benefits of Whole Plant Cannabis vs. Currently Legal Medicines and Intoxicants" section, we explore how each item stacks up against cannabis in terms of safety, therapeutic merit, risks, and side effects.

The second half of the book begins with the "Cannabis Users Guide." This section helps you get into the nitty-gritty of applying knowledge gained in the first part of the book. Here I try to help you understand the different intake methods, risks, how to mitigate them, possible benefits, cannabis selection, cannabis use strategy, establishing serving sizes, and cannabis testing.

The conclusion discusses the "American War on People Who Use Drugs" and "Your Voice Counts." I explore what cannabis prohibition is doing to society and how each of us can be part of the solution.

It is impossible to write a truly conclusive text on this topic. Our knowledge about cannabis and its interaction with human biology is growing quicker than one can capture in a single book. The goal is to offer content that is correctly based on what we know today and will remain relevant in the future. I hope this book makes you laugh, touches your heart, answers your most important cannabis questions, gives you the resources you need to dig deeper where questions remain, and that you are empowered to make choices that help you and those you love live better!

Following the conclusion is a collection of recipes. If you are interested in making edibles, these will help. If cannabis edibles are not your thing, you can enjoy these wonderful recipes non-medicated!

Chapter 1

NADINE:
The Inspiration for Chronic Relief

This book began as a cannabis e-cookbook to help those who are suffering and want the therapeutic benefits of cannabis but don't want to smoke. The inspiration came from my mother's experience at the end of her battle with lung cancer. My mom, Nadine, was one of a kind. She would be delighted to know that she inspired this book and honored that her experience might make someone else's life better.

Mom's death has rocked my, my sister's and my dad's world. There are no words to explain the depth of our loss. As I write those words with tears streaming down my face, I hear my mother's voice say, "Aren't we lucky!" She would often nudge me just before saying those words to make sure I looked up and saw her smiling. Just thinking about this reminds me to find joy in the little pleasures of life and be grateful.

Mom and Dad came from meager rural beginnings, so they had an appreciation for what living without certain comforts was like and were keenly aware of life's important things. This was the root of my mom's gratitude for the life she and Dad intentionally created during the forty-three years they were happily married.

When I was in fourth grade, we moved from the inner city of Austin, Texas to our farm outside Pflugerville twenty miles into the countryside in what then seemed the middle of nowhere. My parents bought the farm to provide a better life for my sister and me. This created financial hardship for my parents, as making the move to the farm took everything they had. For several years we didn't have two nickels to rub together, but we had love, a roof over our heads, and a bounty of wonderful freshly grown food. Mom or Dad would often look across the dinner table at our fabulous homegrown spread and say, "I wonder what the rich folks are eating tonight" as if to remind my sister Shana and me that money couldn't buy what we had. That phrase was frequently followed by my mother exclaiming, "Aren't we lucky!" As I reflect, I realize how very lucky we really were.

Mom reveled in our luck and grace. She savored every incredible moment and, in down times, was able to see and show us that things could be worse and that we should focus on our blessings and privileges. My mom was grateful for big and small blessings alike and often reminded us how important it was to count our blessings. After she was diagnosed with lung cancer, I never witnessed her express self-pity. Two things broke my mother's heart about her disease: she didn't want to leave Dad and she wanted to spend more time with her grandson who was four when she passed. She made me promise to teach my nephew about gardening, plants, flowers, books, and travel to help open his eyes to things she had hoped to teach him. I hope this book is a good step in the direction of keeping that promise. And she asked me to hug Dad often, most especially when he was cranky.

At the time of my mom's illness, many in our community were suffering from some disease. People were dying frequently, and many others in our circle were struggling with health in other ways. It would have been easy for Mom to go the route of doom and gloom. Instead, she focused on how lucky she felt and how lucky we all were. "Aren't we lucky," she would repeat.

Many people who pride themselves on being law-abiding citizens wrestle with the questions of the legality and morality of utilizing cannabis, an illegal and "illicit" (if wrongly classified) drug. I did. By this time, my mom was experiencing horrific side effects from chemo and the rapid progression of her disease. It was difficult to watch. When my sister called to say mom had asked for some Kenny Chesney, our code word for cannabis, I had a Norma Rae, Not Without My Child, Erin Brockovich moment; I was determined to do what was best for my mother and our family regardless of the consequences! My "morality" went out the window and down the street to my "happy" friend where, at forty-one years of age, I acquired my first bag of cannabis. In that moment the only important thing was to make my mother comfortable. Where was the morality in letting her suffer—especially when there was something I could do, and she was willing to try it?

Until that day I had never sought cannabis. I was scared of getting caught. What would people think? Would it damage my professional reputation? I could hear the yet unspoken whispers throughout our small community, "Oh, one of the Whiteley kids (remember, I'm over forty) is into cannabis. She says it's for medicinal use, but she's always been a bit of a loner and rule bender. She just wants to get high. What would you expect from someone who has traveled the world and does that yoga stuff? She has always been a bit strange." Blah, blah, blah. I wondered, "Will I go to jail? Gosh, orange is not really my color, and horizontal stripes make me look fat. Will I have to wear one of those unflattering jumpsuits? Will people think I'm a druggie? What if I want to run for office? Will people vote for me?" These questions and more raced through my head.

I had no clue what we needed or where to start. After a few phone calls and a surprise visit to a friendly neighbor's house, I found someone willing to help. Once I had the medicine, I hit the Internet. Surely I could find someone who could tell me what to do with this magical herb. Time was of the essence because Mom was growing more nauseated, agitated, and miserable by the minute.

I cooked fast and did something I never do: follow the directions of a random stoner on the Internet. I generally cook by taste but thought it prudent to take this guy's advice since I was a canna butter making novice. Mom had no desire for anything super sweet, but she liked the idea of peanut butter cookies. Since my nephew is allergic to peanuts, we thought this would be a good starting place for mom and a good way to make sure the little one stayed away from those cookies. From there I made pizza and savory empanadas and experimented with adding the butter to foods that sounded appetizing to her. The cookies and other foods provided her relief from agitation, nausea, lack of appetite, and pain. Cannabis calmed her and relieved suffering in a way morphine and other prescriptions could not. It gave relief where otherwise there was none. Her relief comforted us all.

At first we were very hush-hush about mom using cannabis. I made my then fiancé swear he would not talk about it with our friends. Frankly, I didn't think people would see the topic as "polite conversation" — especially in Texas.

Yet, after seeing her get relief, we were sold, and so was she. The cat slowly found its way out of the bag. In fact, the day before she died she made sure each of her friends who came to visit and was suffering with pain, disease, or any ailment went home with two peanut butter cookies.

Hollering my name from across the house, my mom summoned me to her room. She told her audience I was preparing a care package for them. She gave strict instructions for how each guest was to consume the cookies and made them promise to report back to me with their experience. I think she knew her final relief was coming in a matter of hours but sensed that this could be the beginning of a new kind of relief for her friends. She laid in her bed with a smile on her face nurturing all of those she would soon leave. She made each person feel safe about trying something otherwise taboo and made them feel at peace about walking away from her for the last time. Every person who went home with a goody bag of cookies reported relief!

After my mother's death, I was trying to find a way to share my knowledge about cooking with cannabis. The e-book craze was just beginning, and I thought it was the perfect platform. I wanted an informative introduction to the book, so I started doing research. The more research I did, the more I realized this is an important story that needs telling.

I didn't know then that there are lots of books about cannabis, cooking with cannabis, and growing cannabis and that many of them are incredibly well done. At the time I needed them, they were not easy to find. They would have been had I known where to look, but I didn't. The same was true for information on-line. As a cannabis novice, I needed someone to explain how it could be ingested, the pros and cons of one intake method versus another, and what to expect. It would have been helpful to know what to ask for, how to evaluate quality, how much plant material or butter I could use safely, and so on. We have come a long way since then. Information about cannabis seems to be everywhere, yet it is hard to find almost all you need in one place. This book would have been useful when I was trying to help my mom.

My family and I are mainstream people with regular jobs and lives probably much like yours. We pay taxes, are active members of our community, and are generally law abiding citizens except for that occasional roll through the STOP sign. While we do not fit the stereotype of "stoners," I think it is worth noting that the majority of people who use cannabis and/or support its legalization don't fit the stereotype.

This book is for people like us, people who know there must be better medicines and therapies beyond the conventional treatments doctors are trained to prescribe.

Moving Nadine Forward

Mom died peacefully at home in her favorite place: Dad's arms. Several weeks before her death, doctors told us the time would come soon and to make necessary arrangements. From the time we were kids, my mom told my sister and me that we better not throw her one of those sad sappy downer funerals or "I'll come back to haunt you," she would say with a wry grin. Instead, she requested a celebration where people would come and laugh and talk about the silly things she had done and their good memories of her. My mom was bigger than life. She made every day experiences fun and wanted her going away party to represent that. She didn't want people to waste money on flowers after she was gone. To honor Mom's wishes, my family sent an email (included in the Appendix) titled "Moving Nadine Forward" to our family and friends before her death to encourage them to honor her while she was still around to enjoy it.

The email generated a wonderful response of flowers, stories, cards, and sweet gestures that uplifted us all. Had it not been for the cannabis, I don't think Mom would have been present enough in the last two weeks of her life to have felt the love, respect, and gratitude with which she was so deservedly showered. Cannabis made it possible for her to witness the contributions she had generously made to the lives of those around her. In the few weeks between that email being sent and the day before she died, over $5,000 was donated in her name to the Travis [County] 4-H Scholarship. That brought her much joy. People crawled out of the woodwork to share directly with her and us how she impacted their lives. It was cathartic for us all. I'm deeply grateful my mom had that experience, and my family and I could witness it together. When the time comes, I encourage you to do something similar to celebrate the life of your loved one.

My biggest regret about my mother's care is that we waited until the end of her battle with cancer to try cannabis. I cannot help wondering if she would have felt better, and therefore lived longer, had we used it from the onset of her treatment. Some of my research leads me to believe that, had she ingested cannabis oil, she might have killed the cancer or prevented its spread. Maybe she would still be alive. No matter what, I know she would have lived better, and that is what this book is about—living better.

My mother's life was dedicated to helping others live better, and now, even though she is not here physically, she is still doing that through this book. I offer this information so you may have the benefit of my mother's experience and my learning to help you and those you love live better and die more comfortably.

Chapter Two

Cannabis Introduction: Is It Snake Oil or Real Medicine?

Cannabis is the single most versatile herbal remedy and the most useful plant on Earth. No other single plant contains as wide a range of medically active herbal constituents.
—Ethan Russo, MD

Cannabis (marijuana) is the most popular "illicit" drug in America and the third most popular drug of choice behind tobacco and alcohol. Twenty-five million Americans admit to smoking or ingesting cannabis at least once a year, and over fifteen million are estimated to use it monthly, which totally negates the poorly constructed argument that cannabis is a gateway drug. If that were true, we would have a much bigger hard drug problem. Over 2.2 million Americans have medical cannabis cards in twenty-five states and the District of Columbia, and almost half of Americans live in states that have some sort of a medical cannabis law. Sadly, over 650,000 people per year are arrested on cannabis related charges, most for simple possession.

Cannabis users are doctors, plumbers, housewives, retired veterans, students, elected officials, blue-collar workers, white-collar workers, rich, poor, disabled and not, gay, straight, black, white, brown, and polka dotted. We are represented in every walk of life, educational background, socio-economic level, ethnicity, and religious group. **It is high time** (pun intended) **that we dissolve the contrived cloud of shame, secrecy, and controversy around the use of this legitimate medicine and bring science to the forefront of our cannabis conversation and policies.**

Cannabis is a flowering plant. When grown for medicine, the flowers (also known as buds) and leaves of the female plant are dried and cured resulting in what we generally regard as cannabis or the more commonly used pejorative term "marijuana." Hemp and medicinal cannabis are in the same genus: Cannabis (*Cannabis sativa, Cannabis indica*, and their hybrids). The difference stems from different uses. Hemp is grown for food, including oil and hemp seeds, and for fiber, which is used to make clothing, rope, paper, etc. Medicinal cannabis (sometimes referred to as drug varieties or marijuana) is bred to have larger buds and more psychoactive compounds.

> ## Top Cannabis Expert – Ethan B. Russo
>
> One of the most prolific and respected medical cannabis scientists is Ethan Russo, MD. He is a neurologist, ethnobotanist, international medical cannabis expert, former Senior Medical Advisor for GW Pharmaceuticals, (an international leader in the development of whole plant cannabinoid medicines) and now the Medical Director of PHYTECS (a U.S. plant-based medical therapeutics company focused on creating products that stimulate the ECS), and the person who has written the Foreword to this book. He and his writings contributed greatly to my understanding of cannabis. Many of his papers can be found at *https://www.researchgate.net/profile/Ethan_Russo/publications*.

The highly versatile cannabis plant provides relief from many different ailments and symptoms with a high degree of safety. Does this sound like snake oil? It's not! The reason the plant benefits so many different illnesses and ailments boils down to the fact that its active pharmacological components mimic an internal chemical harm reduction system in the human body that keeps our health in balance: the *Endocannabinoid System.*

The Endocannabinoid System (ECS) is controlled by chemicals our body produces called endocannabinoids. Endocannabinoids are responsible for keeping our most critical biological functions, such as sleep, appetite, pain, and immunity, in balance. When the body gets out of balance and moves into a state of stress, endocannabinoids fix the problem. Pharmaceutically active components in cannabis mimic endocannabinoids and therefore can be effective in helping the body manage crises and restore itself after trauma when the body's endocannabinoids alone are insufficient. For example, take the case of someone suffering from glaucoma. Pressure builds in the eye causing pain and interfering with vision. Over time, a patient may completely lose their sight. At its root, the cause of glaucoma is inflammation. If the endocannabinoid system were functioning properly, it would prevent this. But in this case, and many others, it is not functioning properly. Some outside assistance from cannabis—regardless of intake method—supports the endocannabinoid system by giving it the chemical support needed to reduce inflammation and give relief from pain and impairments to vision.

You are probably wondering, "Why does cannabis benefit so many different illnesses?" The short answer is that cannabis is highly effective at working with the endocannabinoid system, which controls pain and inflammation. Can you think of a disease that does not come with inflammation and pain? I can't.

The cannabis plant happens to be one of the most (if not the most) pharmacologically active plants on the planet containing over four hundred active chemicals. The unique active components are called *cannabinoids*, which are found alongside active chemicals called *terpenoids* (we also refer to them as *terpenes*) and *flavonoids*. These chemical components work together to provide a wide variety of therapeutic benefits.

Various levels and combinations of cannabinoids, terpenoids, flavonoids, and other chemicals present in the plant provide many benefits such as dilating blood vessels, stimulating bone growth, protecting damaged brain cells, killing certain kinds of cancer cells, preventing seizures, and killing viruses and bacteria. It is the combination of varying levels of cannabinoids, terpenes, flavonoids, and other plant chemicals that seems to make the most effective medicine for specific symptoms and dis-eases. Isolated components appear to be less effective. Whether you are recovering from an injury, living with "dis-ease," fighting it, or dying from it, cannabis may provide partial or complete relief from suffering. Cannabis has been found to ease general pain, chemo-induced neuropathy, and nausea as well as increasing appetite and reversing wasting. It is effective in controlling muscle spasms, certain kinds of seizures, healing damaged brain cells, protecting against the ravages of Alzheimer's, and it is an effective antioxidant. Regardless where you are in your health journey, responsible use of cannabis may improve your quality of life and slow the aging process.

U.S. Cannabinoid Patent

Did you know that several chemicals in the cannabis plant are antioxidants? In fact, the second most common cannabinoid, cannabidiol (CBD), is a more powerful antioxidant than vitamins C and E. (McPartland and Russo 2001) It's true! Our government knows this, too. They have a patent for the antioxidant properties and the neuroprotective properties of cannabis. (Hampson, Axelrod and Maurizio 1999)

Cannabis is commonly (but not exclusively) used by people who suffer from:

- Chemo Associated Nausea and Vomiting
- Epilepsy
- HIV/AIDS
- Migraine
- Rheumatic Diseases
- Premenstrual Syndrome
- Severe Morning Sickness
- Alzheimer's
- Cancer
- Glaucoma
- Multiple Sclerosis
- Chronic Pain
- Ulcerative Colitis
- Crohn's Disease
- Phantom Limb Pain
- Depression
- PTSD
- ALS
- Parkinson's

These, and all other chronic issues, are life altering and can greatly diminish ones quality of life while limiting the ability to work, be social, and care for oneself.

Pharmaceutical drugs prescribed for these and other ailments frequently come with side effects that are as bad as the dis-ease or condition itself. For people who find themselves at the end of their pharmaceutical rope (pun intended), cannabis offers new hope of relief from suffering.

Cannabis: Restorative Medicine

Scientific research indicates cannabis and cannabis-based medicines may be highly effective preventative and restorative medicines altering disease progression in certain illnesses such as cancer, diabetes, and depression.

Cannabis not only gives patients a chance to be in control of their relief, it frequently costs less than manufactured drugs and has **NO** lethal side effects. Now don't get me wrong; cannabis is NOT a cure-all, and it definitely does have side effects for certain individuals. It is neither for everyone nor for every condition. *However, its safety profile is superior to any modern pharmaceutical medicine including aspirin.*

Aspirin, originally a plant-based medicine, is one of the most versatile of modern pharmaceutical medicines and has one of the best safety profiles. *Tetrahydrocannabinol* (THC), the widely recognized component of cannabis that causes you to feel "stoned" and the most prominent cannabinoid in American-grown cannabis, has twenty times the anti-inflammatory power of aspirin (and twice that of hydrocortisone). (E. Russo 2011) Approximately one thousand people die annually from complications related to taking aspirin. There are no known recorded fatal doses of cannabis.

Lester Grinspoon, MD, Associate Professor Emeritus of Psychiatry at Harvard Medical School, has long argued that cannabis is "...less toxic than almost any other medicine in the pharmacopeia: it is like aspirin, remarkably versatile." (Grinspoon 2005) Dr. Grinspoon once set out in his research to prove the damaging effects of cannabis. What he found was the opposite of what he expected and had been trained to believe.

In 1967, Dr. Grinspoon's then ten year old son Danny was diagnosed with acute lymphocytic leukemia. Chemo treatments caused him to vomit violently. Dr. Grinspoon and his wife heard about a boy in Houston who was suffering with the same illness and side effects as Danny but was using cannabis to successfully control the symptoms. From then on Danny smoked cannabis twenty minutes prior to his chemo treatments. For the remainder of his life, a year and a half, Danny did not suffer from nausea or vomiting. Dr. Grinspoon realized that many people facing many types of disease are able to get relief with small amounts of cannabis making it possible for them to do normal activity in comfort. How can this be?

Although cannabis is a safe medicinal plant with low toxicity and broad application, it remains illegal at the federal level. In some states the possession of even small amounts of cannabis plant matter can be a felony. It is important to know your state and local laws. Even in states that do not have medical cannabis laws, there is great variability in terms of how cannabis laws are enforced and the associated penalties. Hopefully, landmark votes in Colorado and Washington, and subsequent votes in Alaska and Oregon for full-scale legalization, will trigger a change in our national drug policy, and this will be a moot point. Until then, know your rights, get active, educate others, and vote!

Many people are unaware of the legal consequences conviction of cannabis possession can bear: revocation of your driver's license, disqualification for federal student aid, ineligibility to apply to certain universities, denial of adoption applications, and social stigma in your community by your employer and potential future employers.

I cannot overemphasize the importance of understanding your rights under the Fourth, Fifth, and Sixth Amendments. Nationally respected criminal defense attorney and former police officer Jamie Balagia shares detailed information on his website *www.420dude.com* about how to handle yourself should you have an encounter with the police. Mr. Balagia is a cannabis activist in his spare time and works closely with the San Antonio, Texas chapter of NORML. He says, "Law enforcement can lie to you to get evidence. That is why it is important to know what to do and say when dealing with law enforcement."

Here are a couple of important things to know about communicating with law enforcement officials should you get caught with illegal cannabis:

- Be polite, and keep your hands where they can be seen.
- If questioned, ask if you are being arrested or detained. If the answer is no, walk away.
- If you are being detained, ask why, and remember the officer's response.
- If questioned, say, "I choose to remain silent. I want to see a lawyer." Repeat this every time the officer asks a question.
- If you are in your vehicle and are asked to step out, be sure to close the door so as to not invite a search.
- Should you be asked if law enforcement can search your property, the answer is "I do not consent to a search." If searched without permission, keep repeating this phrase so possible witnesses can hear you.
- If presented a search warrant in your home, step outside and lock the door. Police, DEA, IRS, and other law enforcement can follow you into any room you enter when they have a warrant.
- If searched, do not resist. Keep hands visible, and do not make fast movements.

These are just a few of the important things you should know about protecting your rights under American law. Learn more on the Americans for Safe Access Security Culture webpage. Find a lawyer in your state by visiting *www.norml.org/legal*. Your financial support of these two organizations helps further national cannabis legalization lobbying efforts and the protection of the rights of cannabis users.

The Difference between Medical Marijuana and Hemp

People are often confused about how hemp differs from medical marijuana (which is generally referred to in this book as cannabis) and whether hemp is psychoactive. Both medical cannabis and hemp are known by the botanical name *Cannabis sativa*. Medical cannabis may also be of the species *Cannabis indica* or *Cannabis ruderalis*, but this is an area about which botanists cannot agree. In the medical context, what differentiates "industrial hemp" (oilseed and fiber varieties) from "cannabis" (drug varieties) is not botanical classification but chemical makeup. Most industrial hemp has a THC (the primary psychoactive component) content of 0.2 – 0.4 percent or less. (Mahlbert 2013) Since only cannabis material containing over 2 percent THC is said to provide a psychoactive effect, it is clear that hemp is not psychoactive. (Mahlbert 2013) The DEA argues that any amount of THC is dangerous.

Hemp is a versatile plant. It can be grown for food, oil, fiber, fuel, and a wide variety of industrial products. Hemp, unlike drug varieties of cannabis, is a poor producer of cannabinoids and therefore is an inferior source for CBD and other cannabinoids. It is an excellent rotation crop and helps remediate soil health. Hemp was once widely cultivated throughout the United States. In fact, the Declaration of Independence was drafted on hemp paper, and there was a time when it was illegal for farmers not to grow hemp. (Sloman 1979) Some of the most famous American hemp farmers include George Washington and Thomas Jefferson. Towns across the country were named after hemp: Hemphill, Kentucky and Louisiana and Hempstead, New York and Texas for example. Unfortunately, hemp production was outlawed in the United States in 1937 with a brief return of strategic production during World War II.

Until the spring of 2014, anyone wanting to grow hemp in the U.S. had to apply to the DEA for a license because hemp was not recognized as different from medical cannabis under the Controlled Substances Act. While it was theoretically possible to get a DEA license to grow hemp, the requirements to do so were so strict and unreasonable that only one permit for a quarter acre research plot was ever granted. The passage of the 2014 Farm Bill signals a significant change in American hemp policy making hemp production legal in states that have a state law permitting it.

Under Farm Bill Section 7607, the following states have passed laws that allow growing industrial hemp for research, pilot programs, and even for commercial purposes: California, Colorado, Hawaii, Indiana, Kentucky, Maine, Montana, Nebraska, North Dakota, Oregon, Utah, Vermont, Washington, and West Virginia. The Farm Bill mandated that the state department of agriculture or a university be the certifying body nullifying the need for a license from the DEA. Thus, only farmers in the above listed states, who have followed their state's certification, registration, or license process, can grow hemp in the U.S. The complicating factors are that it is illegal for growers to import seed for sowing hemp and there is no processing infrastructure in place.

Legal Hemp-States

Laws are different in each state. Visit the National Conference of State Legislators website and search State Industrial Hemp Statutes for a complete list of each state's statues on this issue. *Votehemp.com* is another excellent resource for the latest information on this topic.

"This is the first time in American history that industrial hemp has been legally defined by our federal government as distinct from drug varieties of Cannabis," said Eric Steenstra, president of the advocacy group Vote Hemp. (Vote Hemp 2014)

The folks at *www.votehemp.com* say industrial cannabis (hemp) is an agricultural commodity crop while medical cannabis is a horticultural crop. Commodity crops are grown outdoors on a larger scale. A horticultural crop may be grown outdoors or indoors but requires more specific feeding and care. Although the two plants look similar, a trained eye can differentiate hemp fields from cannabis gardens, as the growing methods are completely different. Medical cannabis plants are generally grown as single plants more like an orchard whereas industrial hemp is grown en masse with the seeds sown close together. Individual medical cannabis plants are given great care with specific amounts of water, nutrients, light, and space to thrive. Male plants are discarded when growing medical or recreational cannabis but not when growing hemp. Only the female flowers are used in medical and recreational cannabis. Without being pollinated by male plants, female flowers continue flowering and producing resin, thus increasing the potency of the medicine.

Federal law enforcement contends hemp fields can be hiding places for medical or recreation cannabis plants and therefore hemp should be illegal. Medical cannabis growers will tell you this is laughable, as the two crops cannot be grown well together or even near each other. While the presence of high THC containing medical plants will not impact a hemp crop, hemp plants will happily cross pollinate with medical/recreational cannabis resulting in lower quality and lower potency medicine. Such a sneaky tactic would not be worth the time, money, and risk it would entail.

Over $500 million worth of hemp products are sold in the U.S. annually. (R. Johnson 2013) Since commercial cultivation was outlawed in the 1950s, nearly all the revenue we spend on hemp products goes to producers in the thirty plus countries around the world that allow production of hemp.

Essential Fatty Acids

Essential fatty acids are the building blocks for our own endocannabinoids, so they help our bodies maintain balance.

Several hemp products have become popular in the U.S. including hemp seed kernels and hemp seed oil. Both are currently enjoying a renewed popularity as health foods—and rightfully so. Hemp seeds, like other nut meats, are primarily made of oil. Most nuts and seeds are high in omega-6 essential fatty acids (EFA) and low in omega-3 EFA. The desired ratio of omega-6: omega-3 EFA intake for optimal health is 4:1, yet Western diets are typically too rich in omega-6 with a ratio of 10:1. Hemp seeds contain a 3:1 ratio of omega-6 to omega-3 EFAs thus approaching the most desirable ratio. (E. Russo 2001) And that is not all! Hemp seeds have approximately 33 percent protein (including all the essential amino acids), are high in fiber, dense in vitamins and minerals, easily digested, and their nutrients are easy to absorb and utilize. (Leson 2011) Consuming hemp seeds can help maintain a balanced intake of EFAs. This contributes to reduced risk of atherosclerosis (buildup of fats and cholesterol on artery walls), sudden cardiac death, certain types of cancers, enhanced mood, and reduction in the symptoms of rheumatoid arthritis. (Leson 2011)

It is important to note that hemp seeds do not contain THC. You are probably thinking that with all those benefits hemp foods may taste bad. No! Hemp seeds and oil have a light, nutty flavor. They should be used cold or in low heat cooking.

THC comes from the glandular trichomes that exist on the exterior of flowers and leaves. These trichomes break off easily and may fall onto hemp seeds during harvest. Nonetheless, the amount of THC that might make its way into a bag of commercial hemp seed is negligible in volume and potency. (Mahlbert 2013)

Online Hemp Resources

If you are ready to learn more about hemp, an excellent resource is the North American Industrial Hemp Council. This section of their website, *http://www.naihc.org/hemp-information/286-hemp-facts*, has interesting facts about the history, ecology, industry, and science of hemp.

An Abbreviated History of Cannabis

Cannabis was first documented as a prescribed medicine in 2737 BC by the Chinese Emperor Shen Neng. (Earlywine 2002) Hemp seed has been documented as far back as 8000 BC at a Japanese archeological site. (Clarke, Personal Communication 2016) The use of cannabis plants is documented in historical medical texts from China, India, Central Asia, the Middle East, Africa, and later Europe for many of the same purposes people use it today.

History of Cannabis

Cannabis in Medical Practice: A Legal, Historical, and Pharmacological History of Therapeutic Cannabis by Mary Lynn Mathre, RN is an excellent resource. The chapter "History of Therapeutic Cannabis" is written by cannabis historian Michael Aldrich, PhD. *Understanding Marijuana: A New Look at the Scientific Evidence* by Mitch Earleywine's, PhD also has an excellent chapter on the history of cannabis. If you want to know more about the history of cannabis as medicine, both books are comprehensive. Additionally, excellent scholarly work has been done by Raphael Mechoulam, PhD and Ethan Russo, MD. A pdf of *A History of Cannabis as a Medicine* by Lester Grinspoon, MD is available on the Internet with a quick search of the title and his last name. For a detailed (and at times humorous) review of modern cannabis history, read *Reefer Madness: A History of Marijuana* by Larry "Ratso" Sloman, former editor of *High Times* magazine.

In the U.S., hemp was an important industrial crop from 1629, when it was introduced in New England, until the invention of the cotton gin in the late 1800s. (Sloman 1979) Hemp was primarily grown for its fiber. Larry Sloman writes, "In fact, in 1762 Virginia imposed penalties on those who did not produce it." (Sloman 1979) Even George Washington grew hemp! In his journal writings he talks about separating male and female plants. Some think this is evidence he partook in the medicinal values of the great herb. Thomas Jefferson was also a fan of hemp. It is widely speculated he may have used the plant for its medicinal purposes; however, his notes are so cryptic it is hard to know. You can read their diary notes on-line via the Library of Congress website or at *www.antiquecannabisbook.com*. (The Antique Cannabis Book 2014)

Irish surgeon W. B. O'Shaughnessy brought medicinal cannabis from India to Britain in the 1840s introducing cannabis as medicine to the Western world. Cannabis was introduced to the U.S. Pharmacopoeia (USP) in 1854 (NORML 2010, 9), and from 1854 to 1942 cannabis preparations were listed in the U.S. Pharmacopoeia for treatment of a wide variety of ailments including asthma, depression, hysteria, and pain. Highly regarded companies such as Eli Lily, Parke Davis, and Squibb produced many prescription drugs with cannabis as an ingredient. (Earlywine 2002) Those drugs addressed everything from pain to anxiety to insomnia and stomach problems. It has been widely reported that cannabis was Queen Victoria's favorite relief for dysmenorrhea (menstrual cramps). Although it is true her physician recommended cannabis for a variety of ailments, it is not known for sure that she used the herb. By the time Dr. O'Shaughnessy became court physician, the queen was likely menopausal. The website *www.AntiqueCannabisBook.com* documents over 2,000 different cannabis-based-medicines in use in America during this time.

Cannabis History Timeline

2700 BCE	*Shen Nong Ben Cao Jing (Chinese book on medicinal plants)* notes cannabis as a hallucinogen, appetite stimulant, tonic and as an anti-senility agent[1]
c. 750 BCE	*Kaneh bosem* (aromatic cane) mentioned as part of holy anointing oil of Hebrews (Exodus 30:22-25)[1]
c. 214 BCE	*Erh-Ya* (oldest known Chinese dictionary or encyclopedia) China describes superiority of female plants for intoxication and males for fiber[1]
c. 1000	al-Mayusi (Arab writer) first mention of cannabis for epilepsy[1]
1200	Anandakanda (Ayurvedic medical text from India) mentions for increasing longevity
1751	*Medicina Britannica (book that outlines medicinal and garden plants from Britain)*, mentions hemp for medical use in menses[1]
1839	O'Shaughnessy, doctor responsible for bringing cannabis to the West studies cannabis in India[1]
1851	Cannabis makes its first appearance in the 3rd Edition of the American Pharmacopoeia (antique cannabis book) [1]
1860s	Used for war injuries in the American Civil War[1]
1899	CBN, is the first isolated cannabinoid[2]
1930	Anslinger appointed first commissioner of U.S. Treasury Department's Federal Bureau of Narcotics
1932	Movie *Reefer Madness* released
1937	Cannabis Tax Act passed, which imposed a $100 per ounce tax
1940	CBD is isolated[2]
1942	Cannabis is removed from the American Pharmacopoeia[2]
1944	La Guardia Committee Report was released; this is the first American scientific investigation on cannabis use in humans
1964	Isolation and synthesis of THC[1]

Cannabis History Timeline continued

1971	Cannabis was listed as a Schedule I drug with the creation of the Controlled Substances Act
1972	National Commission on Marihuana releases the first government sponsored study on cannabis use, Marihuana: A Signal of Misunderstanding
1973	Oregon becomes first state to decriminalize cannabis possession
1975	DEA ALJ Lewis F. Parker 1988 recommends to the DEA to reschedule cannabis to Schedule II
1978	U.S. Government ships its first canister of cannabis cigarettes to the first Compassionate Use Investigational New Drug program participant Robert Randall
1985	Marinol® (synthetic THC) is approved in the US for chemotherapy nausea[1]
1988	Discovery of the CB_1 receptor[1]
1988	DEA's Administrative Law Judge Francis L. Young recommends that cannabis be moved to Schedule II
1992	The endocannabinoid arachadonoylethanolamide (Ananadamide or AEA) is discovered[1]
1993	Discovery of CB_2 receptor[1]
1994	California is the first state to legalize medical marijuana
1995	The endocannabinoid arachidonlylglycerol (2AG) is discovered[1]
1998	"Entourage Effect" of plant cannabinoids is discovered and reported[1]
1999	US researchers file cannabinoid patent on behalf of the U.S Department of Health and Human Services, it was awarded in 2004
2014	Colorado & Washington pass state legislation to legalize recreational cannabis

[1] Russo, Ethan. 2014. "The Pharmacological History of Cannabis." In *Handbook of Cannabis*, by Roger G. Pertwee, 23-29. Oxford: Oxford University Press.

[2] Murray, Robin M., Paul D. Morrison, Cécile Henquet, and Marta Di Forti. "Cannabis, the mind and society: the hash realities." Nature Reviews Neuroscience 8, no. 11 (November 2007): 885-95.

Cannabis Prohibition: Rooted in Fear, Greed, and Misinformation

Until the mid-1900s, cannabis was used around the world medically, spiritually, and socially in a safe and peaceful manner. In thousands of years of cannabis history, there are NO documented deaths associated with its use. You may wonder, since

17

cannabis is so safe, why the big fuss? Why has there been a campaign to demonize this plant? The answer is a topic for another book (and several have been written). I think the answer is one part fear, one part greed, and one part ignorance. I hope this book can help us move past fear and ignorance. I'm unsure what can be done about greed.

The current prohibition on cannabis began brewing between 1910 and 1920. During that time cannabis tinctures and extract medications lost popularity because of the development of injectable medicines and as a result of the varying potency of cannabis preparations. While still widely accepted, cannabis medicines were not prescribed as often.

At the same time, smoked cannabis as a recreational drug grew in popularity in Mexico. The Mexican Revolution, which lasted from 1910 –1920, caused an influx of Mexican immigrants who brought the "evil weed" to the U.S. *Reefer Madness* states that the first American citizens to smoke cannabis flower tops for recreational purposes in the U.S. were likely members of the Black Cavalry stationed along the border. (Sloman 1979) Simultaneously, servicemen were bringing cannabis home from Asia and other countries. Smoked cannabis was used by musicians and artists who enjoyed the creativity it brought. Moving into the Great Depression, fear and suspicion of Mexicans, blacks, and even artists and musicians grew. At this time we see an increase in erroneous news reports that cannabis was causing violent crime and putting women and children at risk.

Enter cannabis prohibition ring leader Harry Anslinger. As assistant prohibition commissioner in the Bureau of Prohibition, he made a name for himself as a reliable bureaucrat. His success as one of the country's top alcohol prohibitionists led to him being appointed the first commissioner of the U.S. Treasury Department's Federal Bureau of Narcotics (later becoming the Drug Enforcement Administration) in August of 1930. Immediately after taking office, Anslinger started aligning with other prohibitionist entrepreneurs, chemical companies, and pharmaceutical companies to coordinate and fund a full-scale political and media assault on cannabis.

The government funded propaganda movie *Reefer Madness* hit screens in 1936 as a way to "educate" people about the dangers of cannabis. The movie is considered a farce now but was taken seriously by many at the time (view the movie at *http://youtu.be/S_jGAC77Tpg*). The movie falsely depicts cannabis use by a group of young, middle-class white people leading to suicide, murder, and rape and created mass public hysteria based on pure fiction. This eased the way for the passage of the 1937 Cannabis Tax Act, which imposed a $100 per ounce tax. The street price for cannabis at the time was $.38 per pound. (Sloman 1979) It went to $1606.08 per pound overnight. Support for the Cannabis Tax Act came from large oil companies threatened by the production of hemp for oil and from chemical companies that feared competition with their patentable drugs. In general, plants, like many natural products, cannot be patented. However, certain preparations or extractive techniques may be patented. This does not provide the kind of competitive protection pharmaceutical companies desire.

In 1942, cannabis was entirely removed from the U.S. Pharmacopeia against the will and advice of the American Medical Association, which testified at the Cannabis Tax Act Hearing that cannabis was not dangerous, was not commonly abused, and had a low addiction rate. (Schaffer n.d.)

In 1939, in response to public outrage at the prohibitionists' unfounded claims about the dangers of cannabis and the passage of the Cannabis Tax Act, New York's mayor Fiorello La Guardia commissioned a medical study on cannabis titled Mayor's Committee on Marihuana but known as the La Guardia Committee Report. The report was released in 1944. It was the first American scientific investigation of the effects of cannabis on humans. *The report concluded that cannabis did not change one's personality and posed no real threat to humans,* contrary to the prohibitionist rhetoric supported by Anslinger and his crew.

Two years before the release of the La Guardia Report, two of the physicians who were part of the committee published a precursor paper in the *American Journal of Psychiatry* stating that cannabis use is not nearly as addictive as tobacco or alcohol. (Stern and DiFonzo 2009) The American Medical Association praised the article. Anslinger responded by coercing the journal and the association to publish renouncements of their statements and publicly support his prohibitionist stance forcing the AMA to call the report and the paper "thoroughly unscientific." (Stern and DiFonzo 2009)

Fast forward to the rise of cannabis use among youth in the sixties. The new social acceptance of cannabis by young people created fear among conservatives that an entire generation would be lost to the drug's supposed negative effects. Prohibition was ruled unconstitutional in 1969 in US vs. Leary. However, because state laws rendering cannabis illegal were still operative in all fifty states, there was little practical effect. *The Comprehensive Drug Abuse and Control Act of 1970* (AKA the Controlled Substances Act) created much of the legal and law enforcement framework for fighting the "war on drugs" that still exists. This legislation also created the Commission on Cannabis Drug Abuse (long referred to as the Schafer Commission after its chairman, Raymond P. Schafer, then governor of Pennsylvania), which was charged with studying the use, abuse, pharmacology, and efficacy of cannabis. The Schafer Commission had one year to execute its first report. When word got out that the commission was going to recommend decriminalization, President Nixon said to Governor Schafer, "...you're enough of a 'pro' to know that for you to come out with something that would run counter to what... we're planning to do would make your Commission just look bad as hell." (Common Sense for Drug Policy 2002)

The Schafer Commission report titled Marihuana: A Signal of Misunderstanding is the first comprehensive American government commissioned and funded investigation of the science of cannabis, its medical potential, and the social phenomenon of recreational use. The Commission states the perceived "cannabis problem" as follows:

> More than anything else, the visibility of marihuana use
> by a segment of our population previously unfamiliar

with the drug is what stirred public anxiety and thrust marihuana into the problem area. Marihuana usage in the United States has been with us for a very long period of time dating back to the beginning of the century. For decades its use was mainly confined to the underprivileged socioeconomic groups in our cities and to certain insulated social groups such as jazz musicians and artists. As long as use remained confined to these groups and had a negligible impact on the dominant social order, the vast majority of Americans remained unconcerned. From the other side, the insulated marihuana user was in no position to demand careful public or legislative scrutiny.

However, all this changed markedly in the mid-1960s. For various reasons, marihuana use became a common form of recreation for many middle and upper class college youth. The trend spread across the country into the colleges and high schools and into the affluent suburbs as well. Use by American servicemen in Vietnam was frequent. In recent years, use of the drug has spanned every social class and geographic region. (Commission on Marihuana and Drug Abuse 1972)

Overwhelmingly, the report considered experimental and intermittent use to have little to no negative impact on human health or society. Going against President Nixon's will, the report recommended decriminalization with "a social control" policy seeking to discourage marihuana use. The following are highlights from the report:

- A large amount of research has been performed in man and animals regarding the immediate effect of marihuana on bodily processes.
- No conclusive evidence exists of any physical damage, disturbances of bodily processes, or proven human fatalities attributable solely to even very high doses of marihuana. Studies seemed to indicate that safe human study could be undertaken over a wide dose range.
- Animal studies illustrated that the margin of safety between active dose and toxic dose was enormous.
- Looking only at the effects on the individual, there is little proven danger of physical or psychological harm from the experimental or intermittent use of the natural preparations of cannabis including the resinous mixtures commonly used in this country. The risk of harm lies instead in the heavy, long-term use of the drug, particularly of the most potent preparations.
- Until recent years, society was operating under an eliminationist policy. The exaggerated beliefs about the drug's effects, social impact, and user population virtually dictated this legal approach.

- In short, personal possession arrests and even casual sales, which account for more than 95 percent of the marihuana arrests at the state and local level, occur too low in the chain of distribution to diminish supply very effectively.
- In addition to the misallocation of enforcement resources, another consequence of prohibition against possession for personal use is the social cost of criminalizing large numbers of users.
- Cannabis was brought into narcotics framework because of unfounded assumptions about its ill effects.
- Considering the range of social concerns in contemporary America, marihuana does not, in our considered judgment, rank very high. We would deemphasize marihuana as a problem.
- The existing social and legal policy is out of proportion to the individual and social harm engendered by the use of the drug.

President Nixon was not concerned with educating people about the truth, and this report did not impact his drug policy trajectory. He wanted stricter laws and control and was determined to get them, regardless of its social impact or financial cost, and so began the "War on Drugs." One could argue that the War on Drugs has been going on since the early 1930s since the inception the Bureau of Narcotics and Anslinger's appointment to head the agency. However, it is more generally accepted that the War on Drugs began in 1970 with the creation of the Controlled Substances Act. While the commission was writing this report, cannabis was temporarily placed in the newly created Schedule I category where it remains today. Nixon wanted to fire the director of the National Institute of Mental Health because that scientist believed that the evidence did not warrant the harsh penalties for cannabis he wanted. (Aggarwal 2014)

To add one more twist of irony to the story, since 1978 the federal government has been supplying cannabis cigarettes to patients who have proven medical necessity. The story begins with a legal battle against glaucoma patient Robert Randall who was arrested for growing cannabis. Mr. Randall successfully proved his medical necessity in court. Cannabis was the only thing that would slow the onset of blindness. Charges were dropped.

Randall first received cannabis from the National Institute on Drug Abuse in 1976. He was encouraged to be quiet about it but felt compelled to help others in need, so he shared how cannabis was helping him. The government responded by stopping his supply. He then sued the federal government for trying to prevent his access to the medicine he had proven was the only thing that would prevent him from going blind. His case was settled out of court. One result of that settlement was the creation of the Compassionate Use Investigational New Drug program. Randall was diagnosed with his disease in his early twenties and told he would be blind by thirty. He died at fifty-two due to the complications of AIDS but maintained his sight. (Russo, Mathre, et al. 2002) Robert Randall and his wife, Alice O'Leary Randall, deserve immense credit for their early role in the cannabis legalization movement. Robert remained a tireless advocate for the clinical use of cannabis until his death in 2001. Alice is still educating lawmakers and firing up crowds across the country.

There are mixed reports of how many people were actually enrolled in this program. Some reports say thirty-four patients while others report only fifteen. New enrollment was halted by the Bush Administration in 1992. (Russo, Mathre, et al. 2002) Approved patients enrolled in the program were grandfathered in, and until recently, seven patients continued to receive medical cannabis cigarettes from the federal government for twenty-two to thirty-one years. As of 2014, there were only three patients left in the program. Two others would qualify if they could find a doctor willing to apply for a license to prescribe Schedule I drugs. Since these two patients have been unsuccessful in finding a doctor, they sold all of their belongings, moved into an RV, and relocated to a medical cannabis state.

It is noteworthy that the government has chosen to not collect data on these heavy clinical cannabis users. Fortunately, third-party research was conducted on four of the patients by a team of highly regarded cannabis science experts as reported in a *Journal of Cannabis Therapeutics* article. "Results demonstrate clinical effectiveness in these patients in treating glaucoma, chronic musculoskeletal pain, spasm and nausea, and spasticity of multiple sclerosis. All 4 patients are stable with respect to their chronic conditions and are taking many fewer standard pharmaceuticals than previously." (Russo, Mathre, et al. 2002) The only negative health effects noted in the investigation were mild changes in pulmonary function of two of the patients. No other negative physiological changes were evident.

Yet, the U.S. Government still claims that "...cannabis has a high potential for abuse, [and] has no accepted medical value in treatment in the United States." (United States Drug Enforcement Agency 2011) U.S. government figures show cannabis as having an addiction rate lower than coffee, but no one is trying to outlaw coffee. The current body of research on this topic challenges the U.S. government's assertion that cannabis has no known medical value. There are over 20,000 research papers from around the world that largely support the medical value of cannabis. You can see this by searching for the word "cannabis" or "cannabinoid" on the Pub Med website *http://www.ncbi.nlm.nih.gov/pubmed*, the National Library of Medicine and National Institutes of Health medical and biological science repository for research.

In 2008, the American College of Physicians (ACP), the second-largest physicians group in the United States, wrote a position paper titled *Supporting Research into the Therapeutic Role of Marijuana*. The paper begins:

> "Marijuana has been smoked for its medicinal properties for centuries. Preclinical, clinical, and anecdotal reports suggest numerous potential medical uses for cannabis. Although the indication for some conditions (e.g., HIV wasting and chemotherapy-induced nausea and vomiting) has been well documented, less information is available about other potential medical uses. Additional research is need-

ed to clarify marijuana's therapeutic properties and determine standard and optimal doses and routes of delivery. Unfortunately, research expansion has been hindered by a complicated federal approval process, limited availability of research-grade cannabis, and the debate over legalization." (American College of Physicians 2008)

The paper goes on to say that the ACP supports funding for "rigorous scientific evaluation" of the efficacy of cannabis as medicine and an evidence-based review of cannabis's status as a Schedule I controlled substance to see if it should be reclassified to a different schedule. (Please see the "Research Conundrum" section of this book for a detailed look at how hard it is to conduct medical cannabis research in the United States.) The ACP proclaims support for an exemption from federal criminal prosecution for prescribing doctors who act in accordance with their state law and for patients who use cannabis as permitted under state law. (American College of Physicians 2008)

The War on Drugs has failed miserably to reduce drug use or keep drugs out of the hands of children. It has been a great success in terms of prospering owners of private prisons, politicians, addiction treatment centers, and encouraging law enforcement agencies to focus their efforts on non-violent drug offenders. In a report published in 2010 by the Cato Institute, Harvard economist Jeffrey Miron, PhD estimates that the national legalization of cannabis would provide a federal savings of $8.7 billion and generate another $8.7 billion in tax revenue. (Miron and Waldock 2010) (Yes, both numbers are $8.7 billion.) According to the Americans for Civil Liberties Union website, 52 percent of all drug arrests in 2010 were for cannabis. The website states that in the same year a cannabis-related arrest was made every thirty-seven seconds, which is over 852,324 arrests, 88 percent of those being for simple possession. (Americans for Civil Liberties Union n.d.)

Note to Reader: Throughout this book several different sources are quoted for the number of people arrested for cannabis. There are discrepancies in those numbers from the various sources ranging from approximately 625,000 to over 850,000 arrests annually. The discrepancies are attributed to different years and basis for record keeping. Regardless, the high number of arrests is not acceptable.

Our prohibition against cannabis is ridiculous, and after reviewing the scientific literature, one could go so far as to say that **prohibition is reckless**. It is a betrayal of the public good. The failed War on Drugs has cost trillions of dollars to implement, trillions in lost revenue, and has prevented significant advances in science and medicine.

The Cannabis Revolution

Public support for legalizing cannabis is growing rapidly in the United States. The 2012 election by the people of Colorado and Washington to legalize cannabis has sparked a level of national comfort in discussing this issue that has never before existed. More and more people are coming out of the proverbial cannabis closet and are willing to be honest about their personal experiences with cannabis and their views on legalization. The mid-term elections of 2014 have ushered in laws for retail cannabis markets in Alaska and Oregon. Florida was two percentage points from the 60 percent margin required to change their constitution to allow for medical cannabis. Washington, D.C. decriminalized cannabis, and California de-felonized simple cannabis possession. We are definitely headed in the right direction!

The landmark special CNN report *WEED* by Dr. Sanjay Gupta, CNN's head medical correspondent, is proof that a groundswell of support exists for cannabis legalization. In an interview on the Piers Morgan show promoting his special report, Dr. Gupta said:

> I mistakenly believed the Drug Enforcement Agency listed cannabis as a Schedule I substance because of sound scientific proof. Surely, they must have quality reasoning as to why cannabis is in the category of the most dangerous drugs that have "no" accepted medicinal use and a high potential for abuse. They didn't have the science to support that claim, and I now know that when it comes to cannabis neither of those things are true. It doesn't have a high potential for abuse, and there are very legitimate medical applications. In fact, sometimes cannabis is the only thing that works. (S. Gupta 2013)

Dr. Gupta is not your average television personality. In addition to being a an Emmy award winning journalist, he is assistant professor of neurosurgery at Emory University School of Medicine, and associate chief of the neurosurgery service at Grady Memorial Hospital in Atlanta, Georgia. It was widely reported that he was favored as President Obama's pick for U.S. Surgeon General in his first term but withdrew his name from consideration. In 2010, Forbes magazine named Dr. Gupta one of their "10 Most Influential Celebrities." His public statement of support for cannabis has helped educate many people who otherwise would not be willing to look at the facts. Additionally, I believe he has helped shape the Department of Justice's new "softer" stance on enforcing federal cannabis laws that are in conflict with the will of the people of Alaska, Colorado, Oregon, and Washington.

If you doubt Dr. Gupta's assertions, read the comments on our Facebook page (*www.facebook.com/MyChronicRelief*) and website (*http://www.MyChronicRelief. com*). In fact, on any medical cannabis website you will see testimonials from person after person describing relief, liberation from pharmaceutical hell, healing, and even remission from cancer as a result of cannabis.

Pioneers of the Cannabis Movement

Despite the oppressive legal situation, there are many people doing great work throughout this country to get cannabis medicine to people who need it. Three examples are the good people of the Wo/Men's Alliance for Medical Marijuana (WAMM) (*https://wamm.org*) in Santa Cruz, California; the Stanley family who started the Realm of Caring (*http://realmofcaringfoundation.org*) in Colorado Springs, Colorado; and Mara Gordon at Aunt Zelda's (*http://www.azcannaoil.com*) in California. These groups are focused on helping the terminally and chronically ill through the use of highly concentrated cannabinoid oil and tinctures.

The Stanley family, who was profiled in Dr. Gupta's two *WEED* specials, operates the Realm of Caring. They have had especially good luck developing cannabis oil that prevents epileptic seizures in children. One of the plants they bred happened to be high in the cannabinoid CBD and had negligible amounts of THC, the intoxicating cannabinoid in cannabis. Through working with the parents of Charlotte Figgy, a child with a severe form of epilepsy called Dravet Syndrome, they quickly discovered that oil made from the high CBD plant material helped prevent seizures for epileptic children who previously had two hundred to three hundred seizures a week. They offer these products at a low cost to their patients.

Valerie Corral, a long-time cannabis advocate, is the co-founder and director of WAMM, the nation's first open cannabis collective. Her organization, which allows members to help grow their own medicine and connect with people, nature, and themselves in a transformative way, is a sanctuary for the ill employing an integrative approach to healing. WAMM provides medicine to their terminally and chronically ill members regardless of their ability to pay. After a traumatic brain injury, Corral was left with residual epileptic seizures. Not long after that, she discovered that cannabis was helpful in controlling them. She, and her former husband, began growing cannabis secretly. According to the WAMM website, "Following a pair of arrests, the Corrals resolved to help others facing similar persecution, and soon local patients started seeking them out." (Wo/Man's Alliance for Medical Marijuana n.d.)

The collective does not buy or sell cannabis. Members of WAMM (who must be California residents) are given cannabis and cannabis products based on their need, and they provide financial support to WAMM based on their ability to pay. Members are asked to help plant, care for, and harvest the crop according to their ability. By working together, members of WAMM have created a deeply loving community of like-minded people. At the core of WAMM's work is compassion. In my first conversation with Corral, she said, "I am not a teacher. I am a servant." WAMM aims to serve their members wherever they may be in their healing or dying journey by providing them moral support and a cannabis regimen that serves their personal goals be they restorative or palliative. Valerie Corral is an angel masquerading as a human. What she has done to advance the cannabis movement is nothing short of amazing! I have the deepest respect and admiration for her.

Mara Gordon, founder of Aunt Zelda's, is a modern-day medicine woman. She is one of the country's premier experts on treating cancer with cannabis. She, like Corral, works with patients to get the result desired by each patient. She develops treatment protocols for children and adults based on their desired outcomes and then develops their medicine—usually some combination of oils, tinctures, extractions and topicals. Gordon has a deep understanding of the origins of disease and how plant medicine works. When asked how her greatest healing successes with patients were different from patients who didn't have great successes, she said, "All medicine works best on the expectation it is going to work." She continued by saying, "…mind, body, spirit—that is how cannabis works best."

One of the things I most admire about Mara Gordon is her commitment to finding the balance between the available science and practical application for every client. She is leading the way with new information on how to treat and kill cancer cells with particular ratios of cannabinoids and order of application. Proof of her commitment lies in the creation of Zelda Therapeutics *(www.zeldatherapeutics.com)*, a company designed to focus on pre-clinical and clinical research in cannabis medicine.

While Valerie Corral, the Stanley family, and Mara Gordon are heroes for all they are doing to advance the cannabis industry and to educate people about cannabis's therapeutic merits, they are not the only ones to breed special plants or make cannabis oil. They are, however, inspiring examples of some of the many "good guys" in this industry who are helping people live better through cannabis.

There are too many cannabis pioneers to mention here: Donald Abrams, Sunil Aggarwal, Michael Backes, Robert Clarke, Steve DeAngelo, Constance Finley, Fred Gardner, Bonnie Goldstein, Manuel Guzman, Mike and Kelly Hyde, Jeffrey Hergenrather, Martin Lee, Richard Lee, Brownie Mary, Mary Lynn Mathre, Rafael Mechoulam, Tod Mikuriya, Dennis Peron, Alice O'Leary Randall, Robert Randall, Amanda Reiman, Ethan Russo, Christina Sanchez, Steph Sherer, Dustin Sulak, and Keith Stroup to name a few. Cannabis pioneers come from all walks of life. We have them to thank for the advances we are seeing in science, laws, and public opinion. These pioneers have started organizations such as the ones listed below, have fought to get the laws changed in their own state (often doing so at great personal risk), and have stuck their necks out to pursue the questions of cannabis science and medicine. We owe a debt of gratitude to these people who have come before us. Because of them, I have been able to write this book, and we all have growing access to information that helps create positive change in our own lives and that of others. The following is a list of organizations that bring together pioneering people and information. This is where the magic is happening:

- Americans for Safe Access *safeaccessnow.org*
- The Marijuana Policy Project *mpp.org*
- The National Organization for the Reform of Marijuana Laws (NORML) *norml.org*
- Patients Out of Time *medicalcannabis.com*

- O'Shaughnessy's The Journal of Cannabis in Clinical Practice *beyondthc.com*
- Multidisciplinary Association for Psychedelic Studies *maps.org*
- The Society of Cannabis Clinicians *cannabisclinicians.org*
- The International Cannabinoid Research Society *icrs.com*
- Project CBD *projectcbd.org*
- International Association of Cannabinoid Medicines *cannabis-med.org*
- Drug Policy Alliance *drugpolicy.org*

These organizations work with a long list of brave physicians and researchers who persevere in recommending and studying the medical benefits of the cannabis plant. Many are quoted and cited throughout this book.

Now that the news is out about the medical benefits of this plant, entrepreneurs are flocking to the cannabis industry and bringing big money with them. All kinds of product companies have emerged to meet the demand from patients who prefer not to smoke their medicine by crafting tinctures, sublingual sprays, topical applications, edible oils, lollipops, baked goods, soft drinks, butters, spreads, chocolates, and nearly anything else you can conjure up. As you can imagine, this boom is creating jobs and opportunities from farms to storefronts in states where cannabis is legal. It makes sense that total legalization of cannabis will result in a medical research and pharmaceutical development boom (if not for Big Pharma, for someone) as well. Cannabis is the new frontier! So I ask, what is in our highest good as a nation—to legalize or not?

Legality

Cannabis is illegal in the United States. At the time of writing this book, twenty-five states and the District of Colombia have some sort of "medical" cannabis law making it possible for doctors to recommend the herb. Another twenty states have decriminalized possession, and four states have laws allowing for recreational use. Visit the NORML website for an interactive national map of which states have legalized and/or decriminalized cannabis. The Controlled Substances Act (CSA), 21 U.S.C 801, et seq, classifies cannabis as a Schedule I (of five schedule classes) drug: the same category as heroin, LSD, PCP, and MDMA.

Schedule I	Schedule II	Schedule III
No accepted medical use *High Potential for abuse*	*Accepted medical use with severe restrictions* *High Potential for abuse*	*Accepted medical use* *Some potential for abuse*
Heroin	Cocaine, PCP	Anabolic Steroids
LSD, DMT	Opium	Codeine
MDMA	Methadone	Marinol®
Cannabis	Cesamet®	Vicodin®

Cesamet˚ (nalbilone) and Marinol˚ (dronabinol) are both synthetic cannabinoids created by pharmaceutical companies. It is important to note that dronabinol and nabilone, two isolated THC pharmaceutical preparations, are approved for treatment of nausea, vomiting, and wasting for cancer and AIDS patients. (Gettman 1999) Marinol˚ is prescribed in a gel cap that combines sesame oil with its active ingredient dronabinol, a Schedule III drug. It is prescribed for chemo-induced nausea and vomiting and appetite stimulation. Cesamet˚ is the prescription name for nabilone, a Schedule II drug also prescribed for chemo-induced nausea and vomiting.

Jon Gettman, PhD is a well-known public policy expert with a specialization in the study of drugs. On his website *www.drugscience.org*, he shares an excerpt from a letter sent to petitioners of the DEA requesting an explanation of the differences between Marinol˚, dronabinol, and delta 9 tetrahydrocannabinol (THC). This is the response provided by the DEA:

> Dronabinol, in its pure form, is a Schedule I controlled substance since it is one of the tetrahydrocannabinols and has no currently accepted medical use in treatment in the United States. See 21 U.S.C. § 812(b)(1); 21 C.F.R. §1308.11(d)(27). Marinol˚, in contrast, has an accepted medical use and is a Schedule II substance [editor's note: Marinol˚ has since been rescheduled to Schedule III]. See 21 C.F.R. 1308.12(f) (1); 51 Fed. Reg. 17,476 (1986) (DEA final rule transferring Marinol˚ from Schedule I to Schedule II following FDA approval of the drug for marketing.) It was approved for marketing by the FDA in 1985 for the treatment of nausea and vomiting associated with cancer chemotherapy. Id. In 1992, FDA expanded Marinol˚'s approved indications to include treatment of anorexia associated with weight loss in patients with AIDS.

In 1999, dronabinol was dropped to a Schedule III classification from Schedule II. It is difficult to understand the rationale that cannabis and its whole plant extracts have NO known medical value when isolated synthetic derived psychoactive cannabis plant ingredients miraculously have medical value as a stand-alone drug—a Schedule III drug no less. This story would not be complete without adding that sometime between 2003 and 2005 the only federally approved grower of cannabis in the U.S. was given permission by NIDA to isolate THC from plant material for pharmaceutical companies.

A whole-plant cannabis extract oral mucosal spray with both THC and CBD named nabiximols (US Adopted Name (USAN) Sativex˚) is on the market in twenty-five countries but not yet in the U.S. The manufacturer of Sativex˚, GW Pharmaceuticals (GWP), received approval in 2006 to start U.S. Phase III clinical trials on the drug for addressing cancer associated pain. Their secondary target for the drug will be to address spasticity in MS. It is important to point out that, while there is a great deal of excitement around this medicine, its potential rise to "pharmaceutical" status approved by the FDA is both ironic and hypocritical as long as cannabis is illegal.

Dr. Sunil Aggarwal (*www.cannabinologist.org*) points out in his paper "Cannabis: A Commonwealth Medicinal Plant, Long Suppressed, Now at Risk of Monopolization," published in the Denver Law Review in 2010, "One need only study the basic details of [GWP's] original process patent filed in 2002, and issued by the U.S. Patent and Trademark Office in 2008, to see how their product is nothing more than a highly characterized, twenty-first century version of hash oil—with peppermint flavoring." Dr. Aggarwal further explains in his paper that the World Health Organization's (WHO) generic name approval of nabiximols is largely suspect as they have convinced the WHO, the British government, and now the U.S. government that somehow the use of CO_2 to extract whole plant cannabinoids changes its illicit nature magically making it worthy of a classification other than Schedule I. Would it surprise you to know that GWP argues that cannabis should remain a Schedule I drug and that their product is "quite different" from "generic and unrefined cannabis" and that "it cannot be said that all cannabis—or all cannabis extracts—are the same." (Aggarwal 2010)

It is worth noting that I requested an interview with one of the top medical researchers at GW Pharmaceuticals. That person was not allowed to grant me the interview because my book advocates the use of what they call "crude" cannabis. That is unfortunate, as I would love to be able to share more about the interesting work they are doing. I think it has great promise for many people.

Let me point out, as will be highlighted with references later, that: A) whole plant extracts have far greater therapeutic benefits than single isolated plant chemicals, and B) dronabinol and nabilone are both processed in the liver thereby possibly increasing the psychoactive effects of cannabis compounds. These are the very effects the DEA considers the danger of consuming cannabis vapor, smoke, or plant material and that land the plant on their Schedule I drug list. Those are your tax dollars hard at work "protecting" the American people. Does this fall into the fear, ignorance, or greed category?

The DEA Ignores Their Own Advisors

The Department of Justice (DOJ) is the premier national law enforcement agency in the United States. The head of that agency is the U.S. Attorney General (AG), an appointee who serves at the pleasure of the president. As outlined in the Controlled Substances Act, the Attorney General has the discretion to change the classification of a Schedule I drug. However, that authority is usually deferred to the Drug Enforcement Administration's (DEA) Chief Administrator. (Aggarwal 2010)

The DEA has twice blatantly ignored their Administrative Law Judge's (ALJ) recommendation to change the schedule classification of cannabis. The first time was in 1975 when ALJ Lewis F. Parker recommended that the DEA Administrator request the Department of Health, Education, and Welfare (HEW), now Health and Human Services, request a scientific and medical evaluation to consider moving cannabis to Schedule II classification. It was ALJ Parker's position that the U.S. could move cannabis to Schedule II and still operate in accordance of international law. The acting administrator ignored all recommendations of ALJ Parker. The National Organization for the Reform of Marijuana Laws (NORML) continues to fight the U.S. government on this issue. It took thirteen years for the DEA to hold another hearing.

In 1988, Administrative Law Judge Francis L. Young recommended that cannabis be reclassified to Schedule II after three days of hearings that included testimony from internationally respected experts and brave patients. In his opinion and recommended ruling, he writes:

> The evidence in this record clearly shows that cannabis has been accepted as capable of relieving the distress of great number of very ill people and doing so with safety under medical supervision. It would be unreasonable, arbitrary, and capricious for DEA to continue to stand between those sufferers and the benefits of this substance in light of the evidence in this record.

He goes further to say:

> The cannabis plant considered as a whole has a currently accepted medical use in treatment in the United States, that there is no lack of accepted safety for use of it under medical supervision and that it may lawfully be transferred from Schedule I to Schedule II.

Ironically, the U.S. government that so vigorously denies the medical efficacy of cannabis holds a patent on cannabinoids from the cannabis plant for their antioxidant and neuroprotective properties. (See U.S. patent #6,630,507 B1.) The patent outlines, in great detail, the possible ways cannabinoids may be used to reduce oxidative stress and create medicines that treat complex conditions such as Alzheimer's, Parkinson's, heart disease, and more. Here is the rub: the patent is held by the U.S. Department of Health and Human Services, the parent agency of the uncooperative National Institute on Drug Abuse that is charged with controlling cannabis for U.S. medical research.

Are you wondering exactly how much research is needed to move cannabis to a different schedule or remove it from scheduling entirely? Dr. Sunil Aggarwal, physician, cannabis researcher, and PhD in Medical Geography (and a great support to me in writing this book) states:

> Despite the political hurdles, published, peer-reviewed scientific research on cannabis and cannabinoids has reached sizable proportions. A 2009 review found that there were over 15,000 articles published on the chemistry and pharmacology of cannabis and cannabinoids and over 2,000 on the endocannabinoid system. A 2010 review counted at least 110 controlled clinical studies of cannabis or cannabinoids conducted around the world, mostly outside the U.S., involving over 6,100 patients with a wide range of conditions. (Aggarwal 2010)

This is with the strict controls on U.S. cannabis research. Imagine what we could learn if cannabis were moved to Schedule II or de-scheduled altogether. How many people could benefit from the new information that would surely come?

Just to recap, pharmaceutical companies have successfully manufactured cannabis medicines that have been approved in the U.S. for prescription. These products are considered medicine and legal for you to use with approval from your doctor even though some of those medicines may provide a psychoactive experience. However, a similar or superior product you might make or use yourself for medicinal use is called an illicit drug, and you can go to jail for possessing it. Please stay safe, know your rights, and make good, well-considered decisions about your medicine.

Chapter Three

The Science of Cannabis

Over the last few decades, many of us have realized that the constituents of the cannabis plant possess major therapeutic properties. Actually, it has been known for millennia that cannabis helps in many diseases states.

–Raphael Mechoulam, PhD (2013)

Note to Readers: This section is intended for my fellow science geeks. You do not have to read this to understand how to utilize cannabis as medicine. Nonetheless, it may give a deeper understanding of how and why cannabis works in the body. For those of you who love science, this section will probably raise more questions. Every effort has been made to heavily reference this information. You can dig deeper where you have the most interest.

Cannabis science is in its infancy. It incorporates the study of the plant, its pharmacologically, active components (cannabinoids, terpenoids and flavonoids), synthetic cannabinoids, the body's endocannabinoid system, the development of pharmaceutical cannabis products, and how these isolated compounds interact with the human body. More questions than answers remain. Cannabis science is an exciting frontier in the field of medicine.

Cannabis is an herb like sage, mint, or oregano. Like those herbs, and thousands of other plants, it is packed with pharmaceutically-active components. There are over four hundred therapeutic chemicals that can occur including cannabinoids, terpenoids flavonoids, and a phytosterol. These compounds are primarily found in the resin produced in the glandular trichomes covering the exterior surface of the flowers and small leaves of female plants.

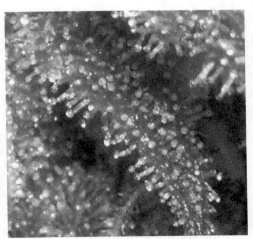

Cannabis trichomes are external plant glands that house therapeutic compounds.

Cannabinoids are a diverse class of chemical compounds that activate cannabinoid receptors found throughout the body. The term cannabinoid encompasses the *endo-*

Cannabis plant

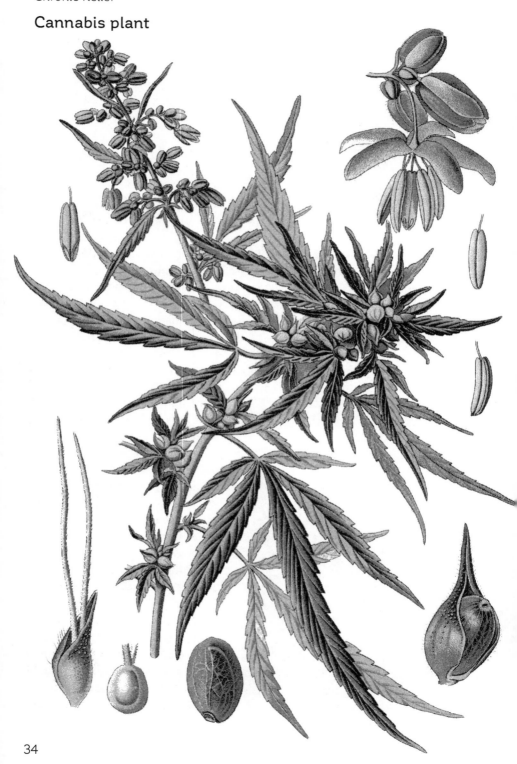

cannabinoids (inner cannabinoids) produced in the human body, *phytocannabinoids* (plant cannabinoids) produced by the cannabis plant, and *synthetic cannabinoids* created in laboratories.

Cannabis flower

Healers have used plants as medicine for many thousands of years. The great healing traditions of the world (Chinese medicine, Ayurveda, and American Folk medicine to name a few) are based on the synergistic use of plants for healing and relief. Doctors and plant experts McPartland and Russo write: "Herbalists contend that polypharmaceutical herbs (herbs with multiple active ingredients) provide two advantages over single ingredient synthetic drugs: (1) therapeutic effects of the primary active ingredients in herbs may be synergized by other compounds and (2) side effects of the primary active ingredients may be mitigated by other compounds." (McPartland and Russo 2001) This is true in the case of cannabis. In their landmark paper "Cannabis and Cannabis Extracts: Greater Than the Sum of Their Parts?" McPartland and Russo cite research indicating that cannabis plant extracts produced effects "…two to four times greater than that expected from their THC content." (McPartland and Russo 2001)

Mojave Richmond

The reason behind this is known as the *entourage effect*. The entourage effect is a scientific hypothesis proposing that combinations of naturally occurring cannabinoids, terpenes, and other active components in cannabis work together to increase the therapeutic benefit of the medicine to the user. Most isolated pharmaceutical medicines, whether they come from a plant or are synthetically created, can be compared to the music of a solo artist versus the more profound effect of a full orchestra, which is whole plant medicine. While the isolated molecule can address a single symptom effectively (sometimes too much so), whole plant compounds are more dynamic. They stimulate the body to address many problems at once in many different biological layers thus bringing not only comfort but restoration in many cases.

In plant-based medicines such as cannabis, when one pharmaceutically active ingredient causes a certain negative effect the same plant often contains the antidote for that very problem! Certain components in cannabis, when present at pharmaceutically-active levels, can reduce the disorientation and *tachycardia* (rapid heartbeat) sometimes caused by THC. (Russo and Guy 2006) This is just one of the advantages of using the whole plant or whole plant extracts over a single isolated chemical such as the isolated synthetic THC product Marinol®.

Cannabis can have seemingly contradictory effects on the body. Users may experience short-term memory loss, yet cannabis helps prevent the formation of amyloid plaques that cause loss of memory in Alzheimer's patients. In addition, cannabis is known for its *biphasic* properties; it creates a certain effect at a low dose while producing a contradictory effect in a larger dose. For example, in some people, low to moderate cannabis use can reduce diarrhea or watery stools while high doses can cause constipation. Similarly, you may find that cannabis is highly effective at managing pain at one dose while actually magnifying it at another.

Another fascinating property of cannabis is its *adaptogenic* nature; it helps balance the body based on the needs of the body's many physiological systems at time of use. You may have heard of other well-known and widely used adaptogenic herbs such as rhodiola, ginseng, and ashwaganda. Adaptogens are known to have antioxidant properties, protect the liver and heart, protect against chemo and radiation, and are anti-cancer and anti-inflammatory in nature. (Winston and Maimes 2007)

Here is an example of the adaptogenic nature of cannabis: imagine two people using the same cannabis tincture made from the same White Widow variety. Their results differ depending on the highest need of each body at the time. The person suffering from depression may feel happy and uplifted. The person with severe pain may feel relaxed and comfortable. While these two medicinal users have consumed the same preparation, the infinite wisdom of their human bodies adapts and distributes the plant cannabinoids and other active components of the tincture to each person's best use.

Michelle Sexton, ND, Medical Research Director at the *Center for the Study of Cannabis and Social Policy* and founder of Phytalab (the first cannabis testing facility in Washington), is a naturopathic doctor, herbalist, researcher, former midwife, educator, and horticultural expert currently writing a book about cannabis as an adaptogen. Here is what Dr. Sexton has to say on the topic:

> Cannabis can be considered an adaptogen because there is a lot of evidence that it meets most of the criteria determined by botanists and researchers who have developed the adaptogen theory. Several of these criteria are:
>
> * Antioxidant and free-radical scavenging activity
> * Modulating the response to stress
> * Having an effect on metabolic regulators
> * Is generally non-toxic
> * Works by normalizing function of an organ or a system in the body
>
> In addition to these criteria, cannabinoids have been shown to be effectors on various biochemical modulators of the stress response including: cortisol, cytokine production,

catecholamines, and sex steroid hormones. Measuring changes in these biochemicals is also a necessary component of the definition of an adaptogen, as these changes define the mechanism by which adaptogens restore balance.

It is the adaptogenic properties of cannabis that make it such a beneficial and broadly useful herb. Because of these balancing properties that affect all body systems and the plant's profound impact on the body's ability to manage the stress response, cannabis is a useful preventative medicine when used appropriately. In our communications, Dr. Sexton expressed concern that the adaptogenic properties of cannabis may be lost at higher doses.

We have much to learn about cannabis and how it can serve the human body. Our current understanding of cannabis and the endocannabinoid system provides profound opportunities for advances in managing and altering the disease process for a wide variety of illnesses. Even though cannabis science is still in its infancy, we know the entire cannabis plant, in all its forms and different preparations, is a treasure trove of healing. **If cannabis were discovered in the Amazon today, it would likely be hailed as a miracle plant.** Instead, this time-tested plant is fighting for legitimacy and its rightful place in modern medicine.

The Endocannabinoid System – The Reason Cannabis Works

The reasons cannabis benefits so many different illnesses and ailments come down to the fact that cannabinoids found in the cannabis plant mimic chemicals in the human body called endocannabinoids or the cannabinoids within. These endocannabinoids, along with a series of enzymes and receptors throughout the body, make up the *endocannabinoid system* or ECS.

The ECS serves as a primary biological harm reduction system tasked with bringing the body back into balance (homeostasis) whenever it is challenged by stress, infection, injury, or lifestyle.

After discovering the phytocannabinoid THC, scientists learned how it functions in the human body and thus identified the ECS. This happened in the early 1990s. Less than twenty-five years ago, the concept of the ECS was completely unknown. (E. B. Russo 2015)

According to Donald Abrams, MD (2001), The ECS regulates, modulates, or plays a role in every major biological function of the human body including, but not limited to:

- experiences of pain and pleasure
- immune function

- newborn suckling
- appetite reward
- temperature regulation
- memory
- inflammation regulation
- neuroprotection

Endocannabinoids are critically important to health, healing, and well-being. They serve as major stabilizing agents at a cellular level as well as within and between different biological systems of the body (endocrine, cellular, musculo-skeletal, cardiovascular, nervous, digestive, excretory, reproductive, respiratory and immune). **Endocannabinoids exist to provide homeostasis.** Said another way, endocannabinoids help balance opposing forces within the body to maintain health. (Melamede 2010) Simply put, health depends on the proper functioning of the endocannabinoid system and balanced levels of endocannabinoids. Italian scientist Vincenzo DiMarzo, PhD explains in simple terms that the ECS affects how we relax, eat, sleep, protect ourselves, and forget (Di Marzo 1998).

The ECS is currently a hot field of study largely because understanding it will lead to better insight into almost all disease causing biological processes such as inflammation, aging and metabolic problems. Advancement in knowledge of the ECS can lead to an array of targeted medicines that will likely be a vast improvement over existing pharmaceutical medicines. Improved understanding of the ECS will also help identify biological red flags that will make it possible to alter the disease causing processes before they actually cause a disease.

Studies on the Endocannabinoid System

A search of PubMed®, an international registry of scientific research, shows 5,036 papers written on endocannabinoids since their discovery in the early 1990s.

As we understand it, the endocannabinoid system includes the following:

- The cannabinoid receptors CB_1 and CB_2
- Several not fully defined cannabinoids receptors that could include GPR18, GPR19 and GPR55 (Atakan 2012)
- Two primary (as we know them now) endocannabinoids: anandamide (arachidonyl ethanolamide or AEA) and 2-AG (2-arachydonoyl glycerol) (Di Marzo 2011)
- Enzymes responsible for the synthesis and degradation of endocannabinoids. The best studied synthesizing hormone is diacyl glycerol lipase (DAGL). The enzymes FAAH (fatty acid amide hydrolase) and MAGL (monoacylglycerol lipase) are

responsible for the degradation of anandamide and 2-AG
(Alhouayek and Muccioli 2012)

The Cannabinoid Receptors

Consider a chemical (natural or synthetic) to be like a key. For the chemical to have an effect on the body, there must be a keyhole, or *receptor*, to which the chemical can bind. Different types of keyholes are found in varying quantities in different parts of the brain and body.

In 1988, the first *cannabinoid receptor*, known as CB_1, was discovered in humans by Allyn Howlett, PhD, and her then graduate student William Devane who were trying to understand how and why delta-9-tetrahydrocannabinol (THC), the primary euphoriant compound in cannabis, works in the brain. (Mechoulam and Hanus 2010)

This was the first in a chain of important scientific enquiries that led to discovering the **endocannabinoid system**. Clint Werner, author of the book *Marijuana Gateway to Health*, describes poignantly the significance of this discovery as, "...one of the most exciting and underappreciated developments in biological science in recent times." (Werner 2011)

CB_1 receptors reside primarily in the brain and spinal cord with the highest concentration in the basal ganglia, the hippocampus, the cerebellum, and in reproductive organs. (Abrams and Guzman 2009) The CB_1 receptor has an affinity for THC, meaning THC molecules most easily fit into CB_1 keyholes. When THC binds to the CB_1 receptor in the body, a euphoric effect is often created. The CB_1 receptor is thought to control appetite, immune function, muscle control, pain, intraocular pressure (pressure in the eye), cognition, reward mechanism, thermoregulation (temperature control), and emesis (nausea and vomiting). (D. Abrams 2011) Since plant cannabinoids fit into CB_1 receptors, they

Cannabinoid receptor

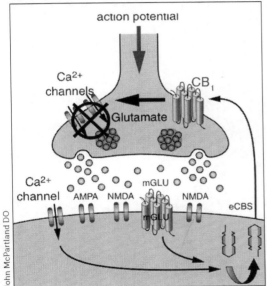

Ca²⁺ influx and upregulation of MGLU receptors in the postsynaptic cell cause DAGL enzymes to synthesize 2-AG. 2-AG moves retrograde across the synapses (opposite the direction of glutamate) to CB1 located on the presynaptic neuron. Activated CB_1 closes presynaptic Ca²⁺ channels, which halts glutamate vesicle release. THC works in a similar fashion by activating CB_1.

CB$_1$ Receptor	CB$_2$ Receptor
More important in neurological events. Assumed to be involved with the transmission of GABA and glutamate. (Mechoulam and Parker 2013)	More important in immune process and inflammation and responsible for reducing pain. (Gerdeman and Schechter 2010)
High concentration in the sensory and motor sections of the brain, which indicates an important role in motivation and cognition. (Mechoulam and Parker 2013)	Highest concentration is believed to be in the immune system with additional receptors throughout the CNS. (Mechoulam and Parker 2013)
Low concentration in the brain stem meaning risk of overdose from receptor activation is extremely low. (Abrams and Guzman 2009)	Suspected to play a major role in an internal system that guards against harmful non-protein attack in the body. (Mechoulam and Parker 2013)
Believed to protect against age-related decline. (Mechoulam and Parker 2013)	Bone growth is controlled through the CB$_2$ receptor, which provides important implications for the treatment of osteoporosis. (Ofek, et al. 2006)
Cannabinoids act through this receptor to initiate a pain killing response. (Skaper and Di Marzo 2012)	2-AG moderate affinity full agonist. (Di Marzo and DePerocellis 2012) This means 2-AG strongly activates the CB$_2$ receptor.
Anandamide is thought to be a high affinity CB$_1$ selective partial agonist. (Di Marzo and DePerocellis 2012) This means anandamide moderately activates the CB$_1$ receptor.	Reduces immune cell migration into the brain which provides neuroprotection. (Hillard 2014)
2-AG is a low-moderate to affinity full agonist. Meaning that 2-AG affects the CB$_1$ receptor in a way that produces a light to moderate impact on that receptor. (Di Marzo and DePerocellis 2012)	Significantly modifies the response to stress and is thought to be a major part of our bodies internal protective mechanism. (Mechoulam and Parker 2013)
Ten times more prevalent in the nervous system than other well studied receptors involved with pain. (Aggarwal 2013)	It is now thought that anandamide is a high affinity, CB$_1$ selective partial agonist whereas 2-AG is a moderate affinity, CB1/CB2 full agonist.
Activation stimulates a chemical reaction that affects synaptic plasticity, cell migration, and possibly neuronal growth. (Howlett, et al. 2002)	
Enhances recovery after flight-or-flight stress response helping bring the body back to balance. (Hillard 2014)	
Helpful in the extinction of fear memories. (Hillard 2014)	

can be effective in controlling nausea and vomiting, pain, eye pressure, spasticity, and can also give you "the munchies."

In 1993, a second cannabinoid receptor, the CB_2 receptor, was found in *macrophage* (a type of white blood cell) cells in the spleen, with the highest concentrations in the natural killer cells, strongly suggesting a role in immune function, cell proliferation, inflammation, and pain regulation. (Abrams and Guzman 2009) It is thought that cannabis reduces inflammation, decreases traumatic injury, and increases cell regeneration by fitting into CB_2 receptors.

The Father of Cannabis Science

Raphael Mechoulam, PhD, the father of cannabis science, deserves a Nobel Prize for his work in this field. His findings have opened the door for understanding the origins and processes for many poorly understood diseases and for incredible advances in new treatment development for a wide group of currently undertreated diseases and symptoms. The movie *The Scientist*, produced by Zach Klein, highlights Dr. Mechoulam's incredible contributions to medical science. Watch it for free at *http://mechoulamthescientist.com*.

Cannabinoids are thought to fit into additional (not CB_1/CB_2) receptors in the body, but they are not yet well understood. These receptors may include a CB_3 receptor, a TRPV1 receptor, and possibly several PPARs receptors. (Hillard 2014) If this is true, it will help add important pieces to the puzzle in our understanding of the endocannabinoid system and how the cannabis plant interacts with it. This could have huge implications for treating and curing disease, managing stress, and slowing aging.

Agonist and Antagonist

A critical component of treating disease is to understand if and where the body is getting too little or too much of a needed chemical. While this is not the only thing at play in the cause of disease, understanding this ballet of chemical interactions makes it possible to prevent, better manage, treat, and in some cases cure the disease.

Chemicals that activate certain receptors to cause a particular biological process to be initiated are called agonists. Chemicals that block a particular biological action are antagonists.

For example, glutamate is an excitatory neurotransmitter that, when produced in too high a volume, can produce cell death. This is an issue in many diseases including autism, epilepsy, head injury and stroke. When glutamate, or any other chemical, is produced in excess, an antagonist, such as certain components of the cannabis plant, can help block the receptor uptake of the glutamate thus reducing the damage done to the cell and therefore reducing the symptoms of the disease. In the case of Alzheimer's, components of the cannabis plant are agonist. They help increase the uptake of acetylcholine, which is needed for memory.

By understanding which part of the biological chemical process is causing the problem, agonists and antagonists can be used to trigger the necessary action or block the offending chemical process thus mitigating the problem. Agonists and antagonists that are naturally produced in the body, such as neurotransmitters or hormones, are referred to as endogenous. Those that are added to the body, such as cannabinoids, cannabinoid-based-medicines, pharmaceuticals, and nutraceuticals are called exogenous agonists or exogenous antagonists.

For example, THC is an exogenous CB_1 and CB_2 agonist. THC activates both these receptors and in so doing, among other things, helps manage pain. CBD is a partial CB_2 agonist but not a CB_1 agonist.

Endocannabinoids: AEA and 2AG

Anandamide (AEA), the name comes from the word *ananda* meaning "bliss" in Sanskrit, was the first endocannabinoid identified. It was discovered in 1992 in Raphael Mechoulam's lab by his postdoctoral researchers Lumír Ondřej Hanuš and William Devane. The second endocannabinoid, *2-arachydonoyl glycerol* (2-AG), was discovered and classified by one of Mechoulam's PhD students, Shimon Ben-Shabat. (The Japanese team of Sugiura, T. et al. made the same discovery simultaneously.)

These endocannabinoids activate the CB_1 and CB_2 receptors and are thought to work in additional ways—possibly through the additional postulated cannabinoid receptors mentioned above or via non-receptor mechanisms. Other possible endocannabinoids have been identified, but research has focused primarily on understanding the function and life cycle of these two endocannabinoids.

AEA and 2-AG are regulated independently from one another and can perform separate functions in the same system, organ, tissue or cell. (Di Marzo and DePerocellis 2012) For example, AEA may be more important in pain mechanisms while 2-AG may be more important in brain injury. (E. B. Russo 2015) Fatty acid amide hydrolase (FAAH) is an enzyme responsible for the breakdown of AEA. FAAH is thought to be linked to emotions and personality expression. (Mechoulam and Parker, The Endocannabinoid System and the Brain 2013) A wide range of animal studies also suggest that FAAH may be useful in treatment of inflammation and increased sensitivity to pain. (Schlosburg, Kinsey and Lichtman 2009)

In a report released by the National Institutes of Health titled *The Endocannabinoid System as an Emerging Target of Pharmacotherapy*, the authors state that, "The growing number of preclinical studies, clinical studies, and clinical trials with compounds that modulate the endocannabinoid system will probably result in novel therapeutic approaches in a number of diseases for which current treatments do not fully address the patients' needs." This study reviews cannabis, cannabinoid, and endocannabinoid research specific to thirty-three major chronic ailments and diseases. Each category reviewed shows cannabis or cannabis-based medicines do or could provide beneficial results.

Many mysteries remain about the ECS. Nonetheless, the new understandings we are gaining are leading to developments that will result in medical treatments that can alter disease progression significantly. Such treatments may include great advances in treating and preventing diabetes, obesity, cancer, Alzheimer's, depression, and many more diseases.

Introduction to the Endocannabinoid System

For additional information about the ECS, see separate essays of the same title "Introduction to the Endocannabinoid System" by Dustin Sulak, DO at *http://www.norml.org* and Dr. Ethan Russo, MD at *http://www.phytecs.com*.

Introducing the Cannabinoids

The primary mind-altering chemical in cannabis is delta-9-tetrahydrocannabinol (THC) discovered in 1964 by Dr. Raphael Mechoulam and his research team. It is one of approximately one hundred plus known cannabinoids in the cannabis plant. (Mechoulam and Hanus 2010) While THC is the primary reason cannabis is popular as a recreational drug, it is but one of over four hundred compounds in the plant. (Abrams and Guzman 2009) How many of these compounds are therapeutic is unknown.

Recent science shows that different cannabinoids and other components in cannabis, which have little to no psychotropic effect, may actually hold more therapeutic promise than the most famous cannabinoid, THC. (Izzo, Borrelli, et al. 2009) A few of the most studied cannabinoids beyond THC are cannabidiol (CBD), canabichromene (CBC), cannabigerol (CBG), tetrahydracannabivarin (THCV), cannabidivarin (CBDV), and cannabinol (CBN). Each of these phytocannabinoids offers multiple benefits to improving health. Let's take a look at what they do.

Delta-9 Tetrahydrocanabinol (THC)

THC, the most common cannabinoid in American grown cannabis, is well known for causing the euphoria people get from inhaling/ingesting cannabis while also relieving pain and inflammation, acting as an anti-spasmodic, and relaxing muscles. The structure of THC was discovered in 1964 by revered cannabis scientists Dr. Raphael Mechoulam and his research partner Yechiel Gaoni, PhD. According to Steep Hill Halent Laboratories of California (*http://steephilllab.com*), THC typically ranges from 5 to 25 percent of a plant's chemical makeup. Mahmoud A. ElSohly, PhD, research professor of the Research Institute of Pharmaceutical Sciences and professor of pharmaceutics, is the project director for the only federally licensed cannabis growing facility in the United States, which is housed at the National Center for National Products Research at the University of Mississippi. He runs the Cannabis Potency Project that tests and tracks the potency of cannabis samples confiscated by the DEA. The project tracks the potency of six different cannabinoids: THC, CBD, CBC, CBN, CBG and THCV. (See below.) Dr. ElSohly reports that on average the THC level of these confiscated samples is 10 percent.

THC is a bronchodilator, anti-spasmodic, muscle relaxant, powerful neuroprotectant, and antioxidant. In fact, it has twenty times the anti-inflammatory power of aspirin and twice that of hydrocortisone. (E. Russo 2011)

Low Doses Can Be Therapeutic

Dr. ElSohly says, "The amount of THC needed to produce a therapeutic effect is much less than needed to get a high." (ElSohly 2013)

THC works in the brain by binding directly to the CB_1 receptor in the body's endocannabinoid system in the same way as the endocannabinoid anandamide (AEA, the bliss molecule), which is produced by the body. When you smoke/ingest cannabis, THC molecules flood the body fitting in the key holes of the CB_1 receptors strongly and CB_2 receptors partially and create many positive harm reduction benefits, along with euphoria and a distinctly "altered" feeling.

In pre-clinical trials, THC has been proven to reduce levels of vascular endothelial growth factor (VEGF) in glioma (brain cancer) cells. A reduction in VEGF means brain cancer tumors are unable to grow the new blood vessels they need to sustain themselves, grow, and spread. This discovery offers great promise in the treatment of brain cancer. (Blázquez, et al. 2004)

Manuel Guzman, PhD, a leading cannabis scientist, studies how cannabinoids work in the body and focuses much of his research on THC and cancer. His work indicates THC can cause cell death in human glioma cancer cells. The paper *"Cannabinoid Action Induces Autophagy—Mediated Cell Death through Stimulation of ER Stress in Glioma Cells,"* for which Guzman was a co-author, cites previous research saying: **"... cannabinoid treatment reduces tumor growth, (specifically, THC administration for 14 days decreased tumour growth by 50%)."** (Salazar, et al. 2009) Guzman's study reviews ways in which animal and human glioma cancer cells responded to cannabinoid "attack" and concludes that: **"... it is clear that THC and other cannabinoids deserve serious consideration and investigation as a strong anti-tumour and anti-cancer agent."** (Salazar, et al. 2009).

As a result of recent success stories about the non-psychoactive high CBD oils being given to children, THC has been under attack. CBD-only legislation has been popping up all over the country. I want to caution you from jumping on this band wagon. THC is a highly therapeutic compound. Let's remember that when it is used in combination with other cannabinoids, terpenes, and chemicals in the cannabis plant, it is far more effective than on its own and potentially negative side effects are mitigated by the other plant chemicals. In 2006, the Laboratory of Physiologic Studies, National Institute on Alcohol Abuse and Alcoholism produced a review paper titled *"The Endocannabinoid System as an Emerging Target of Pharmacotherpy."* This comprehensive review of the research included the following highlights about the benefits of THC:

- THC stimulates appetite in cancer and AIDS patients, which is important in fighting disease related wasting.
- In acute pain, THC is effective against chemical, mechanical, and thermal pain stimuli.
- THC or Sativex® reduces neuropathic pain in patients with traumatic nerve injury or multiple sclerosis in randomized, double-blind, placebo-controlled, crossover trials.
- An analysis of pain questionnaires from 523 patients with HIV infections revealed that 90 to 94 percent of subjects using cannabis experienced improvement in muscle and neuropathic pain.
- Both THC and anandamide exerted CB1-mediated neuroprotective effects in an ouabain-induced rat model of *in vivo* (within a living organism) excitotoxicity. (Ouabian is a plant chemical that is toxic in high doses.)
- The original Cannabinoids and Multiple Sclerosis study of 657 patients showed muscle spasticity measured by the Ashworth scale was significantly improved in the THC-treated group.
- In a pilot study of the safety and tolerability of THC in ALS patients, symptomatic benefits were seen for spasticity, insomnia, and appetite.
- Inhalation of THC also resulted in a greater and longer lasting decrease of arterial blood pressure in hypertensive compared with normotensive individuals.
- Orally administered THC significantly inhibited disease progression [of atherosclerosis in animal models].
- Bronchodilation induced by smoked marijuana and oral THC was also documented in subjects with mild to moderate asthma and in asthmatic patients with methacholine or exercise-induced bronchoconstriction.
- THC or marijuana decreased intraocular pressure whether administered orally, topically, or intravenously.
- While THC has many beneficial traits, it is also largely to blame for what some deem the undesirable traits associated with smoking or ingesting cannabis—most notably dizziness, rapid heartbeat, intoxication, and consciousness alteration such as impaired short-term memory and giddiness. There is a fine balance when it comes to THC; a little can go a long way!

For many conditions, such as autism, cancer, and Alzheimer's, THC plays a critically important role in the effectiveness of medical cannabis treatment. Valerie Corral, co-founder of the Wo/Man's Alliance for Medical Marijuana, wrote to me in an email, "Cancers are being cured, as the body is so willing to heal itself. The success is amazing. But it points much more toward the higher THC cannabis oils and some ration of CBD added to provide the kind of healing that we are looking for." (Corral 2014)

I Don't Want to Get High!

Many people have told me they don't want to get high. They are looking for the benefits whole plant cannabis can provide but either find the high undesirable or are scared of it. I think what these folks are telling me is that they don't want to lose control. You don't have to worry. The mind-altering effects of cannabis can be managed or avoided with just a bit of knowledge and some experimentation with different varieties, intake methods, cannabinoid/terpene profiles, and proper dosing. We will talk later in the book about different varieties and how to select the best ones for you.

Cannabidiol (CBD)

CBD is the second most common cannabinoid in medical cannabis and the most common in hemp plants. (E. Russo 2011) CBD rich cannabis provides potent therapeutic benefits without the euphoria or lethargy caused by many high THC varieties. CBD and THC are believed to have a synergistic effect meaning they are more effective when present at therapeutic levels together than when taken alone. While THC is widely known for its psychoactive properties, CBD may be best known for its ability to counterbalance anxiety, tachycardia (rapid heartbeat), hunger, and the sedation and consciousness alteration caused by THC. (E. Russo 2011)

Project CBD

Project CBD works with seed companies, growers, dispensaries, and patients to identify, track, and spread the gene pool of various CBD rich varieties, catalog their chemical profiles, and gather patients' experiences with them. For more information about how and why CBD works in the body read the article "CBD: How It Works" and for more about the differences between hemp and drug varieties of cannabis, read "Sourcing CBD: Marijuana, Industrial Hemp & the Vagaries of Federal Law", both by Martin A. Lee, and housed on the Project CBD website at *www.projectcbd.org*.

CBD was once considered a minor cannabinoid in comparison to THC. We now know that CBD is as beneficial and versatile as THC in addressing many hard-to-manage conditions such as diabetes, rheumatoid arthritis, cancer, epilepsy, antibiotic-resistant infections, alcoholism, PTSD, and neurological disorders. (O'Shaughnessy's News Service 2011) CBD has very strong *anxiolytic* (reduces anxiousness), anti-convulsant, *antiemetic* (reduces nausea), anti-inflammatory, antioxidant, and anti-psychotic properties. (Fernandez-Ruiz, Sagredo, et al. 2013) One of the most exciting aspects of CBD is its combined powerful anti-inflammatory, antioxidant, and neuroprotective properties that yield great promise for the treatment of Alzheimer's, Parkinson's, and all neurodegenerative-related diseases.

The use of high CBD oil made from the Realm of Caring's medical cannabis variety cultivar, 'Charlotte's Web,' garnered public attention in 2013 when Dr. Sanjay Gupta featured the stories of several children with intractable epilepsy in his documentary *WEED*. Most of these children went from suffering several hundred seizures a week to as few as one a month after beginning high CBD oil treatment. Since *WEED* aired, families are flocking to Colorado from all over the world to get access to the Realm of Caring's high CBD oil for their severely epileptic children. Their stories are as heartbreaking as they are inspiring. Almost every family that seeks this treatment is at the end of their pharmaceutical rope. Their doctors have often given up on finding a solution, but the parents of these suffering children have not! I've heard many a cannabis legalization activist say the therapeutic promise cannabis holds to reduce suffering in children will be the catalyst for national legalization. While the use of CBD holds great promise for epilepsy sufferers and others, it is important to note that many patients will require varying levels of THC to get the desired results. There is so much research needed to understand why and how cannabinoids (and possibly the aromatic terpene compounds) manage disease and which combinations benefit which patients. Two other deeply important questions have entered the conversation as a result of the media attention given to recent successes in treating epilepsy with cannabis: **Why are cannabis or cannabis-based medicines not the first line of treatment for conditions such as Dravet Syndrome (childhood epilepsy) and neuropathic pain? Why are we not doing more and better research into the medical potential of cannabis?** Based on the limited research available, there is significant, compelling evidence leading researchers to believe whole plant cannabis therapeutics offer great promise. One day CBD will likely become a powerful and widely accepted healing agent used for many ailments and delivered in many forms.

CBD balances the body because it:

- Is a potent antioxidant stronger than vitamins C and E.
  (McPartland and Russo 2001)
  - The combination of THC and CBD make an even stronger antioxidant. (Lee 2011)

- Is a powerful analgesic that seems to work especially well for neuropathic pain, chronic pain brought on by damage to the nervous system, which is traditionally difficult to treat. (Lee 2011)
- Is a neuroprotective agent thought to help prevent Alzheimer's and other age related neurodegenerative disorders. (Lee 2011)
- Is a serotonin balancing agent that acts as an anti-depressant and can help reduce anxiety, addiction, appetite, pain perception, nausea, and vomiting. (Lee 2011)
  - As a side note, serotonin also affects your ability to rest, regenerate, and find serenity (Braverman 2004, 138), which is important for anyone but most especially for people trying to heal.
- Regulates blood pressure.
- Has antipsychotic effects. (Fernandez-Ruiz, Sagredo, et al. 2013)
- Facilitates bone reabsorptions.
- Is toxic to breast cancer and other cancer cells while preserving healthy cells. (E. Russo 2011)
- Is an agent against methicillin-resistant staphylococcus aureus (MRSA), the staph infection that plagues many hospitals today. (Lee 2011) However, the cannabinoid cannabigerol is more potent in this regard.
- Animal studies show CBD slows diabetic retinopathy, (damage to the eye's retina due to diabetes) the leading cause of preventable blindness. (Liou 2010)

The National Epilepsy Foundation Calls for Cannabis Research

On February 20, 2014, the National Epilepsy Foundation called for increased research and access to cannabis for people with epilepsy. According to their website, 2.3 million Americans live with epilepsy. One million live with uncontrolled seizures. The cost of a month's supply of cannabis oil for treatment of seizures is approximately $600 per patient. One million consumers would generate an economic stimulus of $600 million per month and $7.2 billion annually to the economy. That doesn't include the domino effect that would occur from families having less stress, more wellness, increased productivity in the parent's workplace, and the economic impact of those families getting out and enjoying their communities. Epilepsy is but one example of how cannabis could revolutionize health and the economy.

Unfortunately, CBD has substantially been bred out of much of the cannabis available in the U.S., U.K., Canada, and Europe. This cannabis is dominated by THC, which is generally preferred by recreational users for its euphoric effects.

However, thanks to the educational work done by organizations such as Project CBD, Dr. Gupta's coverage of cannabis, and increasing positive media attention given to CBD, high CBD varieties are becoming more available in the U.S.

About twelve in every 750 samples being tested in California are found to be **CBD-rich varieties**. (Project CBD 2012) CBD-rich varieties are defined herein as those with 4 percent or higher CBD content. As we learn more about the benefits of CBD, cannabis breeders/growers around the world are striving to grow more CBD rich cultivars. This promotes more diversity in the kinds of whole plant cannabis medicine available, and broadens the range of conditions cannabis medicine can successfully treat.

The Journal of Cannabis in Clinical Practice

One of my favorite resources for the latest advancements in cannabis science is O'Shaughnessy's: The Journal of Cannabis in Clinical Practice. Contributors to O'Shaughnessy's are some of the best and brightest in the medical cannabis industry, and many are supporters of Project CBD. Their website is http://www.beyondthc.com.

In the 2011 *O'Shaughnessy's* autumn issue, a reader wrote to the standing column "CBDiary" to ask: "Why are you trying to do more research on CBD when there are so many journal articles reporting its benefits? Don't we already know that CBD will be effective against a variety of illnesses?" The response (which made me laugh out loud): "We have a key advantage over the academics and corporate scientists when it comes to evaluating drug effects: our input comes from medical cannabis users; theirs comes from rodents." (Lee 2011) In other words, by testing real medicine and learning how patients respond to it, researchers can learn a great deal, even if their research isn't FDA approved.

As a result of the growing attention given to the healing powers of CBD, a handful of companies have emerged marketing their high CBD products made from non-psychoactive hemp. **BUYER BEWARE!** This is a legal gray area, and in most cases really good marketing, but not necessarily good medicine. There can be a big difference between products made from industrial hemp and medical cannabis.

Keep in mind that, because this industry is not regulated, what they claim to put in the bottle, pill, cream, oil, or tincture doesn't have to be exactly correct. Shocking, I know. These products are being marketed through multi-level marketing companies and retail channels alike. While some of these companies are well intentioned and make wholesome products, others prey on desperate people looking for a cure for themselves or their loved one at exorbitant prices.

My biggest concern about these products is their concentration of CBD and purity, which seems to be lost on some of the people doing the marketing. Hemp is a *bioremediator* meaning it absorbs toxins from the soil. The toxins remain in the

Therapeutic Effects of Various Cannabinoids

	THC	THCa	CBD	CBDa	CBN	CBC	CBG	THCV
Analgesic *relieves pain*	✔		✔		✔	✔	✔	✔
Anti-anxiety	✔		✔					
Antibiotic *slows or kills bacterial growth*			✔			✔	✔	
Anti-depressant *alliviates mood disorders including depression*	✔		✔			✔[a]	✔[a]	
Anti-emetic *reduces neasua and vomiting*	✔	✔	✔	✔				
Anti-epileptic *reduces seizures and convulsions*	✔		✔		✔			✔
Anti-fungal *slows or kills fungal growth*						✔	✔	
Anti-inflammatory *reduces inflamation*	✔		✔	✔	✔	✔	✔	✔
Anti-ischemic *reduces artery blockage*			✔					
Anti-insomnia *aids sleep*	✔	✔			✔		✔	
Anti-psychotic *tranquilizing*			✔					
Antioxidant *reduces cell oxidation damage*	✔		✔					
Anti-proliferative *inhibits cancer cell growth*		✔	✔	✔		✔	✔	
Anti-spasmodic *supresses muscle spasms*	✔	✔	✔				✔	
Appetite Stimulant	✔							
Bone Stimulant *promotes bone growth*			✔			✔	✔	✔
Bronchodilator *increases lung air flow*	✔							
Euphoriant	✔							✔
Neuroprotective *protects nervous system*	✔		✔					
Immunosuppressive *modulates function in the immune system*			✔					
Sedative	✔				✔			

[a] in rodent model

plant. Additionally, industrial hemp is sometimes grown with pesticides and other chemicals that can also be transferred during CBD extraction. When someone puts something in their body for therapeutic use, (or for any reason) this should be a major consideration. CBD products from medical cannabis are derived from the flower, which has a higher density of trichomes. Non-drug fiber varieties of cannabis (hemp) are poor producers of cannabinoids in general and therefore not the most efficient source of CBD. If you decide to try any of these high CBD hemp products, please do your homework, and if you are in a state where cannabis is legal, have those products tested! [See, "Cannabis Analysis", on page 225.]

The quality of CBD products on the market is continuously improving. More companies are establishing direct relationships with overseas hemp growers, and in the future more states will pass hemp laws. This is making it possible for more quality oriented companies to get their products on the market. One such brand is SatiVera (*www.sativera.com*), made by SatiMed, Inc., a European Union certified organic hemp producer in Lithuania. At the time of publishing, Kentucky and Colorado are the only states that have legal hemp laws. Entrepreneurial hemp growers are growing drug plants with approximately 6 to 7 percent CBD and negligible THC and calling it hemp. These are steps in the right direction.

There is a craze across the country to implement CBD-only cannabis legislation that legalizes CBD rich oil extracts having negligible amounts of other cannabinoids. While I see those laws can be the first step in opening the door for medical cannabis laws and industry, this approach is narrow-minded and uninformed. Even though CBD holds great therapeutic promise for a wide variety of ailments, the evidence strongly supports THC as equally therapeutic and completely necessary for treatment in a vast number of ailments such as Alzheimer's, autism, and cancer. I repeat: **Multiple cannabinoids, terpenes, and other active components taken together provide a synergistic effect greater than the sum of their parts.** (McPartland and Russo 2001)

Considerably less information is available on the following cannabinoids. As cannabis science advances, we are sure to learn more.

Cannabinol (CBN)

CBN is a less understood plant cannabinoid. It is usually found in older cannabis after the THC has oxidized. A higher concentration of CBN is thought to make someone feel disoriented rather than high, especially when too much is used. Smoked CBN is thought to be mildly psychoactive but alters the effect of THC. CBN also increases testosterone production and plasma concentration of the follicle-stimulating (FSH) hormone. This may be beneficial in men with low testosterone and older women who wish to become pregnant. CBN is an anti-convulsant and an anti-inflammatory. Because CBN has a three times greater affinity for the CB_2 receptor than for the CB_1 receptor, it is believed to have a greater effect on the immune system than the central nervous system. (McPartland and Russo 2001).

Cannabichromene (CBC)

CBC, the fourth major cannabinoid, naturally occurs in tropical cannabis varieties. It is thought to be superior to THC and CBD in antifungal and antibacterial activity showing great promise for topical and internal uses. On the flip side, while CBC does inhibit cellular inflammation like THC and CBD, it does not do so as effectively. (McPartland and Russo 2001) In the mouse model, CBC has been found to reduce inflammation-induced hypermotility in vivo. Further investigation is warranted for relief of irritable bowel syndrome and related disorders. (Izzo, Capasso, et al. 2012)

Cannabigerol (CBG)

CBG is a potent antibacterial superior to THC, CBD, and CBC in fighting gram-positive bacteria, mycobacteria, and fungi. Although CBG exists in very small amounts in cannabis, it is important because it is the biosynthetic precursor to THC and CBD. (McPartland and Russo 2001) This means both THC and CBD begin as CBG. Enzymes in the plant convert CBG to CBD and/or THC. A U.S. patent exists for CBG's potential use in managing mood disorders. (See U.S. Patent 8,481,085.) CBG is also being investigated as a possible tool in fighting prostate cancer. In vivo, CBG has been found to hamper the progression of colon cancer and selectively inhibits the growth of colorectal cancer cells. (Borrelli, et al. 2014) In experimental animal models of Huntington's disease, a neurodegenerative disorder, CBG was shown to be a potent neuroprotectant indicating that further investigation of CBG is warranted. (Valdeolivas, et al. 2015)

Tetrahydrocannabivarin (THCV)

THCV is primarily found in drug varieties of cannabis. It is considered a biochemical marker for drug use because it is not a metabolite of the prescription THC drug Marinol® and is easily detected in drug testing. It can be used to determine if someone has been consuming whole plant (non-FDA approved) cannabis. THCV is an anti-inflammatory agent. It is gaining considerable attention in research circles because it is thought to be a CB_1 antagonist at lower doses thus dampening the negative effects of THC. THCV may also be clinically effective in the treatment of migraine headaches (McPartland and Russo 2001), the treatment of obesity, and metabolic syndrome related fatty liver disease, especially liver disease caused by inflammation (Silvestri, et al. 2015) and as an anti-psychotic. (Cascio, et al. 2015) It inhibits the body's endocannabinoid system and is therefore being researched for weight loss. (Tudge, et al. 2014)

Decarboxylation – How to Activate Cannabis

It is important to note that all cannabinoids exist in raw or dried plant material as *cannabinoid acids*, the chemical precursors to cannabinoids. Cannabinoid acids have a carboxyl group in their chemical structure, which detaches when the material is heated in a process called *decarboxylation*. This process also occurs at any temperature over a long period of time. (Raber 2013) In the case of the medicinal use of cannabis, we generally presume that decarboxylation requires a minimum heat of 100°C or 212°F, the boiling point of water. The higher the heat the quicker the decarboxylation process, although one must be careful not to use heat over 210°C or 410°F or the cannabinoids will evaporate and be lost.

To be clear, heat is required to convert THC-acid (THCA) to THC, the psychotropic compound with many therapeutic benefits. This means you cannot eat fresh cannabis and "get high." Cannabinoid acids do not perform the same way in the human body as decarboxylated cannabinoids, although they are therapeutic in their own right. We are starting to learn that cannabinoid acids are powerful medicines for supporting immunity and reducing inflammation. However, little research exists on cannabinoid acids and how they can benefit the human body. Leaders in cannabis medicine are starting to explore how THCA, CBDA, and other cannabinoid acids play a role in treating cancer and seizures.

Cannabinoid Acid Tea

Cannabis tea is a health tonic with a small amount of cannabinoid acids and traces of neutral cannabinoids. It is widely used in the Netherlands and in Jamaica for its anti-inflammatory and immune boosting properties. Learn more in the "Cannabis Tea" section, on page 208.

Terpenes

Terpenes are chemical components of *essential oils* (EO) that come from plants. Essential oils are used to fragrance and flavor a wide variety of products including shampoos, lotions, face creams, soaps, foods, medicines, air fresheners, household cleaning products, and more. Terpenes make up the largest group of plant (phyto) chemicals with over twenty thousand identified by chemists. Over two hundred terpenes have been identified in cannabis. (Gardner Autumn 2011)

For a terpenoid to be considered relevant in providing therapeutic impact, it is believed it must occur in a concentration of 0.05 percent or more of the plant material. (E. Russo 2011) In medical cannabis states, patients should have access to testing that will indicate which terpenes are present and at what levels. Interestingly, 0.05 percent is a very small amount; nonetheless, it still can contribute to the therapeutic impact and the effects experienced by the user.

Terpenes are found in most herbs, many flowers, barks, some woods, citrus peels, teas, and spices. They give cannabis its unique fragrance and contribute to its taste while providing an important synergistic effect with the *phytocannabinoids* thus making them more therapeutic.

Terpenes are what help the cannabis plant protect itself from disease, animals, and insects. Thus, terpene levels vary in different parts of the plant based on the types of protection needed. It is hypothesized that cannabis plants in different climates evolved to various terpene combinations over the millennia to fight disease and insects in their particular environment.

A Tool of Communication

The PBS documentary *What Plants Talk About* explains that all plants produce green leaf volatiles, chemicals that serve as self-defense and communication tools. This could mean that a better understanding of terpenes produced by cannabis could lead to more environmentally friendly pesticides.

The smell of the cannabis plant largely depends on the terpenes present. It makes sense that cannabis medicines with stronger scents will likely also be medicinally stronger. I argue that when the smell of a cannabis sample is particularly pleasing you are receiving a strong indication the plant will be particularly therapeutically beneficial. This concept, however, has no science behind it.

While terpenes are gaining popularity as an important constituent of cannabis, there remains a lack of scientific information about how terpenes impact cannabinoids and how they work together in the human body. We are, however, learning that terpenes are an important aspect of the therapeutic effects of cannabis. This is another reason why whole plant extracts are better medicines than isolated cannabinoid medicines, which are without terpenes.

Here are some of the believed synergistic effects terpenes have in combination with plant cannabinoids:

- reduce THC induced anxiety
- reduce cholinergic deficits (memory loss)
- suppress the immune system (which is overactive in diseases such as Lupus)
- boost blood flow to the brain and cortical activity (brain activity signaling muscles to act)
- kill respiratory pathogens
- boost anti-inflammatory action of plant cannabinoids
- enhance the anti-viral and anti-bacterial properties of plant cannabinoids

Source: (McPartland and Russo 2001)

The Entourage Effect of Cannabinoids and Terpenes

Dr. Ethan Russo's article "Taming THC: Potential Cannabis Synergy and Phytocannabinoid-terpenoid Entourage Effects," published in the *British Journal of Pharmacology*, gives a great overview of cannabis terpenoids. This article has been particularly helpful in writing this section of the book. It is a must read for anyone interested in cannabis chemistry.

The Werc Shop, a leader in cannabis testing, was the first commercial U.S. lab to test cannabis for terpenes. In their years of gathering data, they have noticed that the terpene makeup of a sample contributes strongly to its therapeutic effect. (Raber 2013)

Terpenes, like cannabinoids, exist in the glandular trichomes on the exterior of cannabis flowers and associated leaves. They compose up to 10 percent of the *trichome* content. Because terpenes are volatile aromatic chemicals, they are degraded by high heat. Most terpenes vaporize at similar but lower temperatures than cannabinoids, which vaporize around 180 to 185°C or 356 to 365°F. Terpenes remain intact in juicing but not in most curative cannabis oils (except the olive oil recipe listed in the "Cannabis Oil" section of this book) or most edibles. (Raber 2013)

If you are buying a high-heat cannabis preparation with the intent of benefiting from the terpenes, it is wise to ask if terpenes were added back for a more complete therapeutic preparation. While this is not yet a common practice, it will likely become so in the near future. Terpene additions must be standardized or they could lead to different therapeutic results each time you consume the medicine. If you are making edibles at home, it will probably be difficult to selectively add terpenes to your edibles or topicals unless you are adding therapeutic grade essential oils (e.g., lavender or peppermint for food, and sandalwood or frankincense for topical) that have a similar terpene profile to those found in cannabis or buying terpenes from a company such as *www.mycannabisterpenes.com* (specializes in cannabis derived terpenes) or *www.cannaroma.com*. The same is true for high dose concentrated cannabis oil. When we have a better understanding of the therapeutic impact of terpenes and how they synergize with cannabinoids, it's likely they will be readily available on the market for cannabis companies to add into products to increase their therapeutic impact. Some people are experimenting with inhaling essential oils vapors prior to inhaling cannabis smoke or vapor and adding them to tinctures and topical applications to enhance the therapeutic impact of cannabis and cannabis products.

The FDA considers most terpenes safe for human consumption. The most common terpenes in cannabis are: *beta-myrcene* (found also in hops), *beta-caryophyllene* (black pepper), *d-limonene* (lemon peel), *linalool* (lavender), *a-pinene* (pine), *caryophyllene oxide* (lemon balm), *nerolidol* (orange), *terpinolene* (tea tree), *humulene* (sage), *ocimene,* and *phytol* (green tea). They are found in a wide variety of other

Therapeutic Effects of Select Terpenes

	Limonene	a-pinene	ß-myrcene	Linalool	ß-caryophyllene	Caryophyllene Oxide	Nerolidol	Phytol
AChE Inhibitor *memory aid*		✔						
Analgesic *relieves pain*		✔	✔	✔				
Anti-anxiety	✔			✔				
Antibiotic *slows or kills bacterial growth*		✔	✔		✔			
Anti-depressant *alliviates mood disorders including depression*	✔			✔				
Anti-emetic *reduces nausea and vomiting*								
Anti-epileptic *reduces seizures and convulsions*				✔				
Anti-fungal *slows or kills fungal growth*	✔					✔		
Anti-inflamatory *reduces inflamation*		✔	✔		✔			
Anti-ischemic *reduces artery blockage*						✔		
Anti-malarial *aids sleep*							✔	
Anti-mutagenic *prevents multiplication of cancer cells*	✔			✔				
Anti-psychotic *tranquilizing*			✔	✔				
Anti-proliferative *inhibits cancer cell growth*	✔							
Anti-spasmodic *supresses muscle spasms*				✔				
Bronchodilator *increases lung air flow*		✔						
Immune Potentiator	✔			✔				
Increases GABA via SSADH inhibition *Modulates function in the immune system*							✔	✔
Sedative			✔	✔	✔		✔	✔

foods, spices, herbs, flowers, and trees throughout the plant world and can be highly effective medicines in their own right.

It is important to note that just because a terpene generally acts in the body in one manner does not mean the same terpene found in cannabis is going to perform the same way. For example, the terpene linalool, common in lavender, works as a sedative, but this does not necessarily mean linalool in cannabis is going to act as a sedative. It may or may not depending on concentrations of cannabinoids, terpenes, and other compounds in the medicine. The truth is that we don't specifically know what cannabis compositions with terpenes are going to do in the body only that they act as important modulators of cannabinoids. (Raber 2013) We can't extrapolate single molecule studies of terpenes, or cannabinoids for that matter, into thinking that because it is simply present in a cannabis product it will do exactly the same thing. The cannabis product composition must be considered as a whole.

Here is a quick overview of what we do know about the primary terpenes available in cannabis:

Myrcene

Myrcene is a mild sedative. It is one of the major essential oils in hops (used to brew most beers) and is widely used in Europe as a sleep aid. In animal models, myrcene has proven to be a strong pain reliever and muscle relaxer. Dr. Russo hypothesizes that myrcene coupled with THC may create the "couch-lock" sensation, or sense of heaviness experienced with some types of cannabis. Myrcene is believed to have a synergistic effect with both THC and CBD in the nervous and immune systems. (E. Russo 2011)

β-Caryophyllene

β (beta)-Caryophyllene is an anti-inflammatory commonly found in black pepper. It has been used in the UK to treat duodenal ulcers and is considered a *gastric cytoprotective* (a compound that protects the mucosal lining of the stomach). (E. Russo 2011) In vitro studies show that β-caryophyllene demonstrates toxicity to breast cancer cells. (Jager 2010) It is also a CB_2 cannabinoid receptor-specific agonist showing anti-inflammatory and analgesic effects in vivo. (Chicca, et al. 2014) As an aside, it is by far the most fun terpenoid to pronounce.

Limonene

Highly bioavailable to the human body, limonene is the second most widely occurring terpene in nature. (McPartland and Russo 2001) When peeling an orange or any other citrus, limonene is one of the terpenes released into the air to create that fresh, uplifting smell. Research on depressed patients shows that the smell of citrus reduces symptoms of depression. This research is supported by other findings showing that terpenes common in citrus increase the activity of the body's serotonin and dopamine systems, both of which play an important role in mood. (E. Russo 2011) Limonene has produced *apoptosis* (death) in breast cancer cells in randomized clinical trials, and research indicates that diets rich in limonene help prevent cancer of the colon, breast, liver, pancreas, and lungs. (McPartland and Russo 2001)

Linalool

Linalool, found in lavender, is thought to work in the body by modulating production of *glutamate* and the neurotransmitter *GABA*, which controls the brain's rhythms so that body and mind can function at a steady pace. (E. Russo 2011) Since linalool increases GABA in the body, it has anti-convulsant, anxiolytic, and sedative properties. (E. Russo 2011) Linalool is suspected to be the acting agent in lavender oil that prevents burns from scarring. (E. Russo 2011)

α-Pinene

The most common terpene in nature, found in pine, cedar, and other evergreen trees, α-pinene is thought to counteract short-term memory loss caused by THC intoxication and to work as an anti-inflammatory. (McPartland and Russo 2001) It is also thought to be a strong antibacterial agent, which may even be effective against MRSA. (E. Russo 2011) At low levels, a-pinene is a bronchodilator. (McPartland and Russo 2001)

Caryophyllene oxide

Here it is folks: caryophyllene oxide is how drug-sniffing dogs identify cannabis. It is an anti-fungal that helps prevent blood cells from clotting and is commonly found in the medicinal herb Melissa or lemon balm. (E. Russo 2011)

Nerolidol

Nerolidol is commonly found in oranges and has somewhat sedative effects. It has been found effective in improving topical penetration of the skin cancer treatment 5-fluorouracil and is thought to inhibit fungal growth. It is an anti-malarial compound and seems to be helpful in controlling protozoan parasites. (E. Russo 2011)

Phytol

Phytol, commonly found in green and white teas, is another sedative. Like linalool, it works by increasing GABA in the brain (E. Russo 2011), which has a calming effect on the body. While Vitamin A is critical to the health of the eyes, skin, teeth, and bones, too much of it in pregnant women can cause birth defects. Phytol has been shown to prevent birth defects associated with too much vitamin A by blocking the conversion of retinol (animal form of Vitamin A) into a harmful chemical. (E. Russo 2011)

Terpenes provide therapeutic benefits regardless of whether they are inhaled, ingested, or applied topically. (Jager 2010) When you smell cannabis, the terpenes immediately activate the limbic system in the brain creating numerous therapeutic effects throughout the body. Highly respected growers and cannabis experts advise that inhaling the aroma of freshly ground dry cannabis five minutes prior to inhalation of cannabis smoke or vapor will increase the quality of the experience and the therapeutic effects.

Fingerprinting

Terpenes are an important marker for cannabis plant variety identification. Plant samples can be *fingerprinted* by analyzing their chemical components thus creating chemical identifiers for each variety. Analysis and record keeping of these fingerprints is in its infancy but is of great interest to many different sectors of the cannabis industry. This data can help medicinal users get exactly the medicine they need and trust that they can buy the same variety month after month and that it will have the same effect. Many terpenes vaporize and evaporate at room temperature. Therefore, total terpene content—how much aroma a sample has—can indicate freshness. The smellier the better in accessing total terpene content and freshness!

Through fingerprinting, growers are beginning to identify unique cannabis terpene profiles and breed accordingly. One of the remaining challenges is to figure out how to create environments that allow plants to express the desired terpene profiles bred into them. Fingerprinting has the potential to help pharmaceutical companies with their product development. Big Brother may be on board, too. Fingerprinting could make it possible for law enforcement to identify where bootlegged cannabis has been imported from, or produced and prosecute accordingly. However, these forensic efforts have failed to bear fruit. (This seems like a waste of resources to me and another good reason to de-schedule cannabis altogether.)

As we expand our understanding of the terpenes present in cannabis, and the public is made aware of their benefits, I expect we will see new highly targeted therapeutic uses for terpenes. Time will teach us how to realize the full benefits of these therapeutic compounds. In concert with new delivery methods, cannabis and its therapeutic compounds will bring individualized healthcare to a new level and create a new world of preventative self-care options.

Chapter Four

Your Body's Control Center

T his section is intended to help you get a feel for how your body responds to cannabinoids and how this impacts your health. The focus is on the brain, central nervous system, and endocannabinoid system. My intention is to help people understand how these systems play an important role in overall health and well-being as well as give simple tips for improving overall health—with or without cannabis. The more we know about how our body works, the better equipped we are to make good decisions for ourselves and help medical providers do the same.

The ECS: Our Internal Harm Reduction System

The father of cannabis science, Dr. Raphael Mechoulam, and his team of researchers discovered the endocannabinoid system (ECS) in the early 1990s. **The ECS is the human body's internal harm reduction system.**

The human body is extraordinarily intricate and well designed. How is it possible that anatomically modern humans have evolved, survived, and flourished as we have over the course of two hundred thousand years? (Clarke and Merlin 2013) The answer is that endocannabinoids in different life forms have evolved over hundreds of millions of years to protect humans from different kinds of imbalances created by the body in response to environmental stress or genetic shortfalls. Robert Melamede, PhD, recently retired associate professor of biology at the University of Colorado at Colorado Springs and retired former president and CEO of Cannabis Science, Inc., says that in the last several hundred years the human body has not evolved quickly enough to keep up with the stresses of our rapidly changing lifestyle and environment. When the body is unable to maintain *homeostasis* (balance), toxicity occurs. Pain, illness, or disease follow. (Melamede 2011)

Chronic illness does not develop overnight. It develops over time when the body exists in a perpetual state of imbalance. Many things contribute to chronic illness including genetics, response to our environment, exposure to toxic chemicals, constant stress, poor sleep quality and sleep deprivation, dehydration, hormonal imbalance, exercise levels, ability to manage oxidative stress, nutrition, weight management, immune system health, rest and relaxation, and the ways we manage our emotions and thought patterns. In many ways, chronic illness is like death by a thousand paper cuts. Small, unrelated decreases in energy, lack of enjoyment of life, inability to bounce back from stress or illness, and so forth add up and compound over time leading to a cascade of interconnected deficits and ailments.

Our bodies are like our cars and houses. If we do not maintain them properly and proactively (that is the key word), increasingly serious and expensive problems arise until fixing them is either too overwhelming or costly to manage. One problem, if not addressed, in your car leads to another. The same is true with your body.

We need not look further than the simple oil change to drive home this point. If you don't change your oil and maintain proper fluid levels, the engine functions are compromised. Oil makes it possible for metal to contact metal at a safe temperature. Without oil, too much heat is generated ultimately seizing the engine. The same is true if the oil is unclean. Dirt and debris accumulate in the engine causing unnecessary wear and tear that ultimately results in engine failure. Then what? Are you going to push your car wherever you go? Probably not!

When the body is unable to make enough endocannabinoids (the oil in the engine) for whatever reason, *phytocannabinoids* (cannabinoids from the cannabis plant) or *synthetic cannabinoids* (made in a laboratory) can be an effective supplement either triggering the previously failed necessary action or enhancing endocannabinoid volume thus balancing the system and "protecting the engine."

The Cannabis Plant Is Over 27 Million Years Old

At the 2016 International Cannabinoid Research Society meeting, John McPartland, DO, reported that the *Cannabis* plant and the *Humulus* plant separated an estimated 27.8 million years ago. This plant does not exist solely for recreational purposes but provides both a window into a greater biological understanding of the human body and a "treasure trove of healing" says Dr. Raphael Mechoulam.

What happens when your body fails? What can you do to prevent this? When balance is compromised, what actions can you take to facilitate restoring balance? Unless you are dead, supporting your endocannabinoid system will always reap benefits—even making the dying process more comfortable—as in my mom's case.

We will talk later about stimulating the ECS to reduce chronic inflammation by improving your diet and exercising. These are powerful tools for creating balance in the body and supporting the endocannabinoid system.

The Nervous System

Consider the nervous system to be your electrical wiring. Like all systems of the body, the nervous system is intricate and complex. The endocannabinoid system and other neurotransmitter systems are intimately involved in all its functions.

The Peripheral Nervous System (PNS) is comprised of nerves and neurons (special cells) that connect the CNS to the rest of the body. These are the switches and wiring that connect to the breaker box and conduit, which sends and receives signals and routes electricity to light switches and appliances.

The Central Nervous System (CNS) is comprised of the brain, spinal cord, and many nerves. The brain is like a breaker box or master control center of the body, and the spinal cord is the conduit through which the brain sends messages to the rest of the body. When there is a problem in the breaker box (brain) or wires (nerves) leading from the breaker box, there will be problems getting electricity in your home (your body) as well. Problems in the breaker box and wires manifest differently depending on the root of the issue. Exposed wires can create a short in the system resulting in intermittent signaling (as in the case of MS), no signaling to certain outlets or switches (as in the case of ALS), and sometimes dead wires (as in the case of Alzheimer's). This in turn shifts the load to other circuits that may be unable to meet the demand for power thus resulting in another layer of problems. The same is true of the body's nervous system. If the protective linings of neurons are compromised, information the brain is trying to send will be interrupted, or not delivered at all, causing crippling effects in motor function, mobility, energy, and eventually leading to involuntary muscle contractions and spasms.

There are two parts of the PNS. Messages are sent to and from the skin, muscles, and skeleton via the **Somatic Nervous System** (SNS). The **Autonomic Nervous System** (ANS) communicates between the brain, glands, and smooth muscles (muscles we do not consciously control such as those in the heart, urinary tract, gastrointestinal tract, and reproductive organs).

In summary, the nervous system includes:

- **Central Nervous System** (CNS) the brain, spinal cord, and retina.
- **Peripheral Nervous System** (PNS) sensory neurons (which transmit sensory information such as sight, sound, and feeling), neuron clusters (ganglia), and nerves that connect the CNS to the rest of the body.
  - The **Somatic Nervous System** is responsible for transporting all sensory information from the skin to and from the CNS and controlling most voluntary muscle movements.
  - The **Autonomic Nervous System** connects the CNS to internal organs that work automatically without thought or direction.
- The **Sympathetic Nervous System** allows the body to function under stress managing the fight-or-flight emergency response.
- The **Parasympathetic Nervous System** is the rest-and-digest system, which helps the body recover after a fight-or-flight response.

The importance of the endocannabinoid system within the nervous system cannot be overstated, as it is the endocannabinoid system that is largely responsible for the nervous system's ability to send and receive signals, and to execute the necessary biological actions based on information received.

Most disease involves the CNS. But some diseases are specifically called diseases of the CNS including:

- Alzheimer's disease (AD)
- Amyotrophic Lateral Sclerosis (ALS)
- Attention Deficit/ Hyperactivity Disorder (ADHD)
- Huntington's disease
- Meningitis
- Epilepsy
- Stroke
- Anxiety
- Insomnia

- Parkinson's disease (PD)
- Arachnoid Cysts
- Locked-in syndrome (LIS)
- Multiple Sclerosis (MS)
- Encephalitis
- Tourette syndrome
- Schizophrenia
- Depression
- Drug Addiction
- Nausea and Vomiting

Research shows us that understanding how the endocannabinoid system is related to the origin of each of these diseases will lead to advancements in treatment. Cannabis is such an effective medicine for many of the ailments listed above because of how it directly activates the endocannabinoid system. In many cases, cannabis has proven the most effective and least toxic medication for treating or managing CNS disorders. Amyotrophic lateral sclerosis (ALS) is a good example of a CNS disorder that is benefited by cannabis. ALS is a degenerative disease that strikes motor neurons in the brain and spinal cord. As motor neurons die, the patient will become unable to send a signal from the brain to control the muscles. Over a period of a few years, the patient becomes paralyzed and ultimately dies of respiratory failure. Currently, there is no cure for this disease and no pharmaceutical has been shown to effectively slow its progress. Cannabis, however, provides great hope for ALS patients. **Because of the neuroprotectant and antioxidant properties of cannabis, it may help slow progression of the disease by protecting motor neurons the disease attacks and kills.** (Carter and Rosen 2001) Additionally, cannabis provides relief for ALS symptoms including spasticity, wasting, depression, and drooling to name a few. (Carter and Rosen 2001) [See "ALS", on page 103.]

Even the U.S. patent for cannabinoids mentions their possible use in helping prevent certain disorders of the CNS. Regardless, if your malady is a CNS disorder, understanding how the central nervous system plays a role in your ailment can be useful in how you choose to utilize cannabis and the benefits you may experience.

Feed Your ECS with Essential Fatty Acids

Endocannabinoids are made in the body from *essential fatty acids* (EFAs). EFAs are fats our body does not produce; we must get these in our food. They are called **essential** because we can't live without them! They are essential to health from conception to death.

You have probably heard from your doctor, and seen in the news, that it is important to consume the right types of fats. If you have not, let me be the first to tell you that **fat matters!** Now we understand why. Good fats are the building blocks for molecules that activate the internal harm reduction system, feed the brain, strengthen the heart, and protect the skin.

Where do we get these critically healthful fats? Dietary *omega-3* fatty acids (alpha-linolenic acids or ALAs) commonly come from cold water fish and certain seeds and seed oils (e.g. borage, flax, and hemp). *Omega-6* fatty acids (linoleic acids or LAs) come from green leafy vegetables, nuts, seeds, and (most prominently in the Western diet-) vegetable oils. (Physicians Committee for Responsible Medicine n.d.) The standard American diet is too rich in omega-6 EFAs. While these are indeed critical to health, Americans generally consume more than ten times as much omega-6 EFAs as they do omega-3 EFAs. As discussed on page 12, the most therapeutic ratio is 4:1 omega-6 to omega-3. Consumption of more therapeutic ratios of essential fatty acids boost the ECS.

Among my favorite sources for EFAs are the widely available hemp seeds and hemp oil. They naturally have the ideal balance of EFAs and blend easily into morning shakes, oatmeal, and salads. Another excellent source of omega-3 fatty acid is the chia seed. Yes, the same chia from the infamous chia pet! The added benefit chia seed provides, which you do not get from other high omega food sources, is that it absorbs over ten times its original weight in water (if soaked in water before you eat it). This is carried directly to the intestines thereby tremendously hydrating the body. If you are looking to hydrate more without actually having to drink more water, chia seed might help! Hemp seeds can also be soaked in water – even if they are dead as proscribed by U.S. law. I try to eat chia and hemp seed (or oil) daily. See the recipe section for a few ideas on how to incorporate both foods into your diet.

The Brain: The Master Organ

The brain is the most important organ in the body and the foundation of the central nervous system. It controls our mental, physical, and emotional health. It makes it possible for us to imagine, learn, think, remember, feel, communicate, move, and experience emotion and pleasure. The book *The Edge Effect* by Eric Braverman, MD. explains that no matter which malady you may have it is somehow connected to brain health and likely originates in the brain (and the gut as we will discuss later).

There is no arguing that cannabinoids (endo-, phyto-, and synthetic) impact the brain, but research shows paradoxical results for how they do so. For example, THC can impair short-term memory but protect long-term memory. CBD can diminish the effects of THC on memory impairment and boost its effects on protecting memory. A healthy, balanced brain has the proper ratio of *neurotransmitters* (chemical keys that fit into receptors to signal the body to take action), nutrients, hydration, and stimulating mental activity, and thus operates with speed and accuracy. When our brain chemistry is balanced, we are more likely to enjoy optimal health and bounce back quickly and fully from the stresses of everyday life; temporary illnesses such as a cold or the flu, or injury. When the brain is not balanced, we may experience subtle declines in health, cognition, energy, inspiration, fulfillment, and immunity. Whereas we once could bounce back quickly, those without balanced brains may find it takes longer to recover from stress; tasks which once came easily now require effort, holiday weight is harder to shed, and words may not come as quickly as they once did.

Neurotransmitters

Let's come back to the topic of neurotransmitters, which we first touched on while discussing the endocannabinoid system (ECS). Neurotransmitters are chemicals generated by *neurons* (brain cells) that send specific signals to other brain cells across *synapses* (space between neurons). (Braverman 2004)

There are many different neurotransmitters including acetylcholine, dopamine, GABA, serotonin, and glutamate. These are fine tuned by the endocannabinoids anandamide (AEA) and 2-AG, which are neuromodulators. These chemicals play a major role in certain functions of our body impacting immunity, personality, movement, cognition, mood, and disease.

To better understand how important a balanced brain is, let's take a basic look at some of the non-cannabinoid neurotransmitters.

Neurotransmitter	Function	Related Diseases
Acetylcholine	Helps brain process and recall information quickly.	Alzheimer's, dementia, and Multiple Sclerosis
Dopamine	Provides the brain power and energy.	addiction, depression, low energy, and Parkinson's
GABA	Brings harmony, rhythm, and calm to the brain and body.	anxiety, hypertension, cystitis, gastrointestinal disorders, tinnitus, and premenstrual syndrome (PMS)
Glutamate	Involved in cognition, memory, and learning mediating most excitatory responses in the nervous system.	Autism, traumatic brain injury, anxiety, psychiatric and mood disorders
Serotonin	Allows the brain to restore itself.	eating disorders, depression sleep disorders, sexual dysfunction and migraine

These neurotransmitters are present in all of us. A balance of them is needed to maintain health. Too much or too little of any neurotransmitters creates a cascade of biological actions that can tip our mind, body, and emotions off kilter increasing susceptibility to disease if balance is not restored. There is strong reason, backed by research, to believe that the modulation of neurotransmitters with cannabinoids can help mitigate disease and possibly change disease progression.

Most neurotransmitters are stored in the body. Endocannabinoids, on the other hand, show up on demand when needed. (Pacher, Batkai and Kunos 2006) When the body needs balancing, endocannabinoids are created and released from post-synaptic neurons to activate the receptor cells in the brain, nervous and immune systems. Different cannabinoids have been shown to help regulate production of other neurotransmitters. They direct or transmit an excitatory or inhibitory response from cells depending on what the body needs at the time. Because of the way our body utilizes endocannabinoids, plant cannabinoids can help balance other neurotransmitters when something is askew. Rather than directly signaling the brain to a certain action, endocannabinoids mostly moderate the activity of other neurotransmitters. (G. L. Wenk 2010)

Here's a story which illustrates how plant cannabinoids (phytocannabinoids) can support the body's endocannabinoid system. You and your best friend have decided to host a party together. Your party planning is going well, but then your best friend gets sick and cannot help anymore. Now you are on your own. The harder you work to make the party a success, the more you feel your energy slip. Things start to fall through the cracks that never would have if the two of you were working together. You find yourself exhausted and not performing optimally. The more stress you feel, the more stressful the whole event becomes. It's a nasty cycle. By the time of the party, you are worn out and racing against time to pull it all together; all the joy of throwing the party feels lost. All you feel is stress! Then several friends come to your aid. You already feel relief! They show up early to set up, bring food, and jump in like superheroes cleaning up behind you. This extra help is just what you need to pull off a great party and keep your health and sanity intact. This is how cannabinoids can interact with neurotransmitters and endocannabinoids in the brain. The endocannabinoids are you and your friend, the two people originally throwing the party. The phytocannabinoids are the friends who show up when needed to provide the right support at the right time allowing you to succeed while not experiencing physical harm from too much stress.

Keeping the Brain Healthy

Regardless of where you are in your health journey, there is always something you can do to nourish your brain and bring it closer to balance. For the vast majority of adults, and for some children, cannabinoids and terpenes may provide long-term benefits to the brain by serving as powerful antioxidants and anti-inflammatories, while supporting the role of the ECS creating balance in the brain and body. These benefits translate to:

- more nerve plasticity (the ability for nerves to respond optimally)
- improved long-term memory
- less depression
- an ability to rest in a more restorative way
- more focus
- management of seizures
- protection of healthy brain cells

My all-time favorite myth about cannabis is that it kills brain cells. Research suggests that is true. Cannabinoids can kill brain cells, but not the healthy ones as we were lead to believe in the famous "this is your brain on drugs" fried egg DARE campaign of the 1980s. Rather, it is highly likely cannabis kills cancerous brain cells and protects healthy ones. Additionally, the cannabinoid CBD is now thought to promote *neurogenesis*, the creation of new brain cells. (Campos, et al. 2013)

What if I told you your brain health was directly related to your gut health? The largest number of cannabinoid receptors exists in the brain. The second largest number is found in the digestive tract. I hypothesize that this is no accident but is instead part of our body's innate wisdom. In many ways, the gut is like a mini-brain. Dr. Ethan Russo proposes that, "the brain and the gut speak the same language." (E. Russo 2008) The language they share is the language of neurotransmitters.

The endocannabinoids 2-AG and AEA are manufactured in the gut. (Massa, et al. 2004) The gut is where nutrients are assimilated from our food to synthesize endocannabinoids, other neurotransmitters, fats, proteins, and other nutrients our body needs to function and protect itself. If the gut is not healthy and able to easily absorb and convert nutrients for the rest of the body's needs, how can the brain function optimally, and how can we be healthy? If only nutrient poor, low-quality food goes into the gut, how can the body produce compounds it needs to feed the ECS and support itself? Garbage in, garbage out.

Medical researcher, neuroscientist, and Ohio State University professor Gary Wenk, PhD writes in his book *Your Brain on Food: How Chemicals Control Your Thoughts and Feelings* that the brain represents 2 to 3 percent of the human body mass but consumes approximately 14 percent of its energy (2010). For the brain to get the right kind of energy and nutrients, doesn't it seem logical that the gut needs to be healthy to properly process food we consume into energy for the brain and body and to convert precursor chemicals into needed endocannabinoids and other neurotransmitters? Based on this, I think we can fairly extrapolate that a healthy gut equates to a healthy brain, and a healthy brain equates to a healthy body. In an interview with Dr. Wenk, he explained that the gut has a complex nervous system of its own—maybe more complex than our autonomic nervous system—and receptors exist in the gut for each neurotransmitter.

Here are five simple things you can do to improve your gut, brain, and overall health:

- **Maintain good intestinal flora** – Eat cultured, fermented foods such as yogurt, kefir, sauerkraut, and kimchee. Cultured foods are packed with probiotics! They're easy to make at home.
- **Add more fresh and raw food to your diet** – Consumption of real food made from scratch dramatically increases your fiber and nutrient intake, which in the long run helps keep the colon clean increasing the absorption of nutrients and decreasing build-up of toxins. Be sure to eat a broad range of colorful foods, and minimize your intake of highly processed foods.
- **Hydrate** – Lack of water in the system is a major contributor to constipation and headaches. Drinking water regularly throughout the day helps flush toxins from the system, enhances digestion, helps maintain muscle tone, and improves brain performance.
- **Get your heart rate up** – Getting your heart pumping and your blood circulating triggers many beneficial chemical and hormonal processes in the body including boosting the ECS. The increase of oxygen throughout the body contributes to healing and distribution of nutrients. If you are physically unable to exercise, use controlled deep breathing to increase your heart rate. It is very effective!
- **Eat quality fats** – Fat and cholesterol have gotten a bad rap. The brain requires fat to function optimally. Quality fats such as wild caught fatty fish, such as salmon or tuna, avocado, coconut oil, grass-fed butter, hemp oil/seeds, chia seed, and Brazil nuts and oil feed your brain, skin, cardiovascular system, and connective tissue. Eat your eggs, too! Cholesterol is a key component of every cell in our bodies.
- **BONUS TIP! – Challenge your brain** – I'm not sure this improves gut health, but challenging yourself is good for the brain. Try brushing your teeth with your non-dominant hand. Learn a new language, dancing, a new skill—something! Work the crossword puzzle daily.

I suspect you are thinking "What does all of this have to do with cannabis?" It's simple: **We cannot rely on cannabis alone to make us well or feel better.** Consider cannabis a part of the support crew for our continually operating innate health balancing, harm reduction system: the endocannabinoid system.

The human body was designed to heal itself. It is a miraculously intricate entity that responds to environment, inputs, and the use and abuse it sustains.

Aging in the Brain and Body

As we age, different systems of the body go through changes in production levels of needed chemicals (hormones, neurotransmitters, etc.). Understanding these natural, age-related declines and how to manage them lets us connect the dots between the natural aging process and how it impacts the process of maintaining balance in the body and reversing or managing disease and helping the body recover from injury.

The majority of age-related changes in the body begin after thirty. Here are some of the effects aging has on the body:

Age   Biological Decline

Age	Biological Decline
20	Hearing declines from age 20–40 affecting cognition and mental health.
30	Bones begin to weaken, which can lead to osteoporosis.
30	Adrenal glands begin to produce less DHEA, an important hormone that boosts immunity, slows cancer growth, and is a precursor to important sex hormones. This decline occurs from 30–60 years of age.
30	Estrogen production decreases in women, which can lead to bone loss, hair thinning, and cognitive decline.
30	Secretion of growth hormone, which is produced in the pituitary and the hypothalamus glands, declines between 30 and 50. This increases fat and decreases muscle.
35	Women begin to experience hormonal changes that can impact ability to bear children, skin quality, cognitive function, hair growth, memory, weight, and menstruation.
40	Slow decline in the sense of smell begins, with a more rapid decline after 65.
40	Ability to see close up begins to decline impairing cognition and mental health.
40	Men begin to experience a decline in the production of testosterone, which impacts energy, drive, and libido.
40	Maximum exercising heart rate begins to decline by up to 20 percent resulting in memory loss and anxiety.
40	Changes in the circulatory system begin including narrowing of blood vessels, stiffening of arterial walls, and a drop in systolic blood pressure.
50	Women experience dramatic decreases in the production of progesterone and testosterone.
50	Between 50 and 70, the average person will lose up to 40 percent of their breathing capacity, which is directly related to longevity.
60	Alzheimer's and dementia affect 10 percent of those over 60 and 50 percent of those over 85.
70	Dramatic increase in the production of cortisol, a stress hormone produced by the adrenal glands. Results can include anxiety, depression, irritability, paranoia, panic attacks, and loss of memory, libido, and attention.
90	Over 40 percent of muscle mass is commonly lost by age 90. This is especially true for those who do not exercise. This impacts strength, memory, and cognitive function.

Source: *The Edge Effect* by Eric Braverman, MD pages 161-172.

All these changes are considered a natural progression of the human experience. What is unnatural is to age before your time and do so gracelessly. This will increase your risk of disease as well as the rate of disease progression, and will generally make any health issues much worse.

Through understanding biology, we have the opportunity to slow the aging process. For most people this can be difficult to do alone. Making sense of how hormones, neurotransmitters, and the ECS work together and how we can use diet, exercise, cannabis, herbs, supplements, and medicines to stay healthy and age gracefully is probably going to take the help of a medical professional or a team of them. Fortunately, the more you know about how your body works, the more quickly you and your medical team can home in on what healing protocols are best.

Protecting the Brain as You Age

In three simple steps you can be on your way to better brain health and, in turn, better health in general.

1. Recognize brain chemistry as an important marker of wellness or biological balance.
2. Understand how that pertains to you specifically and your unique chemistry.
3. Take action! Reduce chemicals in your body that cause harm, and increase those that provide benefits.

This is an oversimplification but, in a nutshell, the path to great brain health.

In addition to protecting the brain, cannabis has also been found to help people recover forgotten memories. In fact, William C. Woodward, a physician and attorney for the American Medical Association, testified during the 1937 Marijuana Tax Act hearings that this was the only irreplaceable use for cannabis in psychotherapy. (Aggarwal 2014) The flip side is that cannabis is also highly effective at destabilizing and eliminating trauma and fear memories. (Marsicano, et al. 2002) Both of these qualities of cannabis have huge therapeutic implications for the successful treatment of post-traumatic stress disorder (PTSD).

Fortunately, more doctors are starting to understand neurotransmitters, hormones, endocannabinoids, and the role they play in our overall health. However, this is such fresh information that you may have to search to find a medical professional knowledgeable about the ECS and cannabis medicine and therefore able to help you. Generally speaking, practitioners who offer integrative or holistic medicine are more likely to be on the cutting edge of preventative medicine and therefore more aware of medicines, diets, and nutrients that support the brain.

To learn more basic information about your brain, visit: *http://www.ninds.nih.gov/disorders/brain_basics/know_your_brain.htm*

Cognition

We have established that cannabinoids can have many different effects on the brain and body. Let's take a deeper look at how they impact cognition. Cognition is our ability to pay attention and focus, make and access memories, problem solve, learn, think, react, process input, and make decisions. The current body of clinical and laboratory research shows that cannabis use results in a small negative effect on neurocognitive performance in people who are actively consuming it, but those effects diminish with abstinence and are completely gone after twenty-eight days. (Pope, et al. 2001)

In their paper "The Endocannabinoid System and the Brain," published in *The Annual Review of Psychology,* Raphael Mechoulam and Linda A. Parker point out that THC can cause impaired ability to form short-term memories and convert them to long-term memory. THC, however, does not interfere with our ability to recall long-term memories that have already formed. They then discuss studies that have shown CBD prevents memory impairment caused by THC in humans. "The relative THC/cannabidiol ratio in cannabis will profoundly modify the effects of cannabis on memory in human cannabis smokers." (Mechoulam and Parker 2013) In other words, measurable amounts of CBD (or other THC modulating cannabinoids or terpenoids) would mitigate the effects of THC on cognition. Fascinating work led by Celia Morgan, published in the *British Journal of Psychiatry,* measured the cognitive function of two different groups of cannabis users. Both groups utilized cannabis with the same THC level, but one group had low CBD and the other high (4 percent) CBD. All subjects were tested while cannabis-free and under the influence. Plant THC and CBD levels were measured, and saliva samples from each participant were taken. Their results show the lower the CBD content in the plant sample, the higher the risk for short-term memory impairment. (Morgan, et al. 2010) Morgan et al report, "Importantly, however, people in our study who smoked higher cannabidiol varieties of cannabis did not show any acute deficit. Indeed, their performance when intoxicated was virtually indistinguishable from that when drug free." (Morgan, et al. 2010)

Amy M. Schreiner and her colleague Michael E. Dunn from the University of Central Florida conducted a review of the literature on the effects of cannabis use on cognitive performance, which was published in the *Journal of Clinical and Experimental Psychopharmacology.* They first reviewed thirty-three studies that tested the long term cognitive effects of cannabis use. They then reviewed thirteen of the original thirty-three studies that evaluated the long term residual effects (after at least twenty-five days of abstinence from cannabis). **Their research affirms "no lasting residual effects on neurocognitive performance as a result of cannabis use."** (Schreiner and Dunn 2012)

Schreiner and Dunn (2012) write that studies of subjects who are under the influence of cannabis have regularly identified "… effects on learning and memory performance with mixed evidence for effects on attention, inhibition, and executive function." It is important to put this in context. First, a broad body of research indicates cognitive disruptions are more pronounced in new or occasional cannabis users, and are more nuanced in moderate to heavy users likely due to the development of tolerance. Second, the cognitive effects associated with acute cannabis intoxication are generally considered safe from a neurocognitive standpoint. (Grant, et al. 2003) Thus, the researchers question whether these cognitive impairments are actually "negative" effects.

The primary cognitive impact of cannabis use is a slowed reaction time. (Schreiner and Dunn 2012) There are many times in my life when a slowed reaction time would have served me well, although there are other times it is a negative. Many agree that the potential short-term cognitive impairments of using cannabis, which are often subtle for the medical user (especially those using a low THC product), are a small price to pay for the incredible antioxidant and neuroprotectant properties of cannabis.

I anticipate that over time we will see that impacts of cannabis on cognition are directly impacted by age, contributing health factors, cannabinoid and terpene profiles, and the amount of medicine consumed. I know a large number of people who consume cannabis all day long every day. My observation is that most of them are as lucid, cogent, and present as their non-cannabis-using counterparts.

Chapter Five

The Common Denominators of Illness

The common denominators of illness are oxidation, inflammation, and pain to one degree or another. Cannabis is extremely effective as an antioxidant, as an anti-inflammatory agent, and in controlling pain— all of which are interconnected. Since it is nearly impossible to keep up with the volumes of medical information coming out about cannabis and how it relates to the management of specific illnesses, I think we should take a look at the common denominators of illness and injury and how cannabis works in the body to help manage them.

Oxidation

One of the most important factors of good health is how our body manages *oxidative stress*. This is a natural process that occurs at the cellular level. When energy is created in the cell, waste products called *free radicals* are generated. Free radicals also result from stress and exposure to environmental toxins such as cigarette smoke and smog as well as ingested toxins such as fluoride.

Free radicals are molecules containing an unpaired *electron*. Electrons are negatively charged particles that like to be paired with other electrons. If an electron is unpaired, it gets "lonely" and pulls a partner off neighboring molecules causing more lonely electrons and more partner stealing from neighboring cells resulting in a cascade.

The body's response to all this is to use *antioxidants* to stabilize the free radicals disabling them from doing damage to the DNA in our cells. However, if there are too many free radicals and not enough antioxidants present in the body, free radicals can go as far as stealing particles from your DNA, which can lead to cancer, Alzheimer's disease, atherosclerosis, autism, heart disease, Parkinson's, and stroke to name a few. This damage is known as *oxidation*. This is the same process that rusts metal or turns an apple brown after it is cut. Too much oxidation is likely to make us sick and old before our time. In the same way that paint protects metal from rusting or lemon juice protects apples from turning brown, cannabinoids protect our cells from oxidation.

Antioxidants come in the form of vitamins, minerals, and flavonoids. Antioxidants are molecules that act as electron donors; they give out electrons to lonely electrons in free radicals creating a pair and preventing the molecule from stealing electrons from healthy neighbors. Antioxidants are produced in the body and occur naturally in food. Commonly known antioxidants include vitamins C and E, Co-enzyme Q10, lipoic acid, ginkgo biloba, and lesser known antioxidants such as glutathione. Much like cannabinoids produce an entourage effect, antioxidants have a "network effect," too. In his book *The Antioxidant Miracle: Your Complete Plan for Total Health and Healing*, noted antioxidant researcher Lester Packer explains that antioxidants work together to support each other and therefore are much more powerful together than on their own. Their cumulative, synergistic effect gives the body the most benefit. (Packer and Colman 2000) Sound familiar? Additionally, research on antioxidants is starting to indicate that whole plant sources are much more effective than extracted supplements in the same way whole plant medicines from cannabis are better than isolated cannabinoids.

Cannabis is a powerful antioxidant—more powerful than vitamin C and E. (Hampson, et al. 1998) In fact, the U.S. Government Patent 1999/008769 is specifically for the neuroprotectant and antioxidant properties of cannabis. The government has known about this for some time. The patent explains that cannabinoids work in different ways to help repair oxidative damage giving the example:

> [T]he ischemic or neurodegenerative disease may be, for example, an ischemic infarct, Alzheimer's disease, Parkinson's disease, Down's syndrome, human immunodeficiency virus (HIV), dementia, myocardial infarction, or treatment and prevention of intraoperative or perioperative hypoxic insults that can leave persistent neurological deficits following open heart surgery requiring heart/lung bypass machines, such as coronary artery bypass grafts. (CABG)

About the antioxidant properties of cannabinoids and cannabinoids compounds the patent states: "*... that includes cannabinoids that act as free radical scavengers for use in prophylaxis and treatment of disease.*" This patent shows that the U.S. government sees cannabis as an effective medicine for treating disease and even preventing it.

This patent was filled by three highly respected government researchers: Aidan J. Hampson, Julius Axelrod (1970 Nobel Prize Winner), and Maurizio Grimaldi. Their work and our patent ("We the People" own the patent) will ultimately serve as a springboard to develop products that help protect the brain and body and reverse oxidative injury.

A diet rich in antioxidant foods such as red beans, cloves, acai, dark chocolate, cranberries, cannabis, blueberries, pecans, other nuts, and garlic to name a few can help reduce inflammation and cellular damage either to prevent disease or help fight it. We have discussed the fact that cannabis alone is not a cure-all for every ailment but an integrated approach of healthy changes for healing mind, body, and soul that increases your likelihood of benefiting from cannabis. I cannot help but wonder: since cannabis is a stronger antioxidant than vitamins C and E, and since antioxidants create a synergistic effect (improving the effects of other antioxidants they are combined with) doesn't combining cannabinoids with other antioxidants stand a good chance of creating great benefit to the body by preventing oxidation and aging? I've not yet found a study reflecting this, but I am willing to place my bet on a favorable outcome when the research is done!

Inflammation

Skeptics often accuse cannabis advocates of presenting cannabis as a panacea, "a cure-all." To some it sounds like snake oil. While cannabis and cannabis-based medicines are not a cure-all, they are effective in providing relief for many people with many problems. As we learned in the "Science" chapter, this is because, among other benefits, cannabis medicines support the body in managing and reducing inflammation. This "simple" benefit can yield huge positive impacts to our overall health and is the foundation for why cannabis is broadly effective as a medicinal agent.

The purpose of this section is to help you understand the role inflammation plays in your experience of health and how to effectively manage inflammation for better quality of life. It will also teach you to recognize when inflammation is an early warning sign of disease helping you to avoid illness in many cases.

One of the common denominators of ALL age-related disease (and many other diseases) is inflammation. Inflammation is a double-edged sword. It is part of the healing, immune, and disease causing process. The word inflammation comes from the Latin word *inflammo*, which means "ignite" or "set alight."

When we think of inflammation, we generally think about our body's response to a stubbed toe, broken bone, cut, or other traumatic physical injuries. The affected area usually swells, turns red, gets warm and stiff, and becomes painful. This type of inflammation is known as *acute inflammation*. The body increases blood flow to the site of the injury to increase oxygenation, nourishment, and immune response. This is the body's way of beginning the healing process after a trauma and is beneficial when it starts and stops as it is meant to do. To learn more, watch an excellent video about the biological process of acute inflammation at *http:// youtu.be/suCKm97yvyk*.

Cannabis supports the body and the ECS in cases of acute inflammation at the cellular and molecular level by reducing swelling and pain, managing spasms, serving as a muscle relaxant, and acting as an antioxidant. Many athletes utilize cannabis to help relieve inflamed, tired, and aching muscles and joints instead of taking an over-the-counter pain killer such as ibuprofen or more toxic prescription painkillers that produce performance dampening side effects. (Loria 2015)

Cannabinoids for Sports Recovery

Beyond a recovery aid, many athletes consider cannabis a performance enhancer. Reasons and results vary from opening one's field of awareness (making it possible to take in more information at once) to improving focus, increasing cellular oxygen, and reducing performance anxiety. Science specific to studying the effects of cannabis on performance and recovery for athletes is almost non-existent. A study conducted on mice in 2012 showed that prolonged oral administration of cannabinoids prevents neuro-inflammation, lowers beta-amyloid plaques (a culprit in the development of Alzheimer' disease), and improves cognitive performance. (Martín-Moreno, et al. 2012)

Chronic inflammation is a different story; it is a silent killer and the culprit behind the majority of chronic and/or age-related diseases. One may not be aware of chronic inflammation until it manifests as a serious condition. Examples of conditions caused by inflammation include all neuro-inflammatory diseases, arthritis, cancer, and heart disease— all of which can sneak up on patients over time.

Inflammation occurs as we age. While this is a natural process, lifestyle indiscretions can worsen it by increasing the level of inflammation or by speeding the onset and progression of disease and premature aging. Either way the outcome is undesirable. In my opinion, many practitioners do not pay enough attention to the underlying role inflammation plays in many different diseases. Thus, it is up to you to get informed and work with practitioners to make reducing chronic inflammation a priority. Research I have read leads me to believe that when inflammation is addressed there is a higher likelihood of managing or recovering from any number of conditions.

Until recently, the general public didn't hear much about inflammation and its role in health. However, the popularity of the books *Grain Brain* and *Wheat Belly*, along with the coverage of inflammation causing foods and anti-inflammatory diets, supplements, and lifestyle by popular physicians such as Dr. Mehmet Oz, Dr. David Perlmutter, and Dr. Andrew Weil, has raised awareness about chronic inflammation. Dr. Perlmutter's recent book *Brain Maker* is a must read to understand the gut-brain connection and how your *microbiome* (bacteria in your gut) contribute to health. Genetics, environment, stress, diet, exercise, injury, and lifestyle all play a major role in inflammation. Understanding that makes it possible for each of us to be proactive in reducing inflammation before disease occurs and actively managing the situation if we don't catch it in time. Do not ignore the little things; they get bigger over time!

Monitoring Inflammation through Blood Testing

There are *inflammation markers* in the blood that indicate chronic inflammation. Because several of these markers can become elevated before the onset of disease, they can predict disease before onset. Be sure to ask your doctor about testing your blood for key inflammation markers.

Cytokines are proteins occurring naturally in the body. They communicate between immune cells to coordinate the body's inflammatory response. Some are good. Some are not. And some can be beneficial or harmful depending on the amount being produced. It's kind of like cabbage. Cabbage is generally considered good, but when you eat too much of it bad things happen (wink).

Elevated levels of *pro-inflammatory cytokines* (the NOT-so-good cytokines) are strong predictors of death in certain types of conditions (including heart attack, stroke, and Alzheimer's disease) because high levels of these cytokines indicate your body is receiving lots of inflammation-causing signals. (Life Extension Foundation 2011) The most important inflammation markers are:

- tumor necrosis factor-alpha (TNF-α)
- interleukin-6 (IL-6)
- interleukin-1 beta (IL-1(6))
- interleukin-8 (IL-8)
- cyclooxygenase (COX-1 and COX-2) enzymes
- lipoxygenase (LOX) enzyme
- nuclear factor kappa-B (NF-kB)

The best place to start is getting your *C-reactive protein* levels tested. C-reactive protein is produced in the liver. It is an inflammation marker that, when elevated, may indicate an underlying chronic inflammatory disorder. A *New England Journal of Medicine* study shows that those with high levels of C-reactive protein are three times more likely to die from a heart attack. (Life Extension Foundation 2003) Another example is from the 2001 study published in *The Journal of American Medical Association* that found women with high levels of the inflammatory cytokine interleukin-6 (IL-6) were at a 2.3 times greater risk of developing type II diabetes, while those with a high level of C-reactive protein were 4.2 times more likely to become diabetic. (Life Extension Foundation 2003)

Other pro-inflammatory cytokines should also be tested, as they are powerful predictors of disease as well. A study of five thousand elderly people published in the *Archives of Internal Medicine* shows that frail seniors generally have higher levels of inflammation than their more active counterparts. (Life Extension Foundation 2011) In addition, those with high inflammatory markers also had more blood clotting activity, disability, fatigue, and muscle weakness than their healthier counterparts.

The Life Extension Foundation (LEF) at *www.lef.org* is an excellent resource for well-researched medical information. Although they have not yet jumped on the cannabis bandwagon, I am hopeful this will change. This organization also has a cost effective blood panel for sale that can be purchased directly.

> **Buy Your Own Blood Test** ——————————————
>
> An excellent resource for you and your doctor to learn more about inflammation markers is: *http://www.lef.org/protocols/ health_concerns/chronic_inflammation_01.htm.*

I bought a series of blood tests from LEF for under $400 during their spring blood test sale. That same test through my doctor (who was sending me to the same lab for the blood draw) was $1,200. And that was with my doctor giving me a pass-through rate from the lab. She would not have made a dime. I had no medical insurance, so my doctor and I looked at the LEF blood test menu together, and she specified what I should order. Saving $800 made a huge difference to me.

When you buy an LEF blood test, they send instructions for how to fast in advance of your blood work and when and where to go. Several days after your blood has been drawn, you receive results via email. With the purchase of the blood panel, you receive a thirty minute phone consultation with one of their technicians to help you understand the results and what you can do (dietary changes, lifestyle modifications, nutritional supplements, and pharmaceutical medicines) to bring your inflammatory markers into balance. Please discuss your blood test results with your physician.

Inflammation Related Disease

The following is a basic (but not comprehensive) list of diseases in which inflammation plays a key role:

For many, it is hard to believe that cannabis may benefit someone with the symptoms of the majority of the issues listed above and may also help stop or alter progression of the disease.

All the different pathways of how the ECS manages, regulates, and participates in the inflammatory response and the interplay between the ECS and other systems of the body that also have a part in the inflammatory response are not fully understood. In part, this is because there are many different scenarios of endogenous and exogenous biological events that can trigger a specific disease and cause an inflammatory response.

Diseases Related To Chronic Inflammation

Disease	Mechanism
Allergy	Inflammatory cytokines induce autoimmune reactions.
Age-related macular degeneration (AMD)	High levels of C-reactive protein doubles chances of developing AMD.
Alzheimer's disease	Chronic inflammation destroys brain cells.
Anemia	Inflammatory cytokines impede erythropoietin production reducing red blood cell count.
Aortic valve stenosis	Chronic inflammation damages heart valves.
Arthritis	Inflammatory cytokines destroy joint cartilage and synovial fluid.
Cancer	Chronic inflammation causes many cancers.
Cardiovascular diseases (CVD)	Inflammatory cytokines predict peripheral arterial disease, heart failure, atrial fibrillation, stroke, and coronary heart disease.
Chronic kidney disease (CKD)	CKD can lead to low-level retention of inflammatory molecules (cytokines, advanced glycation end-products, and homocystine), which can accelerate chronic inflammation in other parts of the body including the cardiovascular system.
Cognitive decline	Chronic low-level inflammation has been linked to cognitive decline including dementia, vascular dementia, and Alzheimer's.
Congestive heart failure	Chronic inflammation contributes to heart muscle wasting.
Depression	Elevated IL-6 and C-reactive protein have been reported in depressed patients.
Diabetes	Pro-inflammatory cytokines increase insulin sensitivity.
Fibromyalgia	Inflammatory cytokines are elevated.
Fibrosis	Inflammatory cytokines attack traumatized tissue.
Heart attack	Chronic inflammation contributes to hardening of the arteries.
Kidney failure	Inflammatory cytokines restrict circulation and damage nephrons, the part of the kidney that produces urine to remove waste.
Lupus (SLE)	Inflammatory cytokines induce an autoimmune attack.
Osteoporosis	Inflammatory cytokines TNF-α, IL-1β, IL-6 are required for normal bone metabolism. When they are chronically elevated, bone loss can occur.
Pancreatitis	Inflammatory cytokines induce pancreatic cell injury.
Psoriasis	Inflammatory cytokines induce dermatitis.
Stroke	Chronic inflammation promotes thromboembolic events in which blood clots block blood vessels.
Surgical complication	Inflammatory cytokines prevent healing.

Source: *Life Extension Foundation (Life Extension Foundation 2003)*

In the past, CB_1 and CB_2 receptors were thought to have an equal role in the attenuation of inflammation. However, evidence is growing that CB_2 receptors play a much more important role in managing inflammatory response than CB_1. (Gertsch 2008) In fact, in certain cases, such as some diseases of the heart, liver, or kidneys, activation of CB_1 receptors increases inflammation and may contribute to tissues injury. (Pacher and Kumos 2013) Practically speaking, this means cannabis high in cannabinoids such as CBD and others that have an affinity for the CB_2 receptor are likely to be more therapeutic for those with diseases of the aforementioned organs than cannabis or cannabis medicines high in THC. THC is a CB_1 and CB_2 agonist with a higher affinity for the CB_1 receptor.

CB_2 receptors, as we learned previously, are most heavily concentrated in cells of the immune system, which are known to naturally manage proinflammatory chemicals. There are a few situations in which activation of the CB2 receptors can actually cause tissues damage or worsen a few particular pathologies. Such is the case in some infections with live pathogens and certain cancers. (Pacher and Mechoulam 2011)

It is suspected that CB_2 receptors' role in managing inflammation is to help regulate the protein *TNFα* (tumor necrosis factor alpha) and the control of its effects on the body. (Gertsch 2008) It is one of the primary inflammatory markers that can be measured in your blood. TNFα has important immune regulatory functions in the body, which includes causing cell death, inducing fever, and preventing replication of cancer cells to name a few. However, when TNFα is overproduced (the ECS is out of balance) for too long, the body will move into a state of chronic inflammation where disease can occur. In this case, cannabinoids and terpenes signal the cells to slow or stop the production of the inflammation causing chemicals. (Gerdeman and Schechter 2010)

Sleep Reduces Inflammation

The production of inflammatory chemicals increases markedly after a single sleepless night. (Irwin, et al. 2006) For people who cannot sleep, a small amount of cannabis may be useful in helping get to sleep and stay asleep.

How Cannabis Reduces Inflammation

Let's look at a few specific examples of how the endocannabinoid system is being manipulated to manage inflammation in different diseases. What is covered here **barely** scratches the surface of research already done and currently underway to better understand the role of the ECS in inflammation and how exogenous cannabinoids can be used to manipulate the ECS to prevent, manage, stop, and cure inflammation- related diseases.

The widespread use of cannabis among those with irritable bowel syndrome (IBS) is prompting more research in this area. A 2011 article published in the *European Journal of Gastroenterology and Hepatology* said, "Experimental evidence suggest that endocannabinoids attenuate intestinal inflammation in animals, and activation of the CB2 receptor has been shown to inhibit the release of the proinflammatory cytokine, interleukin 8, from human colonic epithelial cell lines." (Lal, et al. 2011) The article speculates that both the CB_1 and CB_2 receptors "... play a role in modulating a variety of gastrointestinal responses including motility, secretion, and inflammation." (Lal, et al. 2011)

This helps explain why cannabis use is common among those with IBS and related diseases. When they utilize cannabis, chemical components of the plant support the ECS in doing what it is unable to do for itself thereby reducing spasms, diarrhea and the occurrence of loose stools as well as reducing pain associated with intestinal inflammation. I speculate that this would also result in a positive impact on mood as serotonin, an important mood-enhancing neurotransmitter, is produced in the gut. Additionally, it has to help overall health because slowing the pass-through rate of the stool increases nutritional absorption in the gut.

In disorders of the central nervous system such as Alzheimer's, Parkinson's, and amyotrophic lateral sclerosis, the science has revealed a strong relationship between neurodegeneration and inflammation. Previously, it was thought that one is a result of the other. Now we know they occur in tandem through similar disease pathways and have "mutual influence" on the disease. (Centonze, et al. 2007) Cannabinoids are effective modulators of both inflammation and neurodegeneration (using the shotgun approach as opposed to a rifle shot) addressing multiple disease factors at one time. Additionally, cannabinoids are believed to stimulate *neurogenesis* (growth of new neurons), which is extremely important in CNS related disorders. (Pacher and Mechoulam 2011)

In a 2010 article in the *Journal of the American College of Cardiology*, a strong indication between inflammation in diabetic cardiac dysfunction was indicated in a pre-clinical mouse model. (Rajesh, et al. 2010) The authors wrote specifically about the cannabinoid cannabidiol:

> Remarkably, CBD attenuated myocardial dysfunction, cardiac fibrosis, oxidative/nitrative stress, inflammation, cell death, and interrelated signaling pathways. Furthermore, CBD also attenuated the high glucose-induced increased reactive oxygen species generation, nuclear factor-B activation, and cell death in primary human cardiomyocytes. (Rajesh, et al. 2010)

The article also indicates that CBD shows encouraging signs of being highly effective at treating cardiac inflammation where other antioxidants have not be very effective. (Rajesh, et al. 2010)

A study published in 2008 about the use of cannabinoids in the treatment of pancreas fibrosis and chronic pancreatitis found that "Activation of the endocannabinoid system in chronic pancreatitis-derived stellate cells (PCS) specifically induced a more quiescent phenotype, accompanied by suppression of pro-inflammatory cytokines and extracellular matrix proteins as well as a decrease in invasiveness of PSC." (Michalski, et al. 2008) There is no cure, nor adequate treatment, for this disease. The fact that cannabinoids made the disease go dormant warrants urgent study of cannabinoids as a possible treatment for fibrosis of the pancreas and chronic pancreatitis.

Cannabinoids have also been shown to be effective in helping treat liver disease. In a mouse model of hepatitis, a study of THC was found to significantly suppress inflammatory cytokines and reduce injury to the liver. (Hegde, et al. 2008)

The cannabinoids tetrahydrocannabinol, cannabidiol, cannabichromene, tetrahydrocannabivarin, and the terpenes myrcene and beta-caryophyllene are potent anti-inflammatory agents. (Russo and Hohmann 2013) Research continues to better understand how these cannabinoids can work alone, together, and synergistically with other anti-inflammatory agents to reduce disease and its impact on the individual. The manipulation of the ECS with cannabinoids holds great promise for all inflammatory related diseases.

Anti-Inflammatory Diet Supports the ECS

As you consider ways to reduce unnecessary inflammation, please take a look at your diet. Over consumption of processed foods—most especially foods cooked with high heat, trans-fats, artificial sweeteners, sugar, and alcohol—and certain foods (grains, tree nuts, dairy, soy, and eggs) can cause inflammation or make it worse. A nutritionist or an allergist can help you evaluate your diet to learn what changes would be helpful. The three following resources are good starting points for learning about anti-inflammatory diets: *www.drperlmutter.com*, Sally Fallon's fabulous book, Nourishing Traditions, and the Weston A. Price Foundation at *http://www.westonaprice.org*.

Pain

Cannabis is like Robin Hood because it can give health back to people who have had it taken from them by dis-ease or injury. I know that sounds ridiculous to some of you, but based on the testimonials of the sick and suffering who have contacted me through my website *www.MyChronicRelief.com*, those I have met and interviewed for this book, and from personal experience, I'm here to tell you that this is simply the truth. If you have not lived with great pain or cared for one who has, it is hard to understand how pain robs you of your will to live and your ability to think clearly and be present enough to experience the wonders of being alive. Pain wears you down until there is no more fight left. For many people, cannabis offers a respite from this exhausting cycle.

Fighting for your life, recovering from a severe injury, trying to manage a chronic illness, or being the caregiver is STRESSFUL. There is so much to know and keep up with. There is so much to adjust to: life changes, doctor appointments, raging emotions, the emotions of others, new physical limitations, and so on. No matter how brave, positive, optimistic, determined, or cheerful you or the person you are caring for may be, the rigors of fighting pain and illness take their toll on the mind, body, and spirit. Cannabis helps!

According to the Institute of Medicine's 2011 report *A Blueprint for Transforming Prevention, Care, Education, and Research*, over 100 million adults a year in the U.S. experience chronic pain for a combined cost of $560–635 billion in pain management treatment and lost productivity. The report states: "For many patients, treatment of pain is inadequate not just because of uncertain diagnoses and societal stigma but also because of shortcoming in the availability of effective treatment and inadequate patient and clinician knowledge about the best ways to manage pain." (Institute of Medicine 2011) To say the treatment for my mother's pain was "inadequate" is an understatement.

The American Academy of Pain Medicine states on its website: "More than half of all hospitalized patients experienced pain in the last days of their lives, and although therapies are present to alleviate most pain for those dying of cancer, research shows that 50–75% of patients die in moderate to severe pain." This is not okay with me. What about you? Where is our compassion? **The real crime here is not the use of cannabis, but knowing that cannabis can help and doing nothing!** That is unconscionable.

My Story: Using Cannabis to Manage Pain

As someone who suffered greatly for years with my own undiagnosed and grossly mistreated pain, I am here to tell you that cannabis made it possible for me to work and care for myself at times when NOTHING else worked.

Since I was a child, I have had terrible bone and joint pain attributed to growing pains. Those pains subsided some once I got into my early teen years but never really stopped completely. After taking a popular acne drug during my high school years, I started to experience additional sharp pains all over my body but most especially in my knees and hands. The pain would move around and hit me when I least expected it. Sometimes it was so strong it would take my breath away. It felt as if someone were on the inside of my bones with an ice pick trying to chip their way out. When I went to college it became almost unbearable.

After visiting nineteen doctors over the course of my freshman year in college and receiving no helpful advice, I gave up. I had tried every pain medication available at the time. They all made me sick. After eating ibuprofen like candy (sixteen a day) for several months, I developed stomach problems. I had exhausted my options. I learned that deep breathing, regular sleep, avoiding sugar, and stress management helped but didn't solve the problem. For years I suffered in silence. Some days were so bad I just couldn't get out of bed. Things such as buttoning my pants, picking up change off a counter, or opening a food jar were challenging. I'll never forget having the worst craving for a dill pickle and not being able to open the jar. It was frustrating and disempowering. I suffered in silence for six years before trying cannabis.

The first time I tried cannabis was when my long-time friend Andrea and I were backpacking through Europe after I finished graduate school. We made our way to Amsterdam to see the markets and museums. After a visit to the Red Light district to see what the fuss was about, we landed in a coffee shop and discovered it didn't serve coffee. Since cannabis was legal in Amsterdam, I figured if I was ever going to try it this was the place. And so I did. I didn't get much out of that experience except for the munchies, and I didn't really understand what the fuss was about. Frankly, it was a bit of a letdown.

Fast forward to Budapest. Andrea and I were traveling this leg of our trip with two travelers from California. One night, while we were out exploring the city, they offered us a joint. Since my first experience with cannabis was so benign I thought to myself, "I'm in a foreign country. I'm twenty-five. I am a long way from home. Who is going to know? Maybe I didn't do it right the first time. Surely the whole 'this is your brain; this is your brain on drugs,' mantra was only true for those who smoked in the U.S. Right?" So I tried cannabis a second, and what I figured would be the last, time. Sorry Nancy Reagan, I know you were just trying to look out for me, and you too were brainwashed.

After our meal of fiery Hungarian goulash, we found a bench on a side street where we sat just outside the shine of a street lamp and passed the joint. Andrea did not partake. I was scared to take more than two or three puffs. Since my first experience had been a letdown, I wanted to make sure I was doing it right and not have too much. In a matter of minutes, our two travel buddies were laughing their heads off and acting silly.

My experience was different. I looked at Andrea and said, "Do I look high?" She laughed at me because she didn't know what being high looked like. Then she said, "No. How do you feel?" I looked at my fingers, which two minutes prior were so stiff I couldn't move them, but now I was moving them like I was playing a great Jerry Lee Lewis song on air piano. My fingers moved so freely. My knees, which moments before had been throbbing, felt free and normal. I looked at my friend and said, "I feel normal, like what I think it must feel like to be you. There is no pain." It was incredible. In that moment, for the first time in nine years, I had NO pain. I was relaxed and at peace. I was blown away by the experience. It was as if a one hundred pound backpack of pain had been lifted. I was free in my body and in full control of it and my mind. What a gift! If this is my brain on drugs, may I please have a side of bacon with my fried eggs?

Several years went by, and I continued to power through my pain. I was too scared to admit that cannabis provided me relief (what would people say?) and too afraid to break the law. What if I wanted to run for office one day? I suffered in silence except on the occasion I was outside of the country and smoking with virtual strangers or someone gifted me a joint. When someone did that, I swore them to secrecy. I was a closet toker. I rarely smoked with others and never talked about it. I'd take one or two puffs, feel better instantly, and then save that burned joint for the next time I couldn't move. The memory of saving those burned joints now makes me cringe and chuckle. Yet, I don't think I'm alone in such behavior.

Keep in mind that I had pain around the clock. I would only smoke when the pain was so bad I couldn't function. Getting high was not the objective for me; getting relief and being able to meet my normal work/life obligations were my goals!

Relieving Chronic Pain

Pain is an important indicator that something is wrong in the body, and powering through it is not always a smart move. Unfortunately, there are millions of people (just like me) who live in misery without getting any real help from doctors or pharmaceuticals (which often, in fact, make things worse).

There seems to be a cultural dismissal of the legitimacy of pain when one doesn't respond to traditional treatment. The response of many doctors, rather than striving to understand the pain, is simply to say, "Well, it must be in your head." Or they respond by increasing the dosage of medications or throwing more prescription medications at the problem. I was going to scream if one more person told me the crippling pain I experienced in my bones and joints was in my head. It took all I had not to wish my pain on them. Why would a college student with so much to live for create an ailment that didn't exist? I assure you I was not clamoring for attention. My life was fun and full. I had much better things to do than sit around waiting for my pain to go away or wasting money on fruitless visits to doctors.

The appropriate treatment for chronic pain is different for every patient and condition. Two people with the same illness or injury may have a completely different set of pain symptoms and responses to medications. This is complicated by the fact that most of the current treatments for pain do not provide a satisfactory amount of relief for a large portion of the population. This is just one of the reasons why researching how the endocannabinoid system, which is tied into our experience of pain, works is paramount to advances in pain treatment. (Visit *cannabis-med.org* and type the word pain in the search bar to review a long list of studies that address this.) Study after study shows that the use of cannabinoids and the development of cannabinoid-based-medicines could benefit millions of pain sufferers.

We have a pain epidemic in the United States. Western medicine has overlooked the importance of pain management in treating chronic illness. Hopefully, this may be changing somewhat with the study of cannabis.

Chronic pain often starts as a result of injury or illness or as a side effect of a medical treatment such as chemotherapy. It often starts as acute pain. After six months with a lack of desired response from treatment, pain is considered chronic.

Neuropathic pain is defined as complex, chronic pain usually accompanied by tissue injury. With neuropathic pain, the nerve fibers themselves might be damaged, dysfunctional, or injured. These damaged nerve fibers send incorrect signals to other pain centers. The impact of a nerve fiber injury includes a change in nerve function both at the site of injury and areas around the injury. (American Chronic Pain Association n.d.) Pain can become a disease in and of itself damaging the central nervous system. Over time, pain creates its own side effects that can spiral into a long list of other problems that further complicate treatment and decrease quality of life.

Common effects of chronic pain

- loss of appetite
- insomnia or poor quality sleep
- depression
- a sense of lack of control and helplessness
- exhaustion
- adrenal stress which can turn into hormonal stress and then exhaustion or vice versa
- loss of mobility
- physical weakness – loss of muscle mass
- lowered immunity
- neurotransmitter imbalances (imbalance in brain chemistry)

You **cannot** be well for long without appetite or sleep nor can you get well if you have no will to live. Chronic pain is an insidious evil. It robs people of their personality, joy, purpose, self-confidence, and will to live. The body is designed to manage stressors like pain for short periods of time without negative side effects. Prolonged pain changes your body and brain chemistry setting off a cascade of not yet well understood physiological responses.

As discussed in the "Science" chapter of this book, pain is, in part, managed in our body through our endocannabinoid system. When our endocannabinoid system fails us for whatever reason, leading to an increase in pain, cannabis may be a great equalizer helping control pain and inflammation while balancing other physiological responses caused by pain.

Let us also not overlook the important function of terpenes in controlling pain. While most cannabis samples are going to reduce pain in general, some are going to be more effective than others due to terpene concentration. Each cannabis medicine's effectiveness in treating pain is completely dependent on both the chemical makeup of the plant material and the type of pain.

According to Dr. Russo and his colleague Andrea G. Hohmann, PhD, professor in the Department of Psychological and Brain Sciences and Program in Neuroscience at Gill Center for Biomolecular Science at Indiana State University, "Basic science and clinical trials support the theoretical and practical basis of cannabinoid agents as analgesics for chronic pain. Their unique pharmacological profiles with multimodality effects and generally favorable efficacy and safety profiles render cannabinoid-based medicines promising agents for adjunctive treatment, particularly for neuropathic pain." (Russo and Hohmann 2013)

The endocannabinoid system is designed, in part, to modulate pain. For this reason, cannabinoids seem to be effective in helping manage different types of pain: acute, inflammatory, and neuropathic. Different sensations of pain are processed and controlled differently in the body. Therefore, the body's natural method to manage pain is controlled differently as well. Cannabinoids alleviate pain through a variety of mechanisms: directly through the body's CB_1 and CB_2 receptors as well as through non-receptor mechanisms, neurotransmitter modulation, and interaction with our endogenous (internally produced) opioids such as endorphins. (Russo and Hohmann 2013)

As previously discussed, CB_1 and CB_2 receptors and the endocannabinoids, 2-AG and anandamide (AEA), each have different functions when it comes to pain management. For instance, THC has a relatively high affinity for the CB_1 receptor; it is strongly electrically attracted to fit that receptor. THC is a CB_1 agonist thus increasing the activity of the endocannabinoid system. When a THC molecule fits into a CB_1 receptor, activating that part of the endocannabinoid system, we get the well-known euphoric effects of THC and its powerful analgesic effects. (Russo and Hohmann 2013) When the CB2 receptor is activated, chronic inflammatory and neuropathic pain is modulated. (Russo and Hohmann 2013) THC activates CB_2 receptors as well.

CBD, the second most prominent plant cannabinoid next to THC, is also an analgesic. CBD does not fit into either CB_1 or CB_2 receptors very strongly. Rather, it acts as a stimulant to the endocannabinoid system by suppressing the enzyme FAAH, which breaks down the endocannabinoid anandamide that fits into the CB_1 receptor. Thus, the consumption of plant or pharmaceutical CBD leads to less anandamide breaking down and more remaining in the body for longer. In other words, CBD increases the power of your body's own endocannabinoids. Together, THC and CBD are better pain modulators than they are alone. (E. Russo 2011)

Other phytocannabinoids such as cannabichromene (CBC), cannabigerol (CBG), and tetrahydrocannabivarin (THCV) (E. Russo 2011) as well as the terpenoids myrcene (opioid-type analgesic), beta-caryophyllene (analgesic, anti-inflammatory), alpha-pinene (antibiotic,anti-inflammatory, bronchodialator) and linalool (anesthetic) (Russo and Hohmann 2013) also contribute to pain modulation. While it is true most of these cannabinoids are not likely to occur in high ratios in American grown cannabis, plants can be breed to create higher concentrations of these cannabinoids and terpenes for various medicinal purposes.

Dr. Sunil K. Aggarwal profiles a 2011 review of eighteen randomized clinical trials (RCT) in an article published in the *Clinical Journal of Pain* with 766 subjects who received treatment for pain with oral-mucosal (applied to the gums, and under the tongue), whole plant cannabinoid extracts, inhaled cannabinoids, and single-molecule cannabinoid pharmaceuticals. Trials researching pain killers normally have a dropout rate of 33 percent (Aggarwal 2013) because trial participants cannot withstand the side effects and the harmful effects of the treatment being tested. In the case of the eighteen pooled cannabinoid trials, mild to moderate adverse effects were reported such as dry mouth, dizziness, and poor concentration, but there were NO serious adverse events and no withdrawals from study participation. (Aggarwal 2013)

Of the eighteen trials reviewed, fifteen "... demonstrated a significant analgesic effect of cannabinoid as compared with placebo" with four also reporting "significant improvements with sleep." (Aggarwal 2013) The reviews ultimately concluded, "... that overall there is evidence that cannabinoids are safe and modestly effective in neuropathic pain with preliminary evidence of efficacy in fibromyalgia and rheumatoid arthritis (RA). In patients with RA, the researchers observed lower RA disease activity, which is consistent with pre-clinical research that points to the strong anti-inflammatory benefits of cannabinoids. Also of importance in this review was the fact that the two smoked cannabis trials showed significant pain killing effect on HIV neuropathy. (Aggarwal 2013)

It would be misleading to tell you that every study to test cannabinoids for their effectiveness in treating pain was positive. Dr. Aggarwal researched the National Library of Medicine website *PubMed.gov* for RCTs using cannabinoids in pain management. Thirty-eight RCTs were found and reviewed. Twenty-seven of thirty-eight (71 percent) concluded that cannabinoids had in fact demonstrated pain-relieving effects; eleven (29 percent) did not. (Aggarwal 2013) It should be noted that these studies used varying preparations; dosing may have been inadequate, and other factors likely affected the results.

The growing body of evidence pointing to the pain killing properties of various cannabinoids is clearly statistically relevant. I look forward to the practice of medicine catching up with the science of medicine.

It has been theorized that certain conditions with high rates of pain, such as fibromyalgia, migraine, and irritable bowel syndrome, could be associated with a clinical endocannabinoid deficiency. This could help explain, in part, why cannabis is an effective treatment for these painful conditions. In an article published in the *Neuroendocrinology Letters*, Dr. Russo concludes, "Migraine, fibromyalgia, IBS, and related conditions display common clinical, biochemical, and pathophysiological patterns that suggest an underlying clinical endocannabinoid deficiency that may be suitably treated with cannabinoid medicines." (E. Russo 2008)

William's Pain and Narcotics Story

Everyone's pain story is different but similar. What is shared, sadly, is the suffering and significant loss of quality of life. The following is an email sent to me by one of the people who follow Chronic Relief on Facebook:

By the time I married in my mid to late 20s, marijuana use was a thing of the past for me. I was an electrician, and though my local union didn't require urine screening, certain work places did. Prisons, airports, nuclear power plants, etc. ... After the death of a friend in 1995, and my subsequent marriage a year later, the days of a few beers and burning a joint with friends were becoming far and few between.

In late 2001, I broke my back, but by sheer strength, determination, and stupidity I continued my workaholic ways until my back finally gave out in 2004. Nine surgeries and a few implants later, I was left addicted to narcotic pain medications, which I would often mix in an abusive way with Xanax® or Valium® to gain the desired effects of shutting down the pain. This mixture was akin to death, and death became an option considering my feelings of being totally useless as a father, husband, provider, and employee. The pain was that bad. Now I see so many travel the same road.

Thanks to my wife and a respectable pain doctor, I was able to stabilize my intake of medications, but the pain remained the same. Yes, I did learn to tolerate higher levels of pain, but my quality of life suffered immensely. During this time I became handicapped and unable to perform my above average salary job as a union electrician. The best way to describe my life at this time was a nightmare. Soon my new doctor had me on a stable dose of narcotic pain medication that I still take to this date. On very few occasions I would still use Valium®, as prescribed, to deal with nighttime leg tremors. My life began to turn around, and while still unable to perform my job as an electrician, I became somewhat useful as a stay at home dad. This afforded me the luxury of resting as needed. Still, the upstairs would remain untouched, and laundry piled up as I still have trouble going up or down stairs.

The years passed, and though I followed some news, I looked at the medical marijuana laws as a clever act for the progressive state of California to use as a means of getting stoned! I thought weed was weed and the "good stuff" was skunk bud or the occasional hydroponic buds I would find on tour in my youth.

Then something happened. It was sinister. It was criminal. I would be seen as an outcast in my small community of married parenting youth if my secret got out. I GOT HIGH! I wasn't looking for pain relief nor did I expect it, but it sure as hell found me. I had tears in my eyes mixed with laughter as I phoned my wife from a local store to tell her that even twenty-four hours later I was still almost pain free. The least amount of pain I had felt in nearly ten years and I wasn't nodding off or doped up …Maybe it was just a fluke? I needed further research. So I hit the Internet, and I hit the weed. What did I find?

Well, I didn't get arrested, yet, but I am now a practicing felon. Here in PA, we are at a snail's pace in adjusting our laws to lift the prohibition forced on all to protect the fortunes of a few. I have read so many medical reports from around the world and even here in these United States of America.

Next it was on to trial and error. While some varieties of marijuana worked great for pain, others worked even better. This was NOT the marijuana of my youth. Now, I couldn't constantly be stoned and be a stay at home dad at the same time. My driving duties and other such daily tasks, such as homework help and general parenting, were not acceptable to even myself, never-mind society or, worse yet, my wife. I am kidding about my wife. Sure, she doesn't want a stoned daddy watching our two children, but she is behind me 100 percent when it comes to POT vs. narcotics.

Soon I found that a few tokes after everyone hit the sack would provide pain relief well after the HIGH dissipated. Some varieties were better for nerve pain, and most, if not all, helped with my general outlook on life. Soon I was smiling more. Soon my mind began working and thinking again. I yelled less, and my wife watched as I changed before her eyes. Gone was the miserable curmudgeon who had to be treated with kid gloves. I wasn't a drop out stoner; if anything my thirst for knowledge increased.

I became a casual user of high grade marijuana. It changed my quality of life for the better and in turn helped my family as well. Daily stresses were washed away, the ability to be grateful returned, and my ability to deal with the pain even marijuana couldn't help directly was now being dealt with in an indirect manner. HOW COULD THIS BE ANY BETTER? Well, I guess not being viewed as a criminal would be a start.

I do not wear a T-shirt that reads I SMOKE POT, but I often tell people who suffer in pain of the miracle that took place in my life. In a small town word travels fast. Luckily, I can give a rat's ass. As long as I'm happy with me, I'd even be willing to take a hit for possession. I never own more than an eighth of an ounce anyway.

My hope is that someday in Pennsylvania I will be able to cultivate my own marijuana. I hope someday I can have instant access to tried and tested varieties that help my specific pain. I hope that one day I will not have to provide my pain management doctor with false urine so he won't lose his license. I hope that someday I will be able to forgo narcotic pain medications altogether.

God knows on the days marijuana is involved I take less of my prescribed meds. Gone are the days of Valium, except for the rarest occasions during our harsh winters. There is nothing that marijuana has affected negatively in my life. To anyone who reads my story, there is hope.

This is not a proclamation declaring marijuana as the best thing on the planet. I certainly see no place for pot in the hands of teens. As a youth I smoked weed in excess, and my schoolwork and social life suffered. On the other hand, it was not the gateway to heroin and cocaine. An unskilled doctor and my own decision that more is better lead to my abuse of pain medications.

Thank you marijuana for making my life more beautiful once again.

William from Pennsylvania
April 2013

Relaxation Reduces Pain
Surviving chronic pain of any kind is stressful, which makes the pain worse. Many patients will tell you that stress, anger, and fear increases pain. While I realize I am repeating myself, it is worth saying again: it is important not to underestimate the importance of the physiological benefits of relaxation, which I will argue are grossly undervalued in American culture.

Freedom from Pain Is a Fundamental Right

People are intrigued to learn about the *Chronic Relief* book and project created by me, an openly pro-cannabis Texan. When they meet me, cannabis is probably the last thing they think I'm going to talk about. At a house to house Halloween party in 2013, I met an established lawyer who is also pro-cannabis but thinks legalization will be a long time coming in our state. At the fifth house of the night, after talking about cannabis and this project at every previous stop, I quizzed my new friend to see if he could remember my web address. I really wanted his feedback. When he could not remember my web address, I wrote the URL on his right forearm in one inch letters with a Sharpie. In his follow-up email (after he asked me how to get the ink off his arm) he shared the following:

Somewhere in the arguments for medical marijuana (MM) there must be the proposition that freedom from pain is a fundamental right. So, denying people relief from excruciating pain, especially brought on by diseases any of us can get, is an aggravated case of denying a fundamental right.

Many chronic pain sufferers—and I surely would be one—would happily trade their right to vote, or to freedom of expression and assembly, if that's the price of getting relief NOW from the kinds of pain MM alleviates. Crazy, but probably true.

I bet if you asked people who once experienced severe, continuous, intense, unrelieved pain but then were spared from it by MM, whether they would trade some of their fundamental rights for the relief from pain they got, there are very few who would choose the right to vote.

I agree with my fellow pro-cannabis Texan. Freedom from pain is a fundamental right!

The American Pain Epidemic

In addition to neuropathic pain from treatment for lung cancer, my mother suffered from *spinal stenosis* (narrowing of the spinal column that puts pressure on the spinal cord), which caused shooting pain in her arms and hands. That, coupled with *neuropathic pain* that felt like an itch that couldn't be scratched, plus pin pricks all over her arms, nearly drove her mad. Over time this pain took its toll on her body and spirit. My mother tried many of the "new" pain drugs as prescribed. She HATED the way they made her feel: anxious, forgetful, dry mouthed, and socially removed. The side effects were nearly as bad as the pain itself. How I wish I knew then what I know now. I believe the last three years of my mother's life could have been much better had we tried cannabis earlier. Once she tried it, she got tremendous relief from pain, and it made it possible for her to relax. Normally, my mom would rub and scratch her arms to relieve some of the uncomfortable itching and pin- prick sensations. When she consumed cannabis, she was completely at ease; there was no rubbing and scratching.

Based on figures provided in the previously mentioned study by the American Academy of Pain Medicine, Facts & Figures on Pain, it is estimated that 3 to 4.5 million people suffer from *neuropathic pain* like my Mom. (American Academy of Pain Medicine n.d.) Neuropathic pain is a result of damage or a disease that affects the nervous system. It is characterized as burning or coldness, "pins and needles" sensations, numbness, itching and sometimes both. Dr. Donald Abrams is a well-regarded AIDS specialist and oncologist practicing in California. He is an outspoken yet measured advocate for cannabis as a safe and effective medicine and is vocal about how cannabis has effectively relieved neuropathic pain for his patients.

Dr. Abrams writes about the multi-symptoms common among his cancer and AIDS patients and how cannabis helps: "As an oncologist, I frequently see patients who suffer from anorexia, nausea, pain (despite taking opioids), insomnia, and depression. **Rather than writing them prescriptions for five different medications, all of which have potential toxicity, AEs [adverse effects], and addictive potential, I can recommend just cannabis.**" (D. Abrams 2010) He reiterated this point in a phone interview when I asked him, "What is the most important thing for me to share with others about cannabis?"

According to a U.S. Office of National Drug Control Policy 2007 report, over 27,000 Americans die annually from unintended overdoses, 12,000 of which involve prescription pain relievers. (Office of National Drug Control Policy 2011) Remember that this is not the case with cannabis. In fact, there are no known cases of lethal cannabis overdose because there are few cannabis receptors in the area of the brain that control breathing and heartbeat. The lethal dose is not known but suspected to be approximately eight hundred cigarettes. (D. Abrams 2010) At eight hundred, death would not occur because of cannabis poisoning but because of carbon monoxide poisoning. [See "Why is Cannabis So Safe?", on page 113.]

It is impossible to deny that we have a pain problem in America. The use of cannabis could help millions find some refuge from their nightmare. The tricky part will be for people who have traditionally taken pain pills, at very specific doses, to become empowered to be in charge of their own pain relief. This requires that people have basic information about the chemical components of cannabis that are beneficial for pain, so they can buy medicines that address their symptoms and get relief.

Chapter Six:

Diseases and Symptoms Benefited by Cannabis

Only time and the scientific method will ascertain whether a new paradigm is applicable to human physiology and treatment of its derangements. Our insight into these possibilities is dependent on the contributions of one unique healing plant: for clinical cannabis has become a therapeutic compass to what modern medicine fails to cure.
– Ethan Russo, MD (2008)

As of 2012, half of all American adults, approximately 117 million, have a chronic health condition, with one in four of these reporting having two or more chronic conditions (U.S. Center for Disease Control & Prevention 2014). What is the human and economic impact of that? What if cannabis, in all its possible iterations, could provide relief to even a small percentage of the chronically ill?

The diseases, ailments, and conditions NOT benefited by cannabis would be easier to list than those it does. Let's take a look at just a few medical problems benefited by cannabis: cancer, anxiety, depression, eldercare, Alzheimer's, and PTSD. Scientific articles are being published at an increasing rate about how cannabis works to treat different symptoms and change disease progression. If you don't find what you are looking for here, resources provided at the end of chapter will point you in the right direction. Please see the section on contraindications for guidance on who should not use cannabis (see page 160).

Cancer

The American Cancer Society says that half of all men and one third of women in the U.S. will develop cancer in their lifetime. In 2008, there were an estimated 12.7 million new cancer cases and 7.6 million deaths. (Ferlay, et al. 2010) The term **cancer** includes over one hundred different diseases that occur when cells that would normally die in a natural process not only fail to die but start to spread and grow out of control as abnormal cell groups known as tumors.

It is a rare individual whose life has been unscathed by cancer. How many people do you know who are battling cancer now or have lost their lives to it? The numbers are staggering. How is it possible that the way we treat cancer remains so barbaric? Why are cancer therapies so toxic they create side effects that are sometimes as bad as the disease? Why does the cure rate of these treatments remain so low? And why do many promising cancer treatments never make it to market?

It is well documented and widely accepted among patients and doctors that components of cannabis can help alleviate many side effects of cancer treatment including neuropathic pain, nausea and vomiting, poor appetite, anxiety, insomnia, and depression. Cannabinoid research indicates there is more to the story than just easing side effects and cannabis therapeutics hold the potential of changing cancer progression.

Genetics, environment, and lifestyle are all factors in the generation and spread of cancer cells. Like all other illnesses, cancer is a direct result of imbalance at the cellular level. In fact, some scientists hypothesize that cancer is a disease of the endocannabinoid system. Josée Guindon, DVM, PhD and Andrea G. Hohmann, PhD write in their 2011 paper "The Endocannabinoid System and Cancer: Therapeutic Implication," published in the *British Journal of Pharmacology*, that their observations "...raise the possibility that a dysregulation of the endocannabinoid system may promote cancer by fostering physiological conditions that allow cancer cells to proliferate, migrate, and grow." This certainly seems plausible. Doesn't it stand to reason that protecting the endocannabinoid system may help prevent cancer in the first place and that manipulating the ECS after cancer diagnosis could provide much greater success than we are experiencing with conventional non-ECS targeted cancer therapies?

Bone, brain, breast, colon, lung, prostate, thyroid, and skin cancers are a few of the different cancer types that research has found responsive to cannabinoid treatment. (M. Guzman 2003) How and why cannabinoids work as anti-cancer agents is complex, as cannabinoids work on the body in multiple ways at the same time. According to Guzman (2003), cannabinoids:

- Inhibit tumor growth in animal models by preventing the growth of new blood vessels (angiogenesis) needed to support the tumor.
- Selectively kill (induce apoptosis in) certain types of tumor cells without affecting surrounding healthy cells.
- Are non-toxic (unlike chemotherapy and radiation treatments) and are generally considered to have a favorable safety profile.

Over thirty-five years ago, research found that THC inhibits the growth of lung adenocarcinoma cancer cells in mouse models both *in vivo* (within a living organism) and *in vitro* (in a test tube) thus demonstrating the anti-proliferative effects of cannabis against cancer for the first time. It was two decades later before these findings spurred additional research. (Guindon and Hohmann 2011) Fortunately, research in this area has dramatically increased in the last ten to fifteen years. In the 1980s, as part of prohibition scare tactics, it was widely reported that cannabis causes cancer. This statement has been largely debunked. While some studies show cannabinoid exposure may increase the spread of cancer in a limited number of cancer cell lines, this view is not widely accepted.

It is important to note that inhalation of cannabis vapor and ingesting edible cannabis are the most common intake methods for managing symptoms associated with cancer and cancer treatment. While this is effective for palliative care, it is unlikely either of these ingestion methods provides a high enough concentration of cannabinoids to change disease progression. Success requires a high concentration cannabis tincture, cannabis oil, a cannabis-based extract medicine, or some combination of these with other integrated therapies and/or traditional cancer treatment. See this book's section on cannabis oil for more information on page 196.

Anxiety and Depression

Covering this topic adequately is similar to herding cats—almost impossible. Vastly different scientific models, controls, methodology, variations in cannabis samples, and other differences make it difficult to conclusively review the science on this particular topic. The science is conflicting and complicated but does show that the two primary cannabinoids, THC and CBD, have been shown in animal and human models to have anti-anxiety, and antidepressant effects and also improve mood—most especially in chronically ill individuals. (Patel, Hill and Hillard 2014)

The National Institute of Health speculates that over forty million Americans suffer from anxiety disorders (National Institute of Health n.d.) It is widely reported that there is a high rate of anxiety disorders among chronic cannabis users and a high rate of cannabis use among those with anxiety disorders. (Crippa, et al. 2009) That relationship is not yet understood but deserves a deeper look.

One of the primary reasons people give for utilizing cannabis is to reduce stress/anxiety and improve their mood. At the same time, one of the most common side effects associated with cannabis, and a major reason people stop using cannabis, is anxiety. How can this be? My hypothesis is this: differing effects occur (regardless of ingestion method) based on the chemical content of cannabis medicine used (i.e., plant variety), the volume of cannabinoids/terpenes consumed, the physiology of the consumer (the cause of their anxiety/depression/panic), and the mental state of the individual at the time of use. The biphasic response of THC is also a factor. As reported by the Sumerians over four thousand years ago, THC alleviates anxiety at low doses but promotes it at high doses.

The endocannabinoid system has been proven to have a major role in how the body manages stress. (Hill, et al. 2009) The interplay between the endocannabinoid system, hormones, and other neurotransmitters cannot be overstated in terms of anxiety, depression, and mood disorders. One of the challenges of adequately researching and understanding this topic is the fact that what causes anxiety, depression, and mood disorders is so different for different people, and the biochemical response in the individual can vary greatly. How that plays out in our brain, immune system, cardiovascular system, and hormonal levels, in part, drives how cannabis affects the individual.

Interestingly, the work of Matthew N. Hill et al. (2009) replicates the work of others that shows circulating endocannabinoid levels in depressed persons are lower than in those who are not depressed. This indicates the ECS has an important role in stress response and modulation. It stands to reason that further knowledge of how ECS affects the stress response would make it possible to more accurately manipulate the endocannabinoid system with cannabis therapeutics in order to give people more relief from anxiety, depression, and mood disorders.

Additionally, it makes sense that low doses of cannabinoids would help the ECS bring itself back into balance resulting in a positive, euphoric effect. (Melamede 2015) In my conversations with physicians who prescribe cannabis for anxiety and mood disorders, they generally agree it is reasonable to begin with a higher CBD variety or a straight CBD product, but many patients require the addition of THC, and some will require high doses. What works to manage anxiety and mood disorders is as variable as the individuals seeking relief.

While we see cannabis cause anxiety in some people/situations, we also see it help alleviate depression. Multiple studies conclude that people who used cannabis heavily as teenagers have a higher likelihood of increased rates of depression later in adulthood. That relationship, however, does not prove true for those who are light to moderate cannabis users as adolescents. (Patel, Hill and Hillard 2014) The reasons for this are unknown, but many clinicians are asking if the depression is really caused by the cannabis use or if there are other driving factors. The possibility of pre-existing psychopathology is poorly addressed in such studies.

In a survey of 4,400 subjects that separated users into groups including medical, recreational (daily users, weekly users, and less), and non-users, Thomas Denson, Associate Professor of Psychology at UNSW Australia, and Mitchell Earleywine, PhD, Professor of Psychology and Director of Clinical Training at the University at Albany SUNY, found that cannabis users had fewer and less intense depressive episodes than non-users and medical users had more depression than recreational users. (Denson and Earleywine 2006) Other studies support that cannabis users have less depression, while other studies draw a positive correlation between cannabis use and depression. However, as a practical matter, an overwhelming number of people I have spoken with and interviewed for this book utilize cannabis to lower their anxiety, manage depression, and improve their mood. There is no denying that for certain people cannabis is an effective treatment, and for them it is preferable over conventional treatments and prescription drugs.

It is curious that the vast majority of research in this area has been using THC at the expense of the other cannabinoids. It seems logical that CBD, a well-known modulator of THC induced anxiety, is key to the treatment of depression, anxiety, and mood disorders. I also can't help wondering how the co-administration of key terpenes and other cannabinoids could be used to treat these disorders. The economic impact of helping forty million Americans battle anxiety and mood disorders would be astounding not to mention the positive impact it would create in homes and communities.

Neurodegenerative Disorders

Neurodegenerative disorders include Alzheimer's, amyotrophic lateral sclerosis multiple sclerosis, Huntington's and Parkinson's to name a few.

Many neurological disorders are not well understood. For that reason, effective medicines to address the symptoms associated with them are lacking. In many cases, cannabis has been shown anecdotally to help patients where other medications have fallen short. The science also supports that. One of the driving factors behind why cannabis is a good medicine for neurological issues is the fact that components of the cannabis plant are incredible neuroprotectants. Part of what makes them so is that cannabinoids appear to protect neurons through multiple channels including as an anti-excitotoxic agent that prevents the pathological process that damages or kills nerve cells with too much stimulation by neurotransmitters, as an antioxidant, and as a cellular anti-inflammatory agent. (Fernandez-Ruiz, de Lago, et al. 2014) Additionally, cannabinoids have the ability to be selective in how they target parts of the brain or body that most need their attention and, possibly most important, seem to block or prevent some part or all of the disease causing pathologies at the same time. (Fernandez-Ruiz, de Lago, et al. 2014) Few medicines, if any, work that way. The fact that cannabinoids can act as a protector on different cell killing pathways is in part why they are so effective in treating neurodegenerative disorders.

Additionally, preclinical evidence indicates cannabinoids "...reduce acute neurodegeneration by improving neural repair." (Fernandez-Ruiz, Sagredo, et al. 2013) Serious scientific investigation is warranted for cannabinoids and their role in treating neurodegenerative diseases. Such research could prove useful in the treatment of spinal cord injury, stroke, traumatic brain injury, Alzheimer's, and all other neurodegenerative diseases giving great relief to patients and their families.

ALS

Let's take a look at amyotrophic lateral sclerosis, better known as ALS. This is an insidious disease that kills motor neurons. When motor neurons die, an individual loses the ability to control their limbs and muscles while in most instances the mind remains intact. There is no cure for this disease, and only one medicine is approved by the FDA to help treat its symptoms. This particular medicine has no impact on the rate of disease progression and doesn't significantly slow deterioration or prevent death.

Cannabis, however, has been shown, because of its neuroprotectant and antioxidant properties, to help slow the progression of the disease by protecting motor neurons the disease attacks and kills. (Carter and Rosen 2001) The antioxidant properties of cannabis help reduce the oxidative stress at a cellular level that contributes to cell death.

Animal research shows that both synthetic and plant derived THC counteract neurodegeneration. (Byer and Byer 2013) This research has not yet been conducted in human clinical trials, but a study by Mary Abood, PhD has shown that symptomatic relief was measured for appetite, insomnia, and spasticity in ALS patients. (Byer and Byer 2013) However, from a symptom management or palliative care perspective, cannabis has been shown in practical application to provide great relief for ALS patients. It helps with the following symptoms of the disease: pain, spasticity. drooling, wasting, *dyspnea* (shortness of breath or impaired breathing), *dysautonomia* (the inability for the body to control autonomic functions such as blood pressure, digestion, heart rate, and dilation/constriction of the eyes), and neuronal oxidation. (Carter and Rosen 2001) Gregory Carter, MD, in his presentation to the eighth Conference on Cannabis said that in clinical practice treating neurodegenerative disease, "…cannabis is tailor made for treating ALS." (Carter 2014)

One of the people I know with ALS was diagnosed over twenty years ago. By his doctor's account, he should have died fifteen to eighteen years ago. He credits his life, mobility, and the stalled progression of his disease to his daily cannabis use. When he feels any amount of spasticity, he excuses himself to his vehicle for a smoke and returns moving with greater ease.

One day I had the honor of sitting with a family as they explored the medical merits of cannabis and whether it was a fit for the matriarch of their family who was stricken with ALS and deteriorating rapidly. Her fingers were curling into her palms, and her hands were curling into the forearms. She had to really concentrate to control movement of her hands and fingers. Just to see if there were any benefits, she rubbed her hands with a salve made from cannabis flowers. About five minutes later, her husband asked how her hands felt. She answered, "I don't know, they feel fine." Then she opened and closed all of her fingers freely and easily. Everyone was amazed!

Elder Care and Alzheimer's

Cannabis use is growing substantially among the elderly population to help alleviate or manage challenges of aging. In the documentary *Prescribed Grass* by Zach Klein (available online on the Society of Cannabis Clinicians Vimeo Channel), we see the lives of elderly people in nursing homes in Israel being transformed by medical cannabis. Mr. Klein conducted an observational study that profiled twenty-seven elderly patients who took cannabis for pain, appetite, sleeping, spasticity, *ataxia* (the loss of control of body movements), agitation, depression, inflammation, and movement impediments. Collectively, his subjects discontinued use of thirty-nine different prescription drugs for these symptoms replacing them with cannabis only. Patients report being happier, sleeping and eating better, decreased spasticity and depression, and considerably improved pain relief. (Klein 2014).

Although no valid clinical trials have been conducted on treating Alzheimer's (AD) with cannabis, Jeffrey Hergenrather, MD, president of the Society of Cannabis Clinicians, reports positive, dramatic results using cannabis in treating Alzheimer's patients in nursing homes or Alzheimer's care facilities. (Hargenrather 2014) While there is some concern among physicians and researchers that it may be risky to give a euphoriant to an Alzheimer's patient, making it more difficult for their caregivers to manage them, I think the anecdotal evidence is encouraging and warrants urgent clinical investigation.

Alzheimer's disease is the most common form of dementia. It is NOT a natural part of aging. It is caused, in part, by the formation of tangles and amyloid plaque in the brain that interfere with memory, cognitive abilities, and mood dramatically impacting the quality of life of the patient and their entire family. The origin of Alzheimer's is not fully understood. While there are some medications available to slow the progression of Alzheimer's and manage its symptoms, there is no cure.

Society of Cannabis Clinicians

Cannabisclinicians.org is an excellent resource for doctors and patients alike. The organization strives to offer a platform for doctors to share their clinical experiences with cannabis, so they can collectively learn from their patients and provide them better guidance on medical cannabis use. Their website is packed with evidence based information. Additionally, SCC and The Medical Cannabis Institute offer the first-ever comprehensive clinical cannabinoid medicine curriculum for doctors continuing their education.

According to the Alzheimer's Association, over five million Americans are living with the disease, which is the sixth leading cause of death in America. (Alzhiemer's Association 2014) Twenty-five million people have it worldwide, and that number is expected to increase as the world population grows. (Fernandez-Ruiz, Sagredo, et al. 2013)

As mentioned before, cannabinoids have strong effects against excitotoxicity, inflammation, and oxidative stress associated with neurodegenerative diseases. Additionally, THC appears to inhibit acetylcholinesterase activity (Fernandez-Ruiz, Sagredo, et al. 2013), which directly interferes with the brain's ability to uptake the critical neurotransmitter acetylcholine, which is important for memory, cognition, and movement. CBD will also likely prove a worthy agent in the treatment of Alzhiemer's. CBD has been shown in vitro and vivo to help prevent, among other things, glutamate toxicity, inflammatory responses, and oxidative damage brought about by the presence of beta-amyloid proteins in the brain. (Fernandez-Ruiz, de Lago, et al. 2014) In a rat model, CBD was shown to stimulate *neurogenesis* (growth of neurons), which previously was thought to occur only in pre-natal development. (Romero 2014) This implies that there is an opportunity to not only halt the development of Alzheimer's through the use of cannabinoids but to reverse some of the damage caused by the disease.

Practical data gathered by Dr. Hergenrather not only supports this science but speaks volumes for the use of cannabis in treating Alzheimer's. In one facility, Dr. Hergenrather had fourteen Alzhiemer's patients taking doses ranging from 5 to 60 mg of cannabis derived THC four times per day. Patients and caretakers reported improved sleep, reduced agitation, increased appetite, reduced aggression, reduced pain, and improved mood. **Several patients abandoned prescription medications entirely.** Many prescriptions given to Alzheimer's patients have "boxed warnings" for increased mortality in elderly patients with dementia-related psychosis. (Hargenrather 2014) In a presentation on this topic, Dr. Hergenrather cites work by Lisa M. Eubanks, et al. (2006) stating, "Compared to currently approved drugs prescribed for the treatment of Alzheimer's disease, THC is a considerably superior inhibitor of amyloid B-peptide aggregation." (Hargenrather 2014) *Amyloid B-peptides* are deposits in the brain that are the hallmark Alzheimer's disease. So, in plain English, THC is much more effective at *preventing* these deposits from forming in the brain than all currently prescribed medications. The following are four of fourteen patient summaries from Dr. Hergenrather's independent study. All fourteen patients had similar positive results:

Patient 1 Prior use for agitation after exhausting regular medication. Cannabis is the only medicine that stopped her from loud crying and agitation.

Patient 2 Severe aggression and agitation with direct care. Skin picking and aggression ended on cannabis.

Patient 3 Very petite woman receiving all direct care. Exhausted behavior meds. Thrived on cannabis with spiked appetite and put smile on her face.

Patient 4 Diagnosed with Lewy body dementia (cognitive, physical, sleep, and behavioral symptoms) in his late 60s developed horrible hallucination, delusions, and aggressions. Stopped Haldol to use only cannabis. (Hargenrather 2014)

Post-Traumatic Stress Disorder (PTSD)

According to the National Institute of Mental Health, approximately 7.7 million Americans suffer from *Post-Traumatic Stress Disorder*, which is the feeling of being stressed or in danger when one is no longer in danger. PTSD is most widely associated with war veterans but can include anyone who has suffered a significant trauma such as rape, abuse, surviving a natural disaster, being in a terrifying accident, torture, death of a loved one, or kidnapping. PTSD occurs in people of all ages and walks of life. The information shared in this section specifically refers to the use of cannabis for the treatment of PTSD in adults.

In the past, people with PTSD were treated as if they were weak when they couldn't "just get over it" or "let go" of their trauma or "pull themselves up by their boot straps." Thankfully, society is beginning to recognize that PTSD is real and that it creates a wide variety of disturbances in the mind and body that the sufferer cannot control.

PTSD is characterized in adults by fear, anxiousness, night terrors, night sweats, night crying, rapid heartbeat, flashbacks, scary thoughts, guilt, depression, emotional numbness, emotional outbursts, rage, social disassociation, and being easily startled. It has been linked to inflammation in the brain as well as a misfiring or under/over production of different brain chemicals that affect one's ability to let go of traumatic memories. While PTSD is generally considered an anxiety disorder, I hypothesize that it is also closely associated with adrenal exhaustion.

Adrenal exhaustion occurs when the "fight-or-flight" response is constantly engaged. This response is in large part controlled by the tiny adrenal glands that sit atop the kidneys. Hormones they produce are intended to help manage stressful situations. When these hormones are depleted, other hormones produced in the body and brain try to support the adrenals by doing the job adrenaline was supposed to do. Over time, if the body is unable to rest and recharge, the adrenal glands become exhausted. This negatively impacts the levels of supporting hormones from the pituitary, hypothalamus, and thyroid glands—all which negatively impact neurotransmitter levels as well as other chemicals in the body. This often leads to a variety of additional symptoms including fatigue, headaches, heart palpitations, addiction, weight gain or loss, poor immunity, lack of quality sleep, physical pain, depression, and more. For more information about adrenal exhaustion, visit *http://www.adrenalfatigue.org*.

In the case of PTSD, the endocannabinoid system, which usually helps us forget or deal with painful memories, is somehow overloaded and unable to do that. Because the patient is unable to distance themself from their trauma, they are unable to relax and interact normally. Medical cannabis helps modulate these memories and stimuli enough that the patient can make sense of the memories, begin to integrate them in a healthier and more emotionally sustainable way, and relax the body enough to begin healing.

While cannabis may not work for everyone with PTSD, it deserves serious consideration as a piece of an integrated PTSD treatment including counseling, meditation, exercise, diet, nutritional supplementation, and cannabis. The problems associated with PTSD are as unique as the individuals who suffer from it. Cannabis for PTSD treatment is not a one-size-fits all, but no treatment is.

Raphael Mechoulam, writes the following about cannabis for treatment of PTSD in a blog post on the Veterans for Medical Marijuana page:

> Anecdotal evidence says, by and large, the use of **therapeutic cannabis provides a significant improvement in quality of life both for those suffering from this malady and for their family and friends.** Whether or not this is taking the fullest advantage possible of the ecB [EC] system in the treatment of PTSD is yet to be seen. Mostly the use of cannabis and THC to treat PTSD in humans appears to provide symptomological relief at best. In and of itself, there is nothing wrong with symptomological relief. That's what taking aspirin for a headache, a diuretic for high blood pressure, opiates to control severe pain, or olanzapine for rapid-cycling mania is all about. We do have the potential, however, to do better than just treating symptoms of PTSD via activation of the cannabinoid receptors. With the right combination of extinction/habituation therapy and the judicious administration of a FAAH inhibitor like KDS-4103, we have the potential to actually cure many cases of PTSD. For the time being though, symptomological treatments are all we have for more generalized anxiety and depression disorders.

Veterans and other PTSD sufferers have shared that cannabis makes it possible for them to function in their daily lives, manage pain, and control their depression as well as help manage rage, fear, anxiety, and sleeplessness.

The science in this area has predominantly focused on animal models and has largely been done with THC. THC is widely known to cause anxiety in some patients. PTSD sufferers who choose to engage in cannabis use must keep in mind that subtle differences in the chemical profiles in different plant samples could have different effects on their body and that the same plant sample could have positive or negative effects based on the amount of cannabinoids and terpenes consumed. One last thing to consider is that new research suggests CBD reduces anxiety in humans. (Patel, Hill and Hillard 2014) Increased CBD content is likely to reduce negative side effects caused by THC, which I think are particularly important for those managing PTSD.

Cannabis deserves serious consideration as part of integrated PTSD treatment. The Multidisciplinary Association for Psychedelic Studies (MAPS) received approval from NIDA in March 2014 to move forward with their study of smoked whole plant cannabis for veterans' with PTSD. This research will likely yield important data to help us understand how cannabis helps the brain manage traumatic memories. To learn more and support this research, visit the MAPS website at *www.maps.org*. As of the date of publishing of this book, the lead researcher on this project, Sue Sisley, MD, has been unable to acquire the cannabis necessary for research, yet she has the funding, subjects, and all federal and state approvals needed to conduct her study.

Other Conditions Cannabis Can Help

It is impossible to cover in full all of the different diseases or ailments that can be managed, and possibly treated, with cannabis because research is being published so quickly. The goal here is to provide you with enough information so you know how to seek knowledge that will benefit you most. This section is intended to broadly cover a few of the more common diseases in which cannabis has been found effective in providing relief or otherwise therapeutic. It contains many references to help support you in doing deeper research into your dis-ease and how cannabis and manipulation of the ECS may benefit you.

Conditions Cannabis Can Help

The articles and studies listed can be found easily on-line with a title search.

Condition	How Cannabis Can Help	Source*
AIDS	• relieves nausea and vomiting • stimulates appetite • prevents weight loss • reduces anxiety • may decrease damage to immune tissue of the gut • reduces neuropathic pain	"Marijuana May Smoke Out HIV/AIDS" **Study:** "Short-term Effects of Cannabinoids in Patients with HIV-1 Infection: A Randomized, Placebo controlled Clinical Trial" (Abrams, Leiser, et al. 2003)
Arthritis	• alleviates pain • reduces inflammation • promotes sleep • immunosuppressant	"Medical Marijuana for-Rheumatoid Arthritis?" **Review:** "Efficacy and Safety of Neuromodulators in Inflammatory Arthritis: A Cochrane Systematic. Review" (Richards, et al. 2012)
Asthma	• bronchodilation (expansion of the air passages)	"Can Marijuana Help People with Asthma or Other Breathing Disorders?" **Study:** "Effects of Smoked Marijuana in Experimentally Induced Asthma" (Tashkin, Shapiro, et al. 1975)

Conditions Cannabis Can Help, continued

Condition	How Cannabis Can Help	Source*
Chemotherapy, side effects	• relieves pain • reduces nausea and vomiting • stimulates appetite, increased weight • reduce anxiety • increases sleep • reduces neuropathic pain	"Marijuana" by Cancer.org "Questions and Answers About Cannabis" by National Cancer Institute **Study:** "Multicenter, Double blind, Randomized, Placebo-controlled, Parallel-group Study of the Efficacy, Safety, and Tolerability of THC:CBD Extract and THC Extract in Patients with Intractable Cancer-related Pain" (Johnson, et al. 2010)
Chronic Pain	• substitute for prescription opiates • greater relief from pain when used with opiates	**Study:** "Cannabis as an Adjunct to or Substitute for Opiates in the Treatment of Chronic Pain" (Lucas 2012)
Crohn's, Ulcerative Colitis	• chemicals in cannabis interact with cells in the body that play an important role in gut function and immune responses • phytocannabinoids decrease permeability of the intestines making the intestinal cells bond together tighter • helps regulate bacteria and intestinal function	"Cannabis Hope for Inflammatory Bowel Disease" **Study:** "Pharmacological Effects of Cannabinoids on the Caco-2 Cell Culture Model of Intestinal Model of Intestinal Permeability." (Alhamoruni, et al. Oct 2010)
Concussions, trauma to the brain	• lessens the bruising of the brain • better intracranial pressure control • may help with healing mechanisms after a traumatic injury • neuroprotection	"The NFL Should Combat Concussions with Cannabis" **Study:** "CB_1 and CB_2 Cannabinoid Receptor Antagonists Prevent Minocycline-Induced Neuroprotection Following Neuroprotection Following Traumatic Brain Injury in Mice (Lopez-Rodriguez, et al. 2015)
Depression	• controls anxiety • aids with insomnia • improve appetite • may improve mood	"Cannabis and Depression" **Study:** "Decreased Depression in Marijuana Users." (Denson and Earleywine 2006)
Diabetes	• reduction in weight improves lipids • improves glucose tolerance • better carbohydrate metabolism	"Marijuana: The Next Diabetes Drug?" **Study:** "The Impact of Marijuana Use on Glucose, Insulin, and Insulin Resistance among US Adults" (Penner, Buettner and Mittleman 2013)
Drug addiction	• less adverse side effects • less likely to cause withdrawal problems	**Study:** "Cannabis as a Substitute for Alcohol and Other Drugs" (Reiman 2009)

Conditions Cannabis Can Help, continued

Condition	How Cannabis Can Help	Source*
Epilepsy	• anticonvulsant • controls seizures by binding to brain cells responsible for controlling excitability and regulating relaxation • neuro-protection	"Marijuana and Its Receptor Protein in Brain Control Epilepsy" (Porter and Jacobson 2013) **Study:** "The Endogenous Regulates Cannabinoid System Seizure Frequency and Duration in a Model of Temporal Lobe Epilepsy" (Wallace, et al. 2003)
Fibromyalgia	• reduction of pain and stiffness • enhancement of relaxation • reduction of anxiety • functional improvement	"Medical Marijuana More Effective Than Big Pharma for Fibromyalgia" (Armamento 2014) **Study:** "Nabilone for the) Treatment of Pain in Fibromyalgia" (Skrabek, et al. 2008)
Glaucoma	• decreased pressure inside the eye • lower intraocular pressure (IOP) • may slow the progression of disease preventing blindness	"Glaucoma and Marijuana Use" (NIH National Eye Institute 2005)
Hepatitis C, treatment of	• helps lessen side effects of treatment • allows patients to complete Hepatitis C therapy	"Marijuana Aids Therapy" (Weiss 2006) **Study:** "Cannabis Use Improves Retention and Virological Outcomes in Patients Treated for Hepatitis C" (Sylvestre, Clements and Malibu 2006)
Lupus	• calming effect on immune system • reduces pain and nausea • anti-inflammatory	"Cannabis May Suppress Immune System" (Davis 2003) **Study:** "Suppression of Human Macrophage Interleukin-6 by a Non-psychoactive Cannabinoid Acid" (Parker, et al. 2008)
Metabolism	• healthier metabolism and reaction to sugars	**Study:** "The Impact of Marijuana Use on Glucose, Insulin, and Insulin Resistance among US Adults" (Penner, Buettner and Mittleman 2013)
Migraines	• analgesic • may help modulate pain sign signals • reduces inflammation • may help prevent migraine onset • reduces severity • shortens length of migraine • helps regulate serotonin and dopamine • act as a neuroprotectant antioxidant against glutamate toxicity	"Hemp for Headache: An In-Depth Historical and Scientific Review of Cannabis in Migraine Treatment" (E. Russo 2001) "Marijuana for Migraines" **Study:** "Endocannabinoids in the Brainstem Modulate DuralTrigeminovascular Nociceptive Traffic via CB1 and "Triptan" Receptors: Implications in Migraine" (Akerman, et al. 2013)

Conditions Cannabis Can Help, continued

Condition	How Cannabis Can Help	Source*
Multiple Sclerosis	• THC binds to receptors in nerves and muscles to relieve pain • helps control muscle cramps and spasms • reduces neuropathic pain • reduces inflammation • improves coordination	"Marijuana May Ease Multiple Sclerosis Symptoms" **Study:** "Smoked Cannabis for Spasticity in Multiple Sclerosis: A Randomized, Placebo-controlled Trial" (Corey-Bloom, et al. 2012)
Parkinson's	• reduces pain and tremors • improves sleep • improves fine motor skills • neuro-protection	"Smoking Pot Eases Tremors in Parkinson's" (Susman 2013) **Study:** "Cannabis (Medical Marijuana) Treatment for Motor and Non-motor Symptoms of Parkinson Disease: An Open-label Observational Study." (Lotan, et al. 2014)
Stroke, post	• may help protect the brain from damage caused by stroke	"Cannabis 'May Help Stroke Recovery by Improving Brain Functions after the Attack'" (Huffington Post UK 2013)
Tourette's	• reduces vocal and motor tics • improves obsessive-compulsive behavior (OCD) • serves as a sleep aide	"Tourette's Syndrome" by NORML Study: "Treatment of Tourette Syndrome with Cannabinoids." (Müller-Vahl 2013)

To keep up with the latest scientific developments and research data available about a particular disease, visit the following websites:

Online Cannabis Science Resources

Americans for Safe Access	safeaccessnow.org/medical	Provides useful and comprehensive information for patients and medical professionals.
International Association Cannabinoid Medicines	cannabis-med.org	Geared toward scientists and doctors, it is a wealth of information about the latest research developments.
Patients Out of Time	medicalcannabis.com	Provides continuing medical education conferences to health care professionals and has excellent papers and videos by the world's top experts in cannabis science. Helpful for both individuals and medical professionals.

O'Shaughnessy's: The Journal of Cannabis in Clinical Practice	beyondthc.com	This print and online cannabis news service tracks all major developments and trends in the industry from medical applications of cannabis to laboratory testing of medicine, variety development, and patient stories. An excellent resource. True cannabis science geeks will enjoy backordering previous issues.
PubMed	ncbi.nlm.nih.gov/pubmed	PubMed, the US National Library of Medicine website, comprises more than 23 million citations of biomedical literature from MEDLINE, life science journals, and online books. Citations may include links to full-text content from PubMed Central and publisher websites.
Society of Cannabis Clinicians	cannabisclinicians.org	Frequently updated with the best recent cannabis research as vetted by physicians and with a growing case report library where doctors share stories about treating patients with medical cannabis.
Clinical Trials	clinicaltrials.gov	All recently published clinical trials can be found on this website. See research that is scheduled, in progress, and just completed.
Leaf Science	leafscience.com	Provides short news clips about the politics, science, and trends in the cannabis industry.

Why Is Cannabis So Safe?

Aspirin is considered one of the safest medicines available. Yet almost one thousand people a year die from complications associated with its use. **Remarkably, there are NO known deaths associated with the over-use of cannabis. It has not killed anyone.** Cannabis is considered an extremely safe medicinal plant for the following reasons:

1. **Few cannabinoid receptors exist in areas of the brain that control breathing or heartbeat.** Opiates and many other drugs suppress heart-

beat and/or breathing. When either of those are suppressed too much, the patient dies. This is not a risk with cannabis use. There are not enough receptors in the area of the brain that controls heartbeat or breathing that can be activated by cannabis

2. **Cannabis has an extremely low toxicity rate.** Some medications, such as chemotherapy, can have painful and scary long-term (even permanent) side effects. Cannabis indeed has side effects for some people, but they are considered minimal and temporary. For most people, side effects go away in a number of hours. Regular users of high THC cannabis, as mentioned in the "Cognition" section of this book, may experience changes in cognition up to twenty-eight days after ceasing use.

3. **No Lethal Dose Established.** Most prescription medicines have established lethal doses. Yet no lethal dose has been established in humans for cannabis. No known deaths have been reported associated with overconsumption of cannabis.

The safety of cannabis is unparalleled in medicine. This does not mean cannabis is without risks or side effects. Nevertheless, cannabis and cannabis based preparations/medicines have enormous potential for improving public health because, in part, of their incredible safety profile. Most pharmaceutical drugs are designed to address a primary problem and bring comfort. Cannabis is much more dynamic, stimulating the ECS to address many problems at once in multiple biological layers, not only bringing comfort but restoration in many cases.

The Research Conundrum

Research suggests that cannabis not only can help manage symptoms of a disease but can also positively alter disease progress even fighting cancer by reducing or preventing tumor growth. *Preclinical studies* (studies conducted before the clinical trial phase to prove feasibility and collect drug safety information) strongly suggest that components of cannabis can kill brain, breast, and skin cancer cells. (Salazar, et al. 2009) In addition, one small clinical trial for cancer has been conducted to date using human subjects. In this trial, THC was injected directly into brain tumors with extremely promising results. Two patients with reoccurring *glioblastoma multiforme*, a fast growing and hard to treat form of brain cancer, were selected from nine patients who met the initial parameters of the study to receive a THC injection directly into the brain tumors. The results in both cases showed a reduction in cancer cell proliferation and reduced vascularization. (Guzman, et al. 2006) This is important because without the blood vessels to feed the cancer the tumor cannot survive. While a study of two people does not make a statistically significant result, it does give hope that THC and other cannabinoids have great promise as a cancer treatment possibly as a stand-alone treatment or an integrative treatment. Other cancer studies have been confined to animal models or human cells in test tubes (in vitro). Nevertheless, results strongly suggest the need for further investigation. Other areas where research points to the possibility of altering disease progression include diabetes, Alzheimer's, and anorexia/bulimia.

Sound promising? Are you wondering why this plant is still a Schedule I drug? I'm wondering why it's still scheduled at all.

As you know, the U.S. Government contends there is no known medical use for cannabis. And as you also know, vast amounts of research is being conducted that says otherwise. Unfortunately, much of the current cannabis research is being done outside the United States because of the difficulty our researchers have in getting approval to conduct research on a Schedule I drug. The hoops they must jump through are unbelievable. Can you hear the circus music playing? If cannabis were lowered from Schedule I to any other classification (or better yet declassified), we would see American cannabis research explode and the likely development of important new pharmaceuticals along with gaining a greater understanding of why diseases occur and how to treat them.

Conundrum: a confusing and difficult problem or question.

Conundrum sums up the state of U.S. medical cannabis research. Developing quality research studies is not the problem. Finding participants for studies is not the problem. Funding for these projects is not always the problem. The challenge with conducting medical cannabis research in the U.S. boils down to one thing: getting access to cannabis. Cannabis is grown in every state, and probably every city, in the country, yet researchers cannot acquire it to conduct their research due to legal road blocks.

According to international law, every country must have one governing body that controls the supply of cannabis for medical research. That entity in the U.S. is the National Institute on Drug ABUSE (NIDA). (Not the National Institute on Drug Abuse and Therapeutics because there is no such agency.) Forgive me for repeating myself, but this is really important: the NIDA website states:

> NIDA's mission is to lead the nation in bringing the power of science to bear on drug abuse and addiction. This charge has two critical components. The first is the strategic support and conduct of research across a broad range of disciplines. The second is ensuring the rapid and effective dissemination and use of the results of that research <u>to significantly improve prevention and treatment and to inform policy as it relates to drug abuse and addiction.</u>

Nowhere in that statement is there anything about conducting research into the therapeutic use of drugs. The name, mission, and very nature of NIDA means it is in direct opposition to research that explores the medical efficacy of cannabis and other Schedule 1 drugs.

Now, the content on NIDA's website might lead the unsuspecting to believe otherwise; we call this hogwash in Texas. When you dig a little deeper, a different story unravels.

Why It's Harder to Research Cannabis than LSD

The hurdles medical researchers must go through to access cannabis are extensive and as follows:

Hurdle 1: Any drug study conducted in the U.S. must be approved by the Food and Drug Administration (FDA). The FDA is the federal agency charged with protecting the health of the general public.

Hurdle 2: The research proposal must meet approval of an Institutional Review Board (IRB) whose job it is to ensure that the design of the study is ethical and safe for patients.

Hurdle 3: Researchers must meet any state required standards and procedures.

Hurdle 4: Research studies involving Schedule I substances such as cannabis, psilocybin, LSD, DMT, MDMA, and others have to meet the additional step of getting DEA approval.

Hurdle 5: Cannabis research is the only Schedule I drug research that has to clear a fifth hurdle; it must pass a Public Health Service (PHS is another agency within Health and Human Services) interdisciplinary review process.

Hurdle 6: Once the study has been approved by the above mentioned entities, the research team has to convince NIDA to provide the cannabis. As you might guess, this is more easily said than done.

According to the May 21, 1999 Announcement of the Department of Health and Human Services' Guidance on Procedures for the Provision of Cannabis for Medical Research, "... if NIDA [an agency of the National Institute of Health, which is an agency of Health and Human Services] determines that cannabis is available to support the study, NIDA will provide the researcher with authorization to reference NIDA's cannabis Drug Master File (DMF)." This just means that, if NIDA is so inspired, they will provide cannabis for the study, but if they are not inclined then too bad.

Now, NIDA grows and stores the ONLY herbal cannabis in the United States that is approved for FDA research studies, so Hurdle 6 is getting NIDA to agree to provide the cannabis for the study. Let me repeat that hurdles five and six are not required for conducting research for any other Schedule I drug.

These hurdles have essentially prevented many of our nation's top researchers from carrying out FDA approved cannabis research. These regulations make it especially difficult to get privately funded research approved. NIDA itself happily provides cannabis for its own research studies trying to prove the dangers of cannabis. NIDA has a reputation for incredibly slow responses to requests for cannabis. In the 1990s, NIDA stonewalled noted physicians and cannabis researchers Donald Abrams and Ethan Russo. Dr. Abrams eventually succeeded in getting his study approved because he proposed a study to evaluate the safety of cannabis. Dr. Russo's study was designed to assess therapeutic potential. It was never approved.

The Multidisciplinary Association for Psychedelic Studies (MAPS) tried from 2003 to 2010 to get ten grams (enough to make approximately twelve to eighteen joints) of cannabis from NIDA. The sponsor of their research project ultimately gave up and withdrew. Since that time, MAPS has met many more roadblocks in their quest to get cannabis research approved. Finally, in early 2014, NIDA did approve their study of cannabis for treatment of post-traumatic stress disorder (PTSD). Now, if they could only get the cannabis. You can read more about their frustrating journey on their website under the research section. Other researchers have had similar experiences where they have to poke and prod NIDA for a response. Once they finally get a response from NIDA, they are reminded that NIDA is not directed to support research on drug therapeutics but drug abuse.

There is a deep, rich political story to be told that could easily be the topic for another book, but what is critically important to know is that **cannabis science in the U.S. has been unnecessarily politicized in a way that has retarded nearly all American scientific advancements in our understanding of the endocannabinoid system and both the potential harms and medical merits of cannabis and cannabinoids.** Such behavior is morally misguided and reckless and flies in the face of the advancement of medicine for the public good.

The University of Mississippi holds the only NIDA license to grow medical cannabis; this means "Ole Miss" has a manufacturing monopoly on cannabis for research in the U.S. All other Schedule I drugs have multiple approved private manufacturing sources for research. In 2001, after NIDA refused to supply cannabis for several FDA approved research studies, Lyle Craker, PhD, director of the Medicinal Plant Program in the Department of Plant, Insect, and Soil Sciences at University of Massachusetts–Amherst was approached by the Multidisciplinary Association of Psychedelic Studies (MAPS) to apply to the DEA for a license to grow cannabis for research purposes. He agreed and made an application with the full support of his university.

The DEA ignored his application for three and a half years until they were ordered by a federal district court to show cause as to why they had not ruled. In 2004, the DEA denied his application. In 2005, the American Civil Liberties Union stepped in to help petition the DEA for a hearing in front of an Administrative Law Judge (ALJ). For a play-by-play timeline of this long drama, visit the ACLU website *http://aclu.org* and search "Lyle Cracker."

On August 22, 2005, hearings began in front of ALJ Mary Ann Bittner. Almost two years later her recommendation was made public. In that recommendation she stated that it was in the public's best interest to approve Dr. Cracker's application. This was followed by letters of support from Senators John Kerry and Edward Kennedy and a letter signed by forty-five members of the U.S. House of Representatives in support of Dr. Cracker. Yet four years later, in 2009, the DEA denied the application. Would it surprise you to know that Dr. ElSohly of the University of Mississippi, the holder of the sole U.S. license to grow cannabis, testified against the need to grant another license?

Dr. ElSohly, a well-respected cannabis researcher and expert in forensic toxicology, runs the cannabis growing facility at Ole Miss. He also is the owner of ElSohly Laboratories Inc., a private lab dedicated to "...analytical and advisory service to the drug testing community since 1985." (ElSohly Laboratories n.d.) According to his employer, he is party to over thirty-one patents with twenty-three pending. A web search of U.S. patents, finds at least nine of Dr. ElSohly's patents are directly related to cannabinoid extraction methods or cannabinoid delivery methods including a patch that is placed above the gum line in the mouth to deliver THC and a cannabinoid suppository.

According to testimony provided by Dr. ElSohly, to the Drug Enforcement Administration's Administrative Law Judge Mary Ellen Bittner, in 2005, Dr. ElSohly is able to freely use the cannabis he grows in his university facility for research and development in his private business. As mentioned earlier, he is also allowed to extract THC from the plants he grows under his NIDA license and sell it to pharmaceutical companies for financial gain for himself and the University of Mississippi (United States Department of Justice Drug Enforcement Administration 2005). By all accounts, Dr. ElSohly is an affable man and clearly has expert knowledge of chemistry. However, it is hard to overlook the fact that it is in his personal financial interest—on many levels—for cannabis to remain a Schedule I drug, for access to cannabis for research to remain limited, and for his research to support findings that suggest cannabis is dangerous. While I support Dr. ElSohly's ability to develop cannabis medicines and delivery methods, I cannot help but call out the double-standard at play.

This mess is a political problem that requires a political solution. Recently, I heard someone say that politicians do not change until the people push them to change. It is time to push! Write your national representatives and congressman! Let's ask them to move control of cannabis for research away from NIDA and directly into a department of the National Institute of Health. And let's ask that they drop the additional PHS review requirement for cannabis research thus allowing cannabis to match the same research standards set for other Schedule I drugs. Better yet, let's ask our representatives to legalize cannabis altogether thus allowing researchers to investigate the effects of cannabis as we do alcohol, vegetables, and other food items generally regarded as safe. Should you want to take action, please see our talking points in the last section of this book. Getting involved with Americans for Safe Access, The National Organization for the Reform of Marijuana Laws (NORML), the Marijuana Policy Project, and Patient Out of Time are great conduits for political action.

Thankfully, scientists in other countries do not have the same barriers to cannabis research. Israel, for example, has a vigorous cannabis research program under the leadership of Raphael Mechoulam. There cannabis is considered medicine. The Israeli government strongly supports Dr. Mechoulam's lab in their effort to better understand the different cannabinoids and the endocannabinoid system. Researchers receive funding for their investigations from the government of Israel and the U.S. National Institute of Health. They have minimal barriers to research, as cannabis is widely available from one of eight national pharmacies. Researchers simply call up the pharmacy, order what they need, pick it up, and then conduct research. This open system is yielding rapid advancement in the understanding of cannabis for better living and its benefits and limitations.

Important research is also being done in Spain by Manuel Guzman, PhD, and Christina Sanchez PhD, in Italy by Vincenzo DiMarzo, PhD, and in Canada by Marc Ware, M.D. to name a few.

Chasing the Research Rabbits

While on this soap box, I want to reiterate the point made previously: the vast amount of research done to date has been focused on delta-9 THC. The recreational cannabis market has created the demand for high-THC cannabis. But this is not how cannabis originally existed. It is through the magic of plant breeding that much of the CBD—a critically important balancing and synergistic component of cannabis—has been bred out of most of what is available to recreational and medical users alike. What would the research tell us if we were using 1:1 (THC:CBD) cannabis samples or all research measured more closely the content of all cannabinoids and terpenes?

There are many unanswered questions about how cannabis can serve the human body. Making cannabis accessible for research purposes in the United States is the first step in creating a broader understanding of the power of cannabis plant medicine. It is through such research that we will better understand how to effectively utilize this plant and develop real dosing baselines for all the many diseases and symptoms for which cannabis therapeutics may be an effective treatment.

Autism Spectrum Disorders (ASD) provide an incredible example of how transformative cannabinoid and endocannabinoid research could be to the general population. Autism is the fastest rising developmental disorder in the world. Over the past twenty years, autism rates have increased over 600 percent, and no one knows why. (Suzuki 2013) What was once considered a rare disorder, according to the Centers for Disease Control, now strikes one in eighty-eight children and one in fifty-four boys. There are a couple of riveting theories about what is causing this epidemic. Research shows that 80 percent of children with ASD also have some type of gastrointestinal dysfunction. (Yap, et al. 2010) Another theory hypothesizes that autism is a disorder of the synapses. Regardless, both hypotheses are directly related to the ECS. That knowledge, combined with all the strong anecdotal evidence from parents who have successfully used cannabis to treat their autistic child, leads me to believe it is completely reasonable to assume autism specific research on the ECS to understand what causes autism could lead to clues for its prevention and significantly improved treatment.

Update: On August 11, 2016, during the final production stage of this book, the DEA announced (in response to two petitions) that it would not be rescheduling cannabis under the Controlled Substances Act. Their announcement claimed "it does not meet the criteria for currently accepted medical use in treatment," its "lack of accepted safety," and its "high potential for abuse" as the reasons for their choice not to reclassify the herb.

At the same time, the DEA announced they are expanding the number of federally registered cannabis manufacturers by opening the registration process. This technically could end the monopoly on U.S. cannabis production for medical cannabis research. The rules are such that it is unlikely many entities will apply. It's basically business as usual.

Chapter Seven

The Benefits of Whole Plant Cannabis vs. Currently Legal Medicines and Intoxicants

We know more about cannabis than 95% of products approved by the FDA.

– Gregory T. Carter, MD (2014)

Cannabis vs. Prescription Pharmaceutical Medications

Yes, drugs are bad when abused or misused whether they are illegal, doctor prescribed, or over the counter. However, when used properly, drugs serve a great purpose in individual healing and the public good. Part of the challenge is that a drug having positive effects on one person can be ineffective or even toxic to the next person. And even when a drug is doing what it is supposed to do, it often comes with undesirable side effects, some of which are more bearable than others. In severe cases, if the disease doesn't kill you, the side effects of prescribed pharmaceuticals might!

Many years ago my father was diagnosed with brain cancer. Only after a *craniotomy* (a procedure in which the skull is cut open to provide access to the brain) to culture the tumors did we discover that his "brain cancer" was actually a fungus that could have been identified with a simple $7 skin test. The next twenty-four months were horrible for him and us. He experienced excruciating pain largely brought about by the heavy pharmaceuticals he had to take to kill the fungus consuming his brain and to prevent seizures, which he only began to experience after doctors wrongly cut a hole in his skull. My dad was a very sick man. At night I would pray (not something I was prone to do at sixteen), "God, if you are going to take my dad from us, do it now. There is no reason for him to suffer. If he is going to live with quality of life, let's get on with his healing. Amen." Thankfully, the second part of my prayer was answered, not the first.

After getting some runaround from the doctor about my father's prognosis, I successfully cornered him one afternoon in the waiting room of his private office and forced him to give me an answer about my dad's future. Imagine a sixteen year old 5'10" farm kid holding a 5'7" white-coated doctor up against a glass display case in the lobby of his office by his neck-tie. I wanted answers. During our friendly chat, the doctor confessed that the drugs my dad was taking to kill the fungus were fairly strong. When I pressed him (literally against the glass) about what that meant, he said, "If the disease doesn't kill him, the drugs might."

My dad lost 15 percent of his brain primarily in the areas of motor function. He had to relearn to write and adjust to changes in depth perception and slight changes in his temperament. Getting back to his old self took some time.

Years after my dad's illness, and long after he had ceased taking seizure medications (required when a person undergoes a craniotomy), he found himself a prisoner inside his body. He had stiffness in his muscles and felt generally lethargic and joyless; that is a nice way of saying my Dad felt like SHIT! After a four month detoxification program, my dad recovered his health and the skip in his step. Dad is a sweet, funny, smart, and gentle man. Before the detox program, he was so burdened. The disease, and the effects of medications, robbed him of his quality of life, his sense of humor, and his charm. It was such a relief to all who loved him to see him get back his health and personality.

Could things have been different for my dad had he tried cannabis when he was ill and recovering? I can only imagine how much easier his recovery could have been with cannabis and how it may have greatly lessened his suffering. I hypothesize from all that I have read that cannabis could have been used as a powerful anti-fungal agent had we the right type and preparation available. Based just on the stories I've been told by people who use cannabis for relief, a combination of cannabis sublingual tincture or oil and vaporized medicine would have made my dad more comfortable, and I believe it would have helped repair some of the *oxidative damage* to his brain and perhaps regenerated healthy brain cells to replace those consumed by the fungus. At the very least, cannabis would have reduced his pain and therefore his suffering. Seeing my father have some relief would have made my whole family feel better. Watching Dad suffer was excruciating for all of us. Being helpless to help those you love SUCKS!

We are lucky to have a happy ending. While the situation could have been much better had the doctors been more thorough and thoughtful along the way, it also could have been much worse. We are grateful my dad didn't overdose or get addicted to his pain killers. Such occurrences are more common than you might think and are becoming increasingly serious public health concerns. On their website The Centers for Disease Control and Prevention states the following about the disturbing prescription drug overdose trend:

> Deaths from prescription painkillers have also quadrupled since 1999, killing more than 16,000 people in the U.S. in 2013. Nearly two million Americans, aged 12 or older, either abused or were dependent on opioids in 2013.

For health professionals, policymakers, and legislators, addressing this problem is complicated. While they push for education, prevention, and enforcement to reverse this epidemic, they must also ensure that patients with a legitimate need for these medications still have access to them. (Centers for Disease Control n.d.)

On the CDC website they report:

- Drug overdose rates quadrupled from 1999 to 2014
- Deaths from drug overdoses increased 137 percent since 2000, including a 200% increase in overdose deaths involving opioids
- In 2014, 47,055 people died of drug overdose largely caused by prescription pain killers
- 100 people per day die of drug overdose, 78 specifically from opiates

The CDC lists *opioids*, **benzodiazepines** and **amphetamine**-like drugs as the most abused medicines. *Opioids* are powerful medicines primarily used for pain relief. They are derived from the opium poppy or are created synthetically in laboratories to mimic opium poppy compounds. Common examples of prescription opioids include oxycodone (OxyContin®, Percocet®), fentanyl (Duragesic®, Fentora®) methadone, and codeine. Opiates may be the most dangerous class of drugs for misuse or abuse.

The disturbing recent increase in drug overdoses in this country reflects a tenfold increase in the doctor prescribed use of opioid painkillers such as oxycodone and hydrocodone. The increased availability of such powerful drugs has led to widespread abuse. According to the Centers for Disease Control, nearly two million Americans claimed to misuse prescription painkillers in 2013. And, in the same year (the most recent statics available), there were over seven thousand people treated in emergency rooms for using a drug in ways other than directed. In addition to the risk of overdose, these people face elevated risk of injury, crime-related violence, and suicide.

Oddly enough, cannabis has been shown to increase the effectiveness of opiates making it possible to lower opiate dosage and reduce negative drug effects and the risk of addiction. (Lucas 2012)

Lower Opiate Overdoses in Legal States

Statistics show that in states where medical cannabis is legal, there are 25 percent fewer deaths from opioid overdose. (International Associaton of Cannabinoid Medicine 2014)

Benzodiazepines are pharmaceutical drugs that enhance the effects of the *neurotransmitter GABA*. They are *psychoactive* drugs that depress the central nervous system (CNS) and are generally considered "safe" when used therapeutically for a short time. They are prescribed to induce sleep, prevent seizures, relieve anxiety, and as a general sedative. Examples include alprazolam (Xanax®), diazepam

(Valium®), and lorazepam (Ativan®). The problem with benzodiazepines is twofold: when people mix them with other drugs, the CNS can be depressed, leading to reduced heart rate and breathing, which often results in death. And they come with a long list of negative effects including short and long term memory loss, lowered sex drive, and serious physical addiction.

Can you think of a safe, non-addictive medicine that induces sleep, prevents seizures, and acts as a general sedative? How many soccer moms credit their survival of modern day motherhood to Xanax? They might find that cannabis gives them better sleep.

Amphetamine-like pharmaceutical drugs are highly psychoactive, stimulate the CNS, and increase *serotonin, dopamine,* and *norepinephrine* levels in the brain. They are commonly used to treat attention deficit disorder and ADHD and are often given to young children despite the fact we know little about their long-term effects. Included in this class of drugs are dextoamphetamine/amphetamine (Adderal®, Adderal XR®) and methylphenidate (Ritalin®, Concerta®). Amphetamines are popular street drugs because they stimulate energy, create feelings of euphoria and focus, and lead to increased building of muscle mass. Amphetamine-like drugs are considered to have a high risk of abuse and are classified as Schedule II drugs. Overdose can lead to coma, heart failure, hypertension, psychosis, and even death due to the bursting of blood vessels in the brain. For those who become addicted to amphetamines, recovery can be a fairly long process as the body will continue to crave amphetamines long (sometimes years) after they stop using the drugs.

How would legalization of cannabis impact the problem of prescription drug abuse? As previously mentioned, many of the pain medications available today provide inadequate ongoing relief; maybe this is in part why there are so many accidental overdoses. Additionally, many prescribed medicines come with nasty effects including addiction and overdose death as discussed above. This certainly doesn't mean these drugs should be done away with. It does show that many drugs that are much more dangerous than cannabis have been given FDA approval as safe and effective. And, as Gregory T. Carter said in his presentation at the Eighth National Clinical Conference on Cannabis Therapeutics (2014), "We know more about cannabis than 95 percent of other medicines." Dangerous prescription drugs are widely prescribed and are accepted by the medical community while pharmaceutical companies make bank despite their many dangerous side effects, addictive qualities, and frequent lack of effectiveness. Given all this, it seems high time we give cannabis its rightful place in the pharmacopeia as a safe and legitimate medicine.

Cannabis vs. Alcohol

In November 2011, the *Journal of Psychopharmacology* published a study which assessed the two most prevalent intoxicants used in the UK: alcohol and cannabis. The paper confirms what many supporters of cannabis legalization have long claimed: alcohol is *twice* as harmful as cannabis to the user and five times as harmful as cannabis to others or society in general. The paper goes so far as to say that alcohol is a toxic substance contributing to 5 percent of the "total global disease burden." (Wissenborn and Nutt 2011)

It is ironic that cannabis (non-toxic) is illegal in a country where alcohol (highly toxic) is totally legal and even celebrated by the U.S. Congress during National Craft Beer Week. Yet, according to the Centers for Disease Control and Prevention, an estimated eighty thousand people a year lose their lives as a result of excessive drinking. The CDC also estimates that the total economic cost of excessive drinking is over $223.5 billion annually. While death from alcohol poisoning is rare, it is still estimated to kill over three hundred people annually. (Gable 2006) Compare that to the number of people who die annually as a result of cannabis use, which is ZERO. What is wrong with this picture?

Alcohol consumption is a widely accepted social practice. The federal Substance Abuse and Mental Health Service Administration (SAMHSA) estimates in their 2013 National Survey on Drug Use and Health that approximately 52.2 percent or 136.9 million Americans over the age of twelve are current drinkers. According to the 2014 Gallup Poll, 64 percent of adults drink.

It can be argued that in small amounts alcohol can be therapeutic by helping reduce stress and heart disease. What are those amounts you ask? And what is excessive or binge drinking?

- Standard Drink = 12 oz. beer, 8 oz. malt liquor, 5 oz. wine,
  1.5 oz distilled spirits
- Safe Drinking = 1 per day for women, 2 per day for men. And no more
  than 7 drinks per week for women and 14 for men.
- Excessive Drinking = 4 drinks for women and 5 for men in a day or
  exceeding 7 drinks a week for women or 14 for men.
- Binge Drinking = when one consumes enough alcohol in 2 hours for
  the blood alcohol level to reach .08. That usually occurs after
  4 drinks for women and 5 for men.

The *median effective dose* is the amount of alcohol or any other substance that produces a beneficial effect in 50 percent of the population. Alcohol's median effective does is approximately 33 grams or one shot for a 154 pound healthy adult. On the flip side, the *median lethal dose* is the amount of substance it takes to produce mortality in 50 percent of the population. The median lethal dose is 330 grams of alcohol or 10 shots consumed within several minutes on an empty stomach. Alcohol is considered to be fairly toxic, as the median lethal dose of alcohol is 10 to 20 times the median effective dose, which is similar to cocaine. (Gable 2006)

However, one need not consume that much alcohol for it to have a negative impact on the immune system. This is especially true for anyone with compromised health. Alcohol consumption can impede the body's ability to heal itself and worsen many conditions, especially when one is consuming large quantities or mixing it with prescription or over-the-counter drugs. Additionally, the long-term overconsumption of alcohol has profoundly damaging effects on the brain, heart, immune system, liver, and pancreas. (National Institute on Alcohol Abuse and Alcoholism n.d.)

It is especially interesting to note that research strongly indicates a high correlation between chronic alcohol consumption and lung diseases such as tuberculosis, pneumonia, and lung cancer, diseases more often associated with tobacco use. (Szabo 1997)

Cannabis has not been linked to any such diseases and, in fact, is thought to be beneficial in treating some of them. Please see the "Cannabis vs. Tobacco" section for more detail about how cannabis may protect the lungs.

Another major difference between cannabis and alcohol is how they change people's personalities. It is not uncommon for alcohol to make people volatile, mean or aggressive, or interfere with good judgment. Cannabis may lower inhibitions, and you may find yourself more inclined to be truthful, but it doesn't change your personality and even popular culture is clear that it doesn't lead to aggression. Cheech and Chong may have been lazy, but they weren't known for their quick tempers.

In multiple interviews with law enforcement officers regarding their opinions about legalizing cannabis, the thing that struck me most was that they all said they would rather deal with someone who is high than drunk. They said drunks are more volatile and put officers in much greater physical danger.

Given all this, there is no reasonable argument, especially from a public health and safety point of view, that explains why alcohol is legal and cannabis is not.

While this book is focused on cannabis as medicine, it would be naïve not to address the fact that people are going to enjoy an inebriant from time to time. It is human nature. Even little kids want to alter their consciousness. Just watch them spin on the merry-go-round. They want to go round and round until they are dizzy.

Regardless of one's personal views on drinking, I think we can all look back at alcohol prohibition as a miserable societal failure. It didn't work. Cannabis prohibition isn't working either. It seems especially ridiculous and hypocritical when you compare alcohol and cannabis side by side. The health benefits of alcohol are limited, the therapeutic window is small, the potential for abuse is high, and the side effects are both damaging and costly. Cannabis, on the other hand, is a relatively safe intoxicant with a high degree of medical merit, a large therapeutic window, mild side effects, and low potential for addiction. The most dangerous thing about cannabis use is that it is illegal; getting caught can be costly and dramatically impact your life.

The vast majority of us who drink alcohol do so responsibly. Yet most of us have also consumed alcohol irresponsibly on occasions. As a young adult, I too prayed to the porcelain god, begged for the room to stop spinning, and wasted entire days nursing hangovers. Even if I'm not over-served (wink), alcohol can still make me feel terrible, which is not the case with cannabis. Why not let adults make their own choices as to what kind of altered consciousness experiences they enjoy in their free time if those choices are not harmful to others?

Cannabis vs. Tobacco

According to the Centers for Disease Control and Prevention (CDC), **42.1 million Americans, or one in five adults were tobacco smokers in 2013.** The American Cancer Society says tobacco use is responsible for one in five deaths in the United States. **Around 443,000 Americans die from smoking related causes annually. These numbers are terrifying if you are a smoker or love someone who smokes.**

When my sister Shana and I were little, our family lived in Austin, Texas in a quiet little neighborhood on the east side. Dad had a good job as a scientist and electrical engineer, and Mom stayed home with us. My sister and I thought our parents were the most perfect couple: Dad was so handsome, and Mom so fashionable and beautiful. We adored them (and still do) and wanted to be just like them. They set the bar high for us in terms of who we aspire to be and what we seek in our love partnerships.

I probably would be a tobacco smoker if it hadn't been for my mother. Both of my parents smoked; it was perfectly normal at a time when smoking tobacco was not considered risky behavior, was commonplace in communities, and was not frowned on for teens as it is today.

It was a summer day. My mother was dressed in pretty white hot pants and a pink sleeveless top in the early 1970s fashion. She had her hair all done up in a bouffant and wore cat-rimmed glasses. We needed some groceries, so off to the grocery store we went. The store was so small that it was safe for Shana (age two) and me (age four) to roam the isles. People weren't worried about kid snatching back then. Mom was probably hoping we would wander around so she might have just one minute of silence. But no! We followed her every step. The whole way around the grocery store I was tugging on her shirt tail begging, "Mommy, please can I have a pack of cigarettes? Please? When I grow up I want to be just like you. Please Mommy. I want to smoke with you!" I suspect my pestering began long before we entered the store. When we got to the checkout she finally said, "YES, but under one condition: Whatever you buy you have to smoke today." My eyes lit up, and the cashier looked on in horror as I grabbed two packs of Marlboro Reds. I was going to be just like Mommy! We headed home to smoke!

Once we put the groceries away, my mom put my sister down for a nap, and the smoking party began. Mom opened the garage door, put on KVET (the local country music channel), set out some lawn chairs at the edge of the garage, and commenced to school me in a lady's way of smoking a cigarette. Yes, there were lots of funny looks from the passing cars. She lit herself a cigarette and then lit mine. And for a few puffs I was a big, big girl in my four year old mind. Then the sudden urge to puke up my toenails hit! I spent the remainder of the afternoon curled up on my bed thinking I was dying. I have rarely smoked a cigarette since. (If you were to ever see me with a cigarette in my hand, which is RARE, it is a clear sign that I've been "over-served" whiskey.)

I cannot thank my mom enough for teaching me the disdain for cigarette smoke that ensures I will never become a tobacco smoker! Tobacco smoking is an ugly addiction. Everyone I know who has quit smoking really had to want to do so. It's not easy! Tobacco addiction is physical, mental, social, and emotional. Nicotine is highly physically addictive, and those who stop experience awful withdrawal symptoms and cravings that can be difficult to overcome.

Mom and Dad each tried to quit several times over the years and were finally successful in 1992. It was no small thing. When I texted my dad to ask for clarification on when he quit smoking, he sent back a text that read, "August 16th 1992 4:32 pm."

Kudos to all of you who have quit! Quitting tobacco is not something you can be bullied into doing; it has to be your choice. Sometimes the desire to quit just isn't enough to break the addiction. If you know someone who is trying to quit, the best thing you can do is ask them what they need from you and follow through with their requests.

According to the Federal Trade Commission, over 264 billion cigarettes were either sold or given away by the top tobacco brands in the U.S. in 2014. That's close to 13.2 billion packs if we assume twenty cigarettes per pack. The national average cost per pack is $5.95 for an estimated total of $78.54 billion. The CDC reports on their website that in 2013 states generated $25.7 billion in taxes from cigarette sales. Approximately 1.8 percent of that money was spent on smoking prevention or cessation awareness and support programs—just a drop in the bucket. (Centers for Disease Control 2008)

Smoking is the most common form of cannabis consumption. That is probably because it is the easiest way for the patient to titrate their medicine; it provides immediate relief (but may produce mental effects that might not be necessary to gain symptom relief). The medical and recreational custom of smoking cannabis has been passed down through the ages. When cannabis is inhaled, it moves through the lungs and into the blood quickly passing through the blood-brain barrier to provide relief instantly. However, smoking in Western societies is widely associated with negative health side effects. While there is no exaggerating the side effects of smoking tobacco, the effects of smoking cannabis have been grossly exaggerated.

For years cannabis was erroneously reported to lead to cancers of the head, throat, and neck. There was even a study or two, previously mentioned, that somewhat supported this hypothesis although those studies were not specific to cannabis only. Instead, they mixed cannabis and tobacco. Existing research, however, indicates that while habitual cannabis smoking is associated with the symptoms of acute and chronic bronchitis and some evidence of microscopic injury to the bronchial cells, the link between Chronic Obstruction Pulmonary Disorder (COPD), lung, head, neck, or mouth cancer nor emphysema and cannabis use has not been made in the research. (Tashkin, 2013)

Irritation caused by combusted cannabis material can burn the throat of an overzealous or inexperience smoker. There is no doubt that this causes irritation and coughing. The most well-known authority on the topic of how cannabis affects the lungs is pulmonologist Dr. Donald Tashkin. The results of his research show no measurable link between cannabis smoke and cancer. We will cover this in more detail in the next section.

The latest figures from the CDC are from 2014. They report that tobacco smoking causes $156 billion in annual productivity losses and $300 billion in associated annual healthcare costs. (Centers for Disease Control 2014) If we combine the annual productivity loss and the healthcare cost caused by smoking, we have an annual national expense of $456 billion. This means the real cost of cigarettes to society is approximately $34.55 per pack, which is much more than the average $5.95 people pay. All the while tobacco companies spend $26 million a day in U.S. advertising. These are huge numbers. This is big business.

Commercially available tobacco cigarettes have over seven thousand chemicals in them. (U.S. Department of Health and Human Services 2010) Hundreds are toxic, and at least seventy cause cancer. It is no surprise cigarettes are harmful to one's health. Smoking is the leading preventable cause of death in the U.S. It is responsible for 90 percent of lung cancer in men and 80 percent in women according to the CDC and the American Cancer Society. Don't think for a minute that Ecigs are better. In fact, use of an Ecigs increases one's chance of cancer up to fifteen times that of smoking cigarettes. (Jensen, et al. 2015) As reported by the Surgeon General's *How Tobacco Smoke Causes Disease – What It Means to You*, tobacco negatively affects the body in these ways:

- Increases heart rate ten to twenty-five beats per minute. This makes the heart work harder increasing the chance of heart attack two to four fold.
- Constantly increases white blood cell production making the immune system work in overdrive all the time.
- Increases blood pressure thus increasing chances of stroke two to four times.
- Significantly increases risks of cancer because of the damage it causes to DNA. It especially increases risks for the following cancers: larynx, mouth, esophagus, bladder, pancreas, kidney, cervix, and stomach, and the science indicates it may also increase risk of breast cancer.
- Increased risk of lung diseases such as emphysema and Chronic Obstructive Pulmonary Disease (COPD). Over 90 percent of COPD cases are attributable to tobacco use.
- Increases in periodontal disease and tooth loss due to increased bacteria in the mouth and loss of circulation to the gums.
- Premature wrinkling of the skin due to nicotine interfering with cross-linkage of collagen fibers.

This is just a short list of the negative effects of tobacco on the body. On the bright side, smoking cessation provides immediate health benefits including increased energy, easier breathing, and better oxygen distribution throughout the body. People who quit smoking tobacco will cough less and find it much easier to be active. After two to five years of quitting, the risk of stroke drops to almost that of a non-tobacco smoker. Within five years of quitting tobacco smoking, your chance of mouth, throat, esophagus, and bladder cancer are cut in half. There is even more compelling evidence for quitting, but you get the point.

Cannabis and the Lungs

For years cannabis was reported to lead to cancers of the head, throat, and neck. Several studies were used to support these claims, but they were not on cannabis alone. Rather, subjects in the study were smoking blended cannabis and tobacco. Cannabis smoke has been inhaled medicinally and recreationally by humans for thousands of years. Due to the incredible success of tobacco cigarette marketing in the last one hundred years, most humans now associate the mere act of smoking a plant with the terrible health effects of smoking tobacco. However, as recently as the 1930s smoked plant preparations were regularly used as medicine, especially to treat diseases of the lungs. (Jackson 2010) In more recent years, inhalation of medicine has enjoyed considerable respect in mainstream medicine in the form of steroids and bronchodialators for diseases of the lungs. Granted those medications are for treatment of lung-related issues. Nonetheless, I still think inhalation can be a useful form of medicine delivery—not the best form but a viable option.

Three *epidemiological studies* (the science that studies the patterns, causes, and effects of health and disease conditions in defined populations) showed an association between cannabis use and tobacco-related cancers. (Tashkin 2008) The studies included the following reports and authors: "Marijuana Smoking and Head and Neck Cancer" by Zhang et al., "Etiologic Factors in Primary Bronchial Carcinoma in Tunisia" by Hsairi et al., "A Case-control Study of Lung Cancer in Casablanca, Morocco" by Sasco et al. Research indicates that while habitual cannabis smoking is associated with symptoms of acute and chronic bronchitis and some evidence of microscopic injury to the bronchial cells, it is not associated with COPD, lung, head, neck, or mouth cancer. (Tashkin 2008)

Pulmonologist, Donald Tashkin, MD presented his research at the 2008 Patients Out of Time Conference in Tucson, Arizona. You can see his presentation on the CannabisTherapeutics *YouTube* channel. (Hopefully, that presentation will remain on YouTube; they took my medical cannabis channel down without warning or explanation.) What is most compelling about his presentation is that he compares his findings to the results of other research that also did not show any correlation between cannabis use and cancer. In the end, there was no measurable link showing cannabis smoking causes cancer. (Tashkin 2008) Doctors are often skeptical of cannabis medicine because the most common delivery method is via inhalation. They automatically assume that the dangers of tobacco smoking are the same for cannabis. This is simply not true. The similarities between smoking cannabis (cannabinoids) and smoking tobacco (nicotine) are that both can cause irritation to the lungs and throat and contribute to chronic bronchitis or a smoker's cough. Both release carcinogenic components when combusted, but the way the body activates or responds to each plant is different. (Melamede 2005) In fact, research shows THC in cannabis smoke may prevent carcinogens present in cannabis smoke from being activated in the body whereas nicotine activates carcinogenic processes. (Roth, et al. 2001)

This is not to say that smoking cannabis is without impact on the body. In the 1988 *New England Journal of Medicine* article "Pulmonary Hazards of Smoking Marijuana as Compared with Tobacco," we learn that cannabis smoking is associated with a nearly threefold increase in the amount of tar inhaled and a third more retained tar in the lungs. The authors also observe that cannabis smokers take two-thirds larger puffs with a one-third larger puff volume and have a fourfold longer breath holding time. They conclude that smoking cannabis results in a substantially greater respiratory burden of carbon monoxide and tar versus a similar quantity of tobacco. (Wu, et al. 1988) Additionally, the smoke content of combusted cannabis has higher volumes of two different carcinogenic hydrocarbons than tobacco smoke. (Tashkin 2008) Regardless, it is important to note that tobacco cigarette smokers generally consume with greater frequency and volume versus cannabis smokers. (Tashkin 2008)

Despite this research, which suggests cannabis smokers end up with more tar in their lungs than tobacco smokers, cannabis smoking is not linked with any of the negative health effects of tobacco. This is likely due to the protective nature of the different cannabinoids and terpenoids present in cannabis (Tashkin 2008), which serve as cellular protectants preventing the activation of potentially harmful biological processes, have anti-fungal and anti-bacterial properties that fight lung pathogens, and have bronchiodilating properties that help increase the transport of oxygen throughout the body.

The Truth about Holding Your Breath

It is widely believed among cannabis smokers that holding cannabis smoke in the lungs increases the effect. This is a myth. Longer breath holding just makes you light headed by cutting off oxygen to the brain thus giving a false sense of effectiveness and increasing the amount of tar that stays in the lungs. (Tashkin 2008)

Just as cannabis smoke affects the body differently than tobacco smoke, nicotine and cannabinoids affect the brain in different ways. Cannabis may interfere with short-term memory and disrupt learning after consumption, but it can also provide long-term benefits to the brain because of its strong antioxidant properties, which result in improved memory in mature adults. While there is some evidence that tobacco may have some effect on preventing Alzhiemer's, the potential benefit is not worth the risk.

Here is a mind twister: it is argued that a tobacco smoker who also smokes cannabis is better off than one who does not. Dr. Tashkin's research indicates that the highest incidence of lung cancer occurs in tobacco smokers. The second highest rate of lung, head, neck, and throat cancers occurs in non-smokers. The lowest incidence of lung cancer appeared in habitual cannabis smokers and the second lowest rate in tobacco smokers who also smoke cannabis. This data suggests that cannabis has lung protecting properties. (Tashkin 2008)

It is important to note that most of the negative effects and risks related to cannabis discussed here are greatly diminished if not *entirely eliminated with the use of a vaporizer* or other alternate intake method. Vaporizers gently heat cannabis material releasing the therapeutic compounds into a fine mist or vapor that is inhaled. Since the plant material does not combust, no potentially harmful substances enter the body using this method.

Chapter Eight:

Cannabis Guide

We should be thinking of cannabis as a medicine first that happens to have some psychoactive properties, as many medicines do, rather than as an intoxicant that happens to have a few therapeutic properties on the side.
– Tod Mikuriya, MD

What Is Your Health Strategy?

In all things, including using cannabis as medicine, it is helpful to be clear about your end-game. **What do you want?** This incredibly versatile plant is used differently depending on the health benefits you seek.

It is important to consider your health as a whole and not just the most uncomfortable symptoms. When only the symptoms of a dis-ease are treated, the disease is not cured. That is why it is important to take responsibility for your own health and consider what happened (lifestyle, stress, environment, physical injury, major life events or prior illness) to get your body to this point of dis-ease. In cases such as fibromyalgia, migraine, and other conditions which are not fully understood, while you may not be able to come up with all the answers you seek, there is much to learn that may be useful. As you research your condition, or that of your loved one, you will pick up on little things that are applicable or resonate with you. Don't ignore those things.

Time and again I watch people around me abdicate responsibility for their health by giving their power to their healthcare provider (or to the opinions of loved ones). Your health provider has one important flaw that you must always keep in mind: They are human. They get seven days in a week with twenty-four hours in a day just like the rest of us. Demands for their time, attention, and energy are immense. It's nearly impossible for them to give each patient exceptional care, meet the demands of health care and medical malpractice insurance companies, keep up with all of the regulatory paperwork, and still stay on top of the latest advances in medicine.

Unfortunately, this often leads doctors to use antiquated medical practices; it is not uncommon for it to take ten years for a proven advancement in care or treatment to become an accepted practice. This is why it is important to do your homework about your disease and advances in the treatment of it. Know your body, how it works, what you respond well to, and what you don't. Keep abreast of advancements in treatments for your condition from credible resources such as PubMed® and medical journals specific to your condition.

I am not encouraging you to try every exotic miracle cure from all ends of the earth just because someone on the Internet said it would cure you. This can be counterproductive and even harmful. However, being well informed about your options and what changes you can make to improve your odds of getting the outcome you desire is empowering and the first step towards reaching wellness and relief.

Communication with your provider is key. Remember that doctors do not know what it feels like to live in your body. They are going to treat you based on their knowledge, experience, and biases (both positive and negative). It is your job to speak up, ask good questions, and communicate all your issues and concerns so they can care for you more completely. **If your healthcare providers are not open to questions or your input, fire them and go find someone else.** First and foremost, get your needs met! Listen to your gut. If what you are being told to do concerns you, speak up! Always trust yourself more than you trust anyone else. Your body's inner knowing of what is best for YOU is never wrong. Sometimes our interpretation is wrong because we let our rational brain get too involved, so be sure to truly listen to your intuition. That is Divinity pointing you in the right direction.

If you are new to this, consider taking a meditation, mindfulness, or prayer class. The Heart Math Institute (*www.heartmath.org*) is also a great resource for how to connect mind, body, and soul. Rebecca Hamm, one of my wisest teachers, taught me to seek the truth by listening to what is in my highest good by connecting to, and through, my heart (and therefore the Divine) with this simple technique:

Begin by closing the eyes and focusing on the breath moving in and out. Slowly bring your awareness to the center of your chest, your energetic heart area, and allow your mind to gently, and ever so slightly, bow towards your heart. To be fully present means to be awake within and connected to all that is alive around you. When we are present, we have the opportunity to hear and follow a deeper level of guidance.

Then imagine a situation or question that you are sitting with and ask, "My beloved Source, God, Universe, Spirit, is it true..." Fill in the blank. For instance, "My beloved Source, please show me the truth. Is it true that I can be well?"

Notice what you hear, sense, or feel when asking for the truth. So often we hear or feel the truth, but our minds, perceptions, or beliefs prevent us from trusting and accepting these truths. When you ask for the truth, you'll notice your heart will feel open, expanded, closed, or constricted. A feeling or sense of constriction is often an indication that whatever it is you are considering is not the best choice. The feeling of openness and expansion is often an indication that the truth you are seeking is right in front of you. If you find that you are not hearing anything, or you are not feeling anything in your body or heart, come back to it later in the day or the next day, and keep asking the question until you have a clear response.

Another option is to ask, "My beloved Source, God, Divine world, is it in my highest good to ..." For instance, "My beloved Source, is it in my highest good to continue believing I can't heal?" You would follow the same steps as above listening, feeling, and sensing how it is to hold that question in and from your heart. Time and again we know the truth on some level, but we struggle accepting the truth because of a belief that says or implies we are not worthy of being loved and honored.

These two exercises are a great way to realign and connect to the beauty of who we are and always have been: **a pure and unchanged representation of the quality and essence of Love. Remember: expansion, relief, a feeling of being loved, held, honored, and connected is where we all are meant to live: a state of Grace.**

I have heard from many physicians, chiropractors, acupuncturists, nurses, and other healthcare providers that they are always learning from patients. They take notice when they see something working. This helps them become better informed so they can provide more complete care to all their patients. Many an oncologist will tell you that watching patients successfully use cannabis to relieve vomiting and nausea, pain, depression, lack of appetite, and more helped change their minds about its medicinal value. So share your research and findings with health care practitioners. If you are presenting well-sourced documents, they will probably take you seriously. You may teach them something that benefits you and many others.

Help Your Doctor Get Educated

An exceptional resource for your doctor is *http://www.theanswerpage.com*. This website is free to use and offers comprehensive information about medical uses of cannabis that are transferable to clinical practice.

Whatever your ailment, it is a whole body issue. Your mind, body, and soul are involved and should be considered in your treatment regimen. Take me for example; I shared earlier that I have always suffered from chronic pain. It's taken me years to understand and manage it, and I am still learning. Just addressing the symptoms didn't work for me. Taking high doses of pain killers only addressed the pain not what was causing it. Once I stopped taking painkillers, the pain was still there, and sometimes it was even more intense than before. Painkillers created a whole list of other problems. What I really wanted was to feel healthy, free, powerful, whole, and in full control of my body, and I wasn't going to get that from a pill bottle. I really had to look at my lifestyle, nutrition, stress management, and thought and behavior patterns and take a more integrative approach. By integrating chiropractic, acupuncture, exercise, prayer, meditation, nutrition, and being willing to cut the things from my life that didn't serve me, especially stressful relationships, inflammation causing foods, and harmful thought/behavior patterns, I was able to get control of my situation and feel powerful instead of powerless. Strengthening my physical self required strengthening my emotional self, which required strengthening my spiritual self. This remains an ongoing journey but one that has been deeply rewarding.

Anatomy of the Spirit

If the idea of healing the mind, body, and soul and deepening your connection with the Divine and taking responsibility for thoughts, actions, and behaviors that contribute to your wellness or lack of it is appealing to you, and you want to know more about how to unravel the emotions and thought patterns that hold you back, the book *Anatomy of the Spirit: Seven Stages of Power and Healing* by Caroline Myss is a great place to start. Her book explains in simple language how our thoughts and beliefs create energetic patterns that can contribute to disease and gives the reader great insight into how they got where they are and how to get where they want to go.

Luckily, I have had the counsel of a few incredible healthcare providers who helped me find a holistic approach to living that has significantly reduced my pain and improved my quality of life. I now take quality supplements that are specific to my pain, hormone levels, and body's needs. I exercise regularly in a way that doesn't overwork my joints or muscles, and I eat a clean, healthy, gluten-free diet rich in quality fat, fresh veggies, and grass fed meats. I'm deeply grateful to my acupuncturist Ron Banuelos for being so direct with me about my health. He said he would be happy to treat me, but there would be no real resolution to my health issues until I was willing to go gluten-free and work through unresolved fear. He was right! Once I was willing to do my part, which included some difficult changes to my diet and a willingness to be vulnerable, my health improved tremendously. Twenty-five pounds disappeared, my hormones balanced, I'm generally pain free, and my immunity and energy improved.

I'm not telling you to shave your head, join a monastery, meditate all day, go to a strict raw food vegan diet, and give up everything you love. Of course if that sounds appealing to you then it might be just what you need, but it isn't the cure for everyone. It is up to you to determine what physical and mental health improvements you can realistically make and how to reach your goals. This life is not a dress rehearsal. We get one chance to make the most of it—not just for you, but for everyone who loves you. What are you willing to do to take control? What changes in your physical, mental, and spiritual health are necessary to fully enjoy your life?

How can you make changes that support your body in its healing and still find joy so you can impact the world with your wellness instead of your pain or sickness? If the changes we are making result in a feeling of deprivation or misery, it's unlikely that we will stick with them. **The whole point of making changes is to live better.** What can you do to live better? Here is a short checklist of things that might be helpful:

Checklist for Better Living

- [ ] Spend time looking for things for which to be grateful
- [ ] Hug and touch often
- [ ] Pray or meditate
- [ ] Become aware of your negative thinking patterns and replace them with healthy thoughts and behaviors
- [ ] Exercise
- [ ] Laugh
- [ ] Learn to say no to stressors and yes to fun
- [ ] Get eight hours of sleep a night
- [ ] Balance your hormones
- [ ] Test the inflammation levels in your blood, and take action to reduce them
- [ ] Make yourself the priority
- [ ] Reduce stressors
- [ ] Make decisions and move on
- [ ] Improve your diet
- [ ] Take nutritional supplements that enhance your body's ability to heal itself—get some guidance from a health professional—not all supplements are created equal
- [ ] Take more time to enjoy
- [ ] Learn something new
- [ ] Eat kale and add more greens to your diet
- [ ] Stay hydrated
- [ ] Forgive yourself and others
- [ ] Spend time with people who make you happy
- [ ] Let go of any and all thoughts of victimhood
- [ ] Let go of things not in your control

How does cannabis fit into all of this? The answer is different for everyone. This is why you must be willing to take responsibility for making choices that are in your highest good, and surround yourself with people who support that.

Hindsight Is 20/20: My Mother's Cancer Treatment Program

My mother had tumors in her lung surgically removed. Then she took a pill form of chemo. Although my mom was aware of the benefits of cannabis for managing the effects of chemo, it was not yet something she was willing to consider.

We had a couple of months of respite when she was not being treated, and we thought all was well. A storm was brewing though, and her cancer came back with a vengeance. At that point, we used chemo as advised by her doctor: intravenous vitamin C at the direction of a local integrative medicine expert (MD), a twice daily fresh green juice to increase her nutrient intake and build her immunity, and lots of well-considered supplements. My dad deserves great credit for researching the integrative therapies and doing his homework on how to use juicing effectively as part of her treatment regimen. Making my mother two green drinks daily was not a small commitment. He did it joyfully. The combination of the intravenous vitamin C, the nutrient dense green drink, and the extra dose of love he served with every cup helped my mom tremendously! I credit my dad with buying my mother a few extra months of quality life. Thank you, Dad!

The combination of these treatments worked well for a while. The drawback was that the vitamin C made her very thirsty, which my mom found uncomfortable, so she opted out of continuing the treatment. However, that regimen brought about a significant reduction in her tumors. The chemo alone was simply not as effective. She did try different types of chemo, but ultimately the neuropathy it caused was so bad she was unwilling to continue. It's possible that, had we tried cannabis sooner, it would have provided enough relief that my mom could have continued treatment.

I cannot help wondering: Would my mother's disease have progressed differently if we had access to high quality cannabis oil rich with some combination of high THC and high CBD? There is really no way of knowing. Nonetheless, I believe there is a high likelihood cannabis oil could have been effective and bought her more time and a better quality of life at the least. I'm haunted by the discovery that in test tubes with human cell cultures cannabinoids have proven effective at causing death in lung cancer cells and slowing tumor growth. (M. Guzman 2003)

Hindsight is 20/20. For that reason, I encourage you to talk to people, be it in person or on the Internet, who are in your shoes. Ask lots of questions about the experiences of others and what worked for them. Ask your doctors, "If this were your mother or child, what would you do?" Ask other patients and loved ones what they would have done differently if they had it to do over again. This feedback will help you make better choices for yourself or loved one.

The following section describes five different health plans where cannabis can be integrated.

Prevention Plan

Any intake method of cannabis can be utilized as a proactive part of one's health regimen. Two cannabis naïve Texan friends of mine, Chaul and Pad (wink), who now live in Palm Springs, California, told me a funny story about their adjustment to life in the Golden State. They started to notice a "funny" smell every afternoon around the same time. They thought the smell might be cannabis but were not sure. For the longest time they could not figure out where the smell was coming from and were totally shocked that anyone in their neighborhood would partake. Keep in mind they are Texans, and until recently, that was a taboo topic in Texas. Finally, one of them figured out that the smell was coming from the house next door. The next question was which one of the three people who lived there was smoking? Was it the matriarch, her daughter, or the grandson? It was like a modern day Palm Springs "who done it" mystery. One day Chaul was up on his roof putting up Christmas lights. He was not sure who was more shocked when his eyes met those of the cannabis smoker—the matriarch of the house—who was lighting a pipe. With a chuckle, my friend said hello to his neighbor, and she quickly put her pipe and lighter behind her back like a kid who just got caught with their hand in the cookie jar. That was several years ago. Chaul says she still lives next door and still smokes daily at the same time. For their neighbor, a daily toke is considered an important part of a healthy lifestyle.

One day I was trying to find something to share on our Chronic Relief Facebook page. On my feed there was an excellent picture of Willie Nelson with a joint in his hand. The caption reads, "Willie is 80! If weed is a gateway drug, it better hurry." I couldn't help but giggle.

Neuroscientist Dr. Gary Wenk, PhD says in his TED talk *Life Depends on This*, that a puff of cannabis a day for adults will help people live better by reducing inflammation and keeping the brain nimble. (2012)

Because of social stigmas surrounding cannabis, society as a whole has not embraced the role it could play in preventative health care. I predict that, as we advance our knowledge and acceptance of the medicinal benefits of cannabis, it will become a well-regarded component of healthy living and a proactive healthcare regimen in the same way walking and taking fish oil are considered integral parts of a healthy lifestyle. People will use cannabis in its raw form as juice to boost immunity, components of cannabis will show up in topical anti-aging and beauty care products, and various preparations of whole plant cannabis will be available at health food stores as a nutritional supplement to help build immunity, strengthen the brain, ease the aging process, support relaxation, and so on. A variety of sophisticated whole plant cannabis medicines will also be available at your local pharmacy. One day cannabis will be appreciated for its full utility. Society will look back on this time of prohibition as laughable and un-evolved. Thankfully, we have pioneering growers, activists, entrepreneurs, scientists, doctors, and patients who are currently laying the groundwork for all aspects of cannabis for better living to become mainstream in the not too distant future. It's coming! When it does, it will be a great wealth generator much like the dot com era.

Recovery Plan

For someone trying to recover from injury, illness, or surgery, cannabis can help with pain management, bone healing, controlling or reducing muscle spasms, and reducing swelling and inflammation. For acute pain, small amounts of vaporized cannabis can help take the edge off without the nasty side effects of heavy pain killers such as methadone, codeine, and hydrocodone. Cannabis can be integrated with painkillers such as opiates as a way to boost pain killing power while lowering the dosage of potentially addictive painkillers and managing side effects. Many people have found cannabis a useful tool in weaning themselves off physically addictive drugs such as Oxycontin® and methadone.

Nationally known cannabis activist and injured Vietnam veteran Clif Deuvall used cannabis to wean himself off opiates and methadone prescribed for pain due to the loss of one eye as a result of injuries from an airplane explosion caused by a mortar round. Over time, the pain from these injuries took over Clif's life. From 1975 –2005, he took heavy prescribed opiate drugs. Eventually, they were not enough. In 2005, his prescription was changed to methadone (a potentially very nasty drug). That same year he was declared 100 percent disabled.

The result of changing his prescription was a different kind of pain. Clif says, "I became a shell of a human being as a result of methadone." He felt drugged all the time and spent large amounts of time bedridden and unable to function.

Clif wanted his life back. After researching alternative treatments, he discovered cannabis was an effective substitute to methadone. He decided to give it a try. The effects were felt immediately, as his pain levels were much better managed. He was able to spend time with his family again, and he eventually no longer needed the methadone that robbed him of his quality of life. Clif used cannabis successfully to recover from a methadone addiction, to manage pain, and he has successfully used cannabis to aid in his recovery after a knee replacement and another surgery to place a titanium rod in his arm. He even used a cannabis salve to help heal the incisions on his knee and arm. His doctor remarked that the incisions healed better than anything he had ever seen. It is noteworthy that when Clif began his cannabis regimen he had many lesions on his brain that were confirmed via an MRI. A latter CAT scan showed the lesions had decreased significantly. Clif's health continues to improve.

For those of you taking prescribed opiates to aid your recovery, consider that the co-administration of cannabis and opiates could have many benefits. Dr. Donald Abrams says in his paper *Cannabis in Pain and Palliative Care* that co-administration of cannabis and opiates magnifies the effect of the opiate while often making it possible for the patient to take a lower dose. (D. Abrams 2010)

In May 2013, I officially came out of the cannabis closet in a big way. I testified to the Texas House of Representatives Public Health Committee in favor of a bill that would make it possible for doctors to visit with their patients about cannabis without fear of retribution from the Texas Medical Board and for judges to dismiss cannabis possession charges for medical patients if the judge was so inclined. Clif and I, and seventeen others, testified in favor of the bill. No one spoke out against it. Many who spoke told deeply personal stories of pain, misery, and how cannabis delivered them from their pharmaceutical hells to a better place. I was struck by the number of people just like Clif who told prescription drug horror stories. Drugs prescribed to them were robbing them of their life, and they felt like they were slowly dying more from the prescription drug side effects than from their disease or ailment. Speaker after teary-eyed speaker explained with great passion that if it were not for cannabis they would not even have been able to show up to testify. In 2015, over sixty people testified for the same bill.

A large number of those testifying in 2013 and in 2015 had used cannabis to get off of **all** pharmaceutical medications. With that accomplishment came empowerment to live better, fuller, happier lives!

Among the benefits of using cannabis for recovery is that it has a **VERY LOW risk of addiction and low toxicity** unlike many prescription drugs.

Maintenance and Management Plan

Since I began this project, people of all ages, shapes, sizes, ethnicities, and socioeconomic and religious backgrounds have come out of the woodwork to share their stories with me. Many contact me under secret email accounts and fake names for fear of their cannabis use being discovered. The people who have graciously shared their stories have multiple sclerosis, muscular dystrophy, failed disc fusions, insomnia, depression, PTSD, autism, cancer, Parkinson's disease, fibromyalgia, diabetic neuropathic pain, and the list goes on. Their stories are both sad and inspiring because almost every one includes a history of getting lost in the cracks of the medical system, being so doped up on pharmaceuticals they couldn't function, or finding that pharmaceuticals didn't work for them or made things worse.

One of the lovely people I've met through my cannabis advocacy is a brilliant businessman I'm going to call Ed. He and his wife Melanie have four sons ages late teens to early twenties. Ed is a software engineer with several patents to his name and has led several high-tech companies. In his early thirties he was diagnosed with hereditary degenerative arthritis. He was in excruciating pain for which his doctor prescribed a variety of medicines until he settled on Vicoprofen®. What started as joint pain quickly progressed to pain throughout all the joints and the muscles eventually leading to an additional diagnosis of neuropathic pain, which is extraordinarily difficult to treat. Most people with neuropathic pain will tell you the prescriptions often make it worse. This was the case for Ed. His doctor's response to his increased pain was to increase the dosage. He was taking two to four 750 mg doses of Vicoprofen® every six hours.

Ed was no longer able to get out of bed or off the toilet alone as a result of the pain and weakness in his knees. It took ten minutes to walk down a single flight of stairs in the morning to get to his home office. He found that the prescriptions interfered with his ability to think and do his job, caused major mood changes, led to gut problems, and still there was no relief. Ultimately, his doctor suggested Ed move his family from the northwest to a warmer climate.

They decided to move to Texas. The milder climate made it possible for him to cut his dose almost in half. While that was good news, a new hurdle emerged. Ed could not find a doctor who was willing to prescribe Vicoprofen®. It wasn't long before he had to switch his pain medicine to gabapentin and tramadol. Two years into taking that combo, he had a seizure while driving. After digging deep into the FDA trial vaults about these two medicines, Ed discovered information about the drugs that led him to stop the medication for fear of a more serious reaction. He says the withdrawal "… was unspeakable—it's worse than opiates." Withdrawal took eighteen months. He was still in pain, his mood was affected, his job performance questionable, and his marriage and relationship with his children were rocky.

With his future in the balance, a family friend suggested to Ed's wife that he use cannabis and sent home a cannabis brownie for him. She made Ed promise he would do so. Out of sheer desperation, he tried the brownie. Ed is a cautious guy. He also is a label reader and studies anything he puts in his mouth before he does so, as all of us should. He ate one quarter of the medicated brownie on an empty stomach. Thirty minutes later he found himself on his bed in disbelief and wonder alternating between laughing and crying because for the first time in fifteen years he **wasn't** in pain. At some point he realized he needed to go to the bathroom. He was half way there before it dawned on him that he had gotten off the bed on his own. Can you imagine what that must have felt like?

He is three years into managing his condition with cannabis. He takes approximately 25 milligrams of THC and other cannabinoids per day via brownie in three doses throughout the day, and he smokes a pipe. When I asked him what it has done for him, he looked me square in the eye and said with great emotion, "It gave me my life back." He pointed out that one of the ironies of the effects of the prescription pain killers he was taking is that they turned him into the person who is the typical stereotype of a "stoner"—unmotivated and apathetic.

Since switching to cannabis to manage his chronic illness, his blood pressure dropped from 180/110 to 150/95, he lost thirty-five pounds and is still losing, his asthma has disappeared, he can work and be clear headed, and most importantly his marriage and his relationship with his children have rebounded and are stronger than ever. Ed was extremely candid with me. He said that one of the horrible side effects of heavy pain medication is that you lose your sex drive. For many this causes great stress in the marriage and affects the self-esteem of both partners. Now that Ed is off prescription pain meds, his sex drive has returned. He credits cannabis with enhancing his experience. He said, "I feel like a man again!"

You may need to experiment with different plant samples and intake methods to figure out the best way to manage your chronic condition with cannabis. There are many intake methods and preparations to consider as will be discussed later.

Some people drink cannabis tea or enjoy a nightly edible while others find that a combination of a variety of intake methods best meets their needs. There isn't necessarily a right and a wrong way to use cannabis. The point is to find what works best for you. I'm especially a fan of tinctures, juices, and cannabis tea for people who are holding a day job, as dosages are easy to control, and it is easier to control chronic disease and function as normally as possible when using cannabis in these ways.

Disease Curing Plan

You can only believe in a cure to disease if you believe in the miracle of healing. I know the title of this section is going to make doctors and researchers nervous and readers hopeful. While there is strong anecdotal evidence (including a long list of people who claim they have cured their disease with cannabis oil) and some very compelling research that indicates components of cannabis may cure or change disease progression for cancer, diabetes, multiple sclerosis, and Alzheimer's, to name a few, there simply isn't enough evidence yet for me to tell you conclusively, "Here is how you can cure disease with cannabis." The evidence we do have warrants serious and vigorous investigation, yet there is still a considerable amount of research to be done.

Please keep in mind that curing a disease is not just a matter of taking a few pills or one specific treatment. It requires a determined mindset, opening the heart to healing and being healed, and most likely making some changes in lifestyle.

Vaporizing cannabis and eating edibles will likely give you relief from some of the symptoms of your condition, but they are unlikely to change the progression of it. Current research and anecdotal evidence indicates high doses of cannabinoids are needed to cure certain diseases. If you are looking for a cure, please do your homework. Using a highly concentrated cannabis oil and/or raw juiced cannabis should be at the top of your list of things to investigate.

The tricky part of using cannabis oil to change disease progression is that if you do not have access to the cannabinoid profiles of your medicines you are flying blind. Fortunately, cannabis oil will likely provide a healing benefit to you regardless of its chemical profile. However, if you have the luxury of working with tested material, I strongly encourage you to do so because it will allow you and your doctor to treat your condition much more directly and effectively.

Palliative Care Plan

Palliative care helps patients manage the pain and stress of serious illness for improved quality of life especially during the death transition. Cannabis is a wonderful medicine for this purpose! It can help take the edge off of the pain, stress, and suffering that come with any serious illness. One of the first times my mother had a peanut butter cannabis cookie, my dad and I hesitantly joined her. It had been a stressful day. It was the day the hospice people came for their initial visit. Everyone was trying to be strong for my mom and each other, but no matter how well you handle such a situation, it's hard to look your loved one's mortality square in the eye. Even when you are putting up a brave front and have a smile on your face, there is a lump in your throat or heaviness in the pit of your stomach that just won't go away. That kind of stress takes its toll on your body and spirit.

The house had been full of activity all day, but finally it was quiet. My four year old nephew was sleeping soundly in his bed. Mom and Dad were sitting peacefully in their matching recliners, and I was on the couch. We were reflecting on the highlights of our day and how lucky we were to have this special time together. My sister had just come in from a long day of work at her young restaurant. She could feel the Zen-like calm in the room and immediately asked if we had been in the cookies. We all had a big, guilty laugh. It was nice to sit in that moment and be together and present with each other. One cookie offered subtle relief from the stress of the day— just what each of us needed.

Our lives are so fast. I believe there is real value in the slowing effect many people experience when using certain varieties of cannabis. Slowing down opens the mind to new possibilities, perspectives, and ways to solve problems. It can be especially good for those of us who might otherwise be a little high strung and have a hard time relaxing or turning off our brains. Who knows, you might even find yourself laughing freely, which is good medicine!

We are all going to die or at least our physical body will expire. It is one of the few guaranteed parts of the human experience. There are no words to convey the depth of healing and peace that comes from watching your loved one die on their own terms. I regret that Mom died at what I consider a young age, and Dad is spending his golden years without her, but I'm deeply grateful she did not linger in an undignified state or great pain.

There is peace and joy to be had even in the dying process. Cannabis can be a therapeutic part of this process facilitating healing and relief on the physical, as well as emotional and spiritual level.

Risks, Side Effects, and How You Might Feel – What to Expect

Cannabis, just like foods we eat and other medicines we take, affects everyone differently. One of the greatest challenges of utilizing dried cannabis as medicine is the large number of medically active ingredients occurring in varying levels in different plants, even in different parts of the same plant! Different combinations of cannabinoids and terpenoids drive the effects of a particular cannabis medicine and how your body responds. And, due to differences in our individual endocannabinoid systems, two people can take the same medicine in the same way and have different experiences.

Risks and Harm Reduction

Regardless of your cannabis experience, here are three points that should be a part of any cannabis harm reduction strategy:
1. Start low and go slow.
2. If one variety causes bad effects, try a different one. Keep a variety journal.
3. If you have a bad reaction, stop use and get help.

The following is a list of the most common negative effects experienced by cannabis users and suggestions for managing or mitigating them.

Most Common Risks	Harm Reduction Option
Risk of Arrest	Risk of arrest is the single biggest danger. Until cannabis becomes legal or is decriminalized, please be discreet—especially in places that do not have medical cannabis laws.
Chronic Bronchitis or Lung Irritation	Regular cannabis smokers sometimes have a nagging cough. Use a vaporizer, or take edibles or tinctures to mitigate the harm smoke may cause. Draw vapor/smoke in for a five to ten count and release. Holding smoke in longer may contribute to trapping tar in the lungs thus creating irritation. This also gives a false sense of being high due to lightheadedness caused by holding the breath.
Tachycardia – (increased heart rate)	Interviews with smokers and scientists indicate that the higher the THC level, the higher likelihood of experiencing heart palpitations. If you are in a state where you have access to chemical analysis at the site of purchase, select cannabis with a moderate THC level and at least 4 percent CBD or a balance of THC and CBD. Palpitations will most likely stop within an hour. If you have any sort of heart issue, be sure to visit your doctor and seek cannabis material with a balance of THC and CBD or lower THC and higher CBD.

Most Common Risks	Harm Reduction Option
Adverse Mood Reactions – panic, depression, dysphoria, depersonalization, delusions, illusions, and hallucinations	Among regular users, 17 percent report experiencing some type of adverse mood reaction typically early in their smoking experience. (Joy, Watson and Benson, Jr. 1999) Such reactions are more common in beginners. Wait fifteen minutes after each puff until you know how the herb is going to affect you. This will prevent getting too high a dose as the effects of smoked cannabis can come on slowly.
Sedation	Many people report feeling tired or sleepy after consuming cannabis. If sedation is not what you want or need, try another plant sample with a different terpene profile; one that doesn't include myrcene is preferable.
Irritated throat or lungs from heat	Non-smokers may find that smoking cannabis through anything other than a vaporizer (special equipment that heats the material enough that it releases medicine into an inhalable vapor without combusting it) will irritate their lungs. Use a vaporizer to reduce irritation and prevent carbon monoxide from entering the lungs. If you don't use a vaporizer, try a water pipe, which will cool the air before it reaches your throat. If you use a water pipe, be aware that, in exchange for the cooling effect, you will give up some efficiency; some THC remains in the water. If you are using a pipe, pack it tightly—especially when using a screen at the base of the pipe. A screen in the bowl protects you from inhaling hot plant material but also increases the volume of air pulled through the pipe. This increases the heat of the smoke, which can burn your lungs. Additionally, this will burn your cannabis more quickly. If you decide not to use a screen, lift your tongue to the base of the gums just behind your front teeth as a shield to protect your throat as you inhale. This will ensure that you stop loose plant material from entering your throat. You can find pipes designed to prevent inhalation of plant material. Do not hold a flame to the plant material the whole time you are taking a drag from a pipe. Pass the flame quickly over a small section while inhaling, and remove the flame as soon as it is lit so the temperature can drop. Don't try to light the whole bowl. Keep your thumb on the carburetor (the hole at the side of some pipes) to reduce air flow, and keep the ember alive at a lower temperature. The pretty orange or red ember can be kept alive for several consecutive puffs, which are increasingly medicinal, cool, and easy on the throat and lungs. If your throat gets burned, it may take a day or so to heal completely. Chamomile, peppermint, and lavender teas can be soothing.
Addiction	Addiction is a relatively small risk. A 1999 Institute of Medicine report states the probability of becoming dependent on various abuse-able substances is as follows: cannabis 9 percent, alcohol 15 percent, cocaine 17 percent, opiates 23 percent and nicotine 32 percent. The figure for cannabis is skewed. The majority of people receiving treatment for cannabis dependency do so because of a legal mandate not because of true addiction.

Addiction or Habituation?

The accuracy of the 9 percent figure for cannabis has been criticized by Dr. Aggarwal and other cannabis experts. In Dr. Aggarwal's Huffington Post article, "'9 Percent of Those Who Use Cannabis Become Dependent' Is Based on Drug War Diagnostics and Bad Science," he explains that the data surrounding this particular statistic is grossly out of line.

Most Common Risks	Harm Reduction Option
Addiction, continued	Actually, cannabis addiction is rare. In a 2002 review, cannabis ranked eleventh in dependence potential after heroin, cocaine, tobacco, methadone, barbiturates, alcohol, benzodiazepines, amphetamines, buprenorphine, and ketamine. (Holland 2010, 138)
	While some people may experience habituation to cannabis, withdrawal symptoms are far less serious than severely physically addictive drugs such as heroin and prescribed opiates and benzodiazepenes. Withdrawal symptoms may include restless sleep and agitation and are gone in a matter of days. In many cases, withdrawal symptoms may be the reemergence of disease symptoms the cannabis was treating.
	Take regular breaks if possible, taking the lowest possible dose, and doing other things that stimulate the endocannabinoid system, such as acupuncture/massage, exercise, and supplementing the diet with essential fatty acids, may help lower one's risk for addiction.
Constipation	Certain varieties will slow bowel motility, which is good for people with irritable bowel syndrome and related issues. Try to discover if a particular terpene is to blame. If you get constipated, drink plenty of water and eat high fiber foods. For some, cannabis may make you feel dehydrated. While that is a benefit to patients who drool and have watery stools, it is not to others. If drinking sufficient fluids is a problem, consider adding chia seed to the diet to help intestines get access to water for a sustained period of time. Chia seed also give the added benefits of fiber, essential fatty acids, and other nutrients from the soil.
Cannabinoid Hyperemesis	A small number of regular cannabis smokers report symptoms of cyclical vomiting now known as cannabinoid hyperemesis. It is rare and usually occurs in people who have been smoking for two or more years and regularly smoke large amounts. The cause of this is either a manifestation of a *biphasic response* (where low and high doses produce divergent effects) to THC or a downregulation of the CB_1 receptors due to chronic use. It is more common in men than women. It may be caused by plant quality, contamination, or a biological reaction in the body. If you experience vomiting, stop using cannabis and see your doctor. Unlike cyclical vomiting,

Most Common Risks	Harm Reduction Option
Cannabinoid Hyperemesis, continued	cannabinoid hyperemesis may be relieved somewhat by a hot bath. However, discontinuing cannabis use for a period of time is required. If it is medically necessary to continue cannabis use, it is important to resume with very low doses.
Dry Mouth and Thirst	Dry mouth and thirst are common side effects of cannabis use. Chewing gum or sucking on hard candy can help. If you get thirsty, drink water. In palliative care, water sponges on a stick can be used to keep the mouth moist. Consider trying a different variety of cannabis if you experience unbearable dry mouth.
Itching or Tingling	Some varieties of cannabis cause itching or tingling all over the body or in a specific area. The cure to this is time. Try a different variety, which may not cause you to feel itchy.
Hallucinations	Hallucinations are rare and usually come along with high volume consumption of high-THC material. They will pass in time. Unpleasant hallucinations are a sign to back off your dose, and use cannabis with lower THC content.
Intoxication	Intoxication is considered a desired effect by some but not by others. Terpene and cannabinoid levels, and the amount of cannabis consumed, directly impact your intoxication level and experience. If you do not like the way your medicine makes you feel, experiment with backing off your dose, trying a different intake method, and trying different plant material.
Intense Psychoactivity	This most commonly occurs due to over consuming edibles or consuming high levels of cannabis oil in an attempt to change disease progression. Bob Melamede, PhD turned me on to a supplement called citicholine or choline CDP that helps mitigate unpleasant psychoactivity. It is available on-line or in local health food stores. Dr. Melamede suggests five times as many mgs. of citicholine be taken as mgs of THC. Dr. Melamede has seen people get to the commonly accepted one gram dose believed to be needed for serious disease treatment in one week with citicholine where otherwise it takes three to four weeks. Citicholine can be taken preemptively to make a high dose experience more pleasant and as a remedy if you find you have accidentally overdosed. Lemonade has also been mentioned in historical literature as an antidote to cannabis intoxication. (E. Russo 2011)
Dizziness	Dizziness may occur when consuming cannabis containing THC. It is a serious consideration for elderly patients and the very frail. Use only small amounts until you know how you are affected by a particular variety. If you use a cane or walker to support your mobility, make sure it is within arm's reach should you need it quickly.

Most Common Risks	Harm Reduction Option
Loss of Balance/ Motor Skills	Loss of balance is also of greatest concern in elderly and frail users. Start with a low dose, and build up slowly. Keep in mind that different varieties may impact you differently. If you experience loss of balance or motor skills, please do not drive, operate heavy machinery, or use power tools.
Short-Term Memory Interruption	If you find your short-term memory is affected by cannabis, experiment with different varieties, especially those with a higher CBD ratio if available or increased alpha-pinene content. (Piomelli and Russo 2016) Writing reminders on sticky notes, your phone, or your computer can also help.
Impairment of Cognition	If you find cannabis is interfering with your ability to complete cognitive tasks, try a different variety with a different terpene profile or cannabinoid profile.
Heaviness – Couch Lock	Oh, the famous "couch lock!" That's the street term for the feeling of body heaviness often wrongly associated with certain varieties of cannabis. If you have a product that is giving you unwanted couch lock, consider using it only before bedtime, as it will likely provide nice sleep quality. Find a different variety for the daytime. Cannabis with a higher concentration of the terpene myrcene is thought to cause feelings of couch lock. Many people enjoy the couch lock feeling, as it helps them slow down. Once couch lock sets in, only time will relieve it. I suggest listening to good music, watching a movie, meditating or closing your eyes, observing the experience, and being open to what it can teach you.
Expanded Sense of Time	Time flies when you are having fun, and cannabis can make everything fun! Setting timers on your phone to help you remain conscious of your obligations may help you keep track of time when necessary. If you have no pressing responsibilities, letting go of your sense of time can be freeing and relaxing.
Adrenal Fatigue or Protection	Long-term use may stress the adrenal glands, which are important for energy and stress management. My chiropractor, Hollis Wilson, DC, was the first to mention this to me. Dustin Sulak, DO agrees and explained that in other cases it can help protect the adrenals by modulating adrenal hormone release and overall stress response when used correctly. As always with cannabis, this depends on the person, style of use, and the variety. Talk to your nutritionist, acupuncturist, chiropractor, or integrative medicine doctor to learn more about adrenal balancing herbs.
Shame	Many patients share with me that they feel a sense of shame about using cannabis. Most feel guilty for using an illegal substance. Many have family members who are vocal about their disapproval. This all stems from fear, ignorance, and misinformation. Trust that you are making a choice in your best interest and the best interest of those

Most Common Risks	Harm Reduction Option
Shame, continued	who love you. NEVER fear speaking truth to power. You can say anything to anyone as long as you do so with respect, love, and kindness. To heal you must be willing to be your own top priority and not allow others to talk you out of doing what is best for you.

Recreational Versus Medicinal High

I've always wondered if the experience of a recreational user is different from that of a medicinal user. Personal observation leads me to believe that the experience can be very different. While there is no science to back me up, I do think intention matters. If you want to get what recreational users call "hella high" or "stoned out of your mind," you are likely to have that experience. Yet, if a medicinal user just wants to feel better, they may not get that "hella high" feeling nor need to get really high to get a benefit. That doesn't mean they won't experience a high of some sort; it just means the experience may be different.

Possible Positive Effects

Cannabis can provide a wide array of pleasant sensations and results. This is true for the sick and suffering and their caregivers as well as recreational users.

Being sick, operating with diminished capacity due to pain or discomfort, and being a caregiver are stressful experiences. Even outside of these experiences life can be stressful. Sometimes slowing down and being present helps reduce stress. Cannabis helps us slow down, relax, and bond with others through the sharing of the medicine and the experience it helps create.

We have spent lots of time talking about medical cannabis for the management of disease symptoms. I argue that responsible use of cannabis can also provide important proactive benefits for health, happiness, and successful aging.

Some quality of life benefits you may experience with cannabis include:
- Relaxation
- Better sleep
- Focus
- Sexual arousal, better sex, and greater sensuality
- Sense of peace
- Euphoria
- Heightened awareness of sensations, music, emotions, beauty, and self

- Creativity
- Enhanced spirituality
- Enhanced body consciousness
- Forgetting trauma and unnecessary details
- Remembering buried memories
- Improved sense of hope and optimism

This is a compelling list whether you enjoy complete health or seek it. Joy, laughter, pleasure, peace, focus, and the other positive items listed contribute to good quality of life. Life is meant to be good! Cannabis is a great medicine for those who are ailing as well as those who want to bring even more enjoyment and health into their lives.

Healing Magic of Cannabis

The book *Healing Magic of Cannabis* by Beverly Potter and Dan Joy offers a broader perspective on how cannabis can benefit mind, body, and soul.

Here are a few elaborations on how cannabis can enhance overall well-being.

Sexual Enhancement

My friend Melissa has been a great support throughout this project. She tried cannabis in college but didn't use it much because it wiped her out. Her interest was piqued when I told her that cannabis can increase sexual pleasure. She said, nearly in the same breath with excitement and some disbelief, "Really? How and why? I gotta get me some of that."

Melissa is a middle-aged woman who is an independent business person and active in her church community. Instead of taking my word for it, as she normally does, Melissa decided it was time to do her own field study. She acquired a small amount of cannabis edibles on a night she and her husband, of thirty plus years, had plans for a nice dinner. Just before dessert, she excused herself to the ladies' room where she consumed her edible in secret; she wanted to give the edible enough time to do its thing. The next morning, I received a phone call from her that began, "GIRRRRRRLLLLLL! That cannabis stuff works!" She reported that she and her husband had a most fulfilling evening! The best part was that her enhanced pleasure made her husband feel good, too. (Keep in mind that if she had consumed too much of the edible her evening might have had a very different outcome. Sometimes less is more.)

Are you wondering why cannabis enhanced Melissa's sexual experience? The answer is simple: cannabis is a *vasodilator*, meaning it increases blood flow, which increases sensitivity in all the right places allowing for more pleasure. Who can say no to that?

In addition to increased blood flow, I argue that cannabis relaxes people in a way that allows them to be more in the moment with their partner and in-tune with their own body allowing a deep and sensual connection. Pressure to perform subsides, and anxiety and inhibitions dissolve.

On the flip side, regular cannabis use can be drying to tissue and body fluids, in some people, which can impact the body's ability to lubricate for sexual pleasure. Visit with your acupuncturist, herbalist, nutritionist, or integrative medicine specialist, and ask them how to keep the body in balance when using cannabis.

Creativity

Many a creative person credits cannabis for their genius saying cannabis makes it possible to get out of their own way and let what already exists inside flow to their page, canvas or instrument. It is true that if you consume too much cannabis you may not have much creative motivation or initiative. Conversely, those who consume the right amount will tell you it lowers inhibitions, self-judgment, and angst that can stifle one's creativity. The sweet spot is different for everyone, but when you find it, it may help you share the most beautiful parts of yourself. Additionally, cannabis can help provide new perspectives, which contributes to creative problem solving.

Willie Nelson recently celebrated his eightieth birthday. He has probably smoked cannabis daily for sixty-five of those eighty years. While I am not suggesting everyone consume like Willie (all day every day) I do find it curious he is as healthy, mobile, creative, and musically prolific as he is with no signs of slowing down.

Relaxation and Heightened Senses

Relaxation is another valuable benefit of cannabis. We all need to relax. It is a critical part of managing human biology and wellness. If you are constantly stressed, you will get sick. As discussed in the "Cannabis Science" chapter, the endocannabinoid system keeps the body in balance by managing stress responses. When there is too much stress over too long a period of time, the endocannabinoid system cannot keep up. This is when we get sick.

Relaxation means different things to different people. Whether you like to relax with friends and loved ones or on your own, cannabis may help you relax more deeply and in a more fulfilling way enhancing experiences of nature, music, film, connection with friends and family, and your own body and senses. For many people, small amount of cannabis can strongly enhance the benefits of any relaxing activity making it more restorative to our bodies and minds.

Sleep

It is impossible to get well without sleep. I've always found it strange how hospitals poke and prod patients all the time and never give them a moment's rest. It is nearly impossible to get six to eight hours of continuous sleep in a hospital. Yet, all research points unequivocally to the correlation between getting enough continuous quality sleep and good health and healing.

The American Psychological Association (2014) reports on their website that forty million Americans have one of seventy different sleep disorders, over 60 percent of adults report sleep problems three or more nights a week, and over 40 percent of adults experience afternoon sleepiness strong enough to interfere with their work. Which comes first: sleeplessness or a commonly associated condition such as stress, hypertension, or depression? Sleep can be affected by our emotions; foods, exercise, biological systems in the body (brain, nervous system, cardiovascular system, etc.), stress. prescription medicine, over the counter drugs, nighttime habits, sleeping environment, pain, caffeine, alcohol, and many more things.

Cannabis is an excellent sleep aid for many people. Certain varieties are better for sleep than others, so find one that works for you. You may find some varieties are stimulating and interfere with your ability to sleep. Vaporization and edibles are the most common intake methods for sleep, and tinctures are gaining popularity.

If you are using cannabis in edible form for sleep, don't overdo it. A little bit goes a long way. If you ingest too much, you may wake up feeling stoned or fuzzy, and who knows what kind of dreams you might have? The point is to get quality, deep sleep and wake up rested. [See "Dosing & Titration", on page 214.]

There has not been much research into how cannabis impacts sleep, but what does exist indicates acute cannabis use (THC ingestion) has a minimal effect in sleep disruption. (Carskadon and Dement 2011) What disruption does occur exists as a reduction in the rapid eye movement (REM) phase of sleep for acute cannabis consumption and a reduction in deep sleep for chronic users. (Carskadon and Dement 2011) In a 2007 review of the science on the topic of sleep and cannabis, Russo and colleagues published in *Chemistry & Biodiversity*, that a survey of two thousand Sativex® users with pain disorders such as multiple sclerosis, cancer pain, neuropathic pain, and arthritis "...showed a marked improvement in subjective sleep parameters" with 40 to 50 percent improvement in sleep quality, which seemed to be related to symptom reduction not a hypnotic effect. (Russo, Guy and Robson 2007) A research study with rats suffering from sleep apnea in the REM state shows cannabinoids greatly reduce apnea. (Dempsey 2002)

Next to unrelenting pain, the next most common complaint I hear from people fighting chronic or terminal illness is lack of sleep or lack of restful sleep. The majority of medical cannabis users I've interviewed value cannabis as a sleep aid. Most agree it helps them sleep longer and deeper helping them to wake rested. For this reason, I believe regular cannabis use for improving sleep quality and duration is good for sick people as well as those who want to maintain good health but might be having trouble getting the sleep they need. Regardless, cannabis seems like a safer alternative to prescription sleep aids.

Forgetfulness

The mind is designed to remember and forget. Forgetting things you want or need to remember is not good. Not being able to forget things that serve no purpose is just as bad. What if we remembered everything? Our minds would become cluttered, and I imagine we would exist in a constant state of overstimulation and anxiety. It would be impossible to stay present and live in the moment. One of the functions of the endocannabinoid system is to help us forget that which doesn't serve us.

Awareness

We all experience a full spectrum awareness and consciousness throughout our lives. Sometimes our thoughts are in the past but other times in the future. It takes practice and discipline to cultivate awareness of the present and live in the moment. I have found, as I think many cannabis physicians and patients have, that cannabis expands awareness of the body, mind, and soul. This increased connectedness to the whole self paves the way for patients to make better choices and care for themselves in a holistic, sustainable way.

A father of a four and a six year old shared with me that in college he had been a cannabis connoisseur. At some point he decided his relationship with cannabis was unhealthy, and he put it down. He got a job, got married, and had children. He found himself carrying the weight of the world on his shoulders, bringing his work home, and generally being in a grumpy mood with his wife and children. He said, "I wasn't being a good dad or husband, and I was angry all the time." After trying cannabis again to see if it would help him relax, he discovered it did that but more importantly made it possible for him to be fully present with his wife and children when he came home at night. He said, "It makes me a much better dad! Now I am able to give them my full attention."

In my experience, cannabis brings peace and relief while expanding ones consciousness so we can see ourselves in a new light, make better sense of our current circumstances, and connect with our inner experiences with balance and clarity regardless of how happy or sad we may feel. This is especially helpful when I feel worn out from dealing with difficult situations. I consider this an expansion of myself that has incredible health benefits and improves my quality of life in general.

In my work as a business consultant, I help entrepreneurs and leaders identify and resolve things that they cannot see on their own. I've also been teaching yoga for over fifteen years and regularly work to help my students improve their self-awareness. The transformation that takes place in my clients and students, as their self-awareness grows, is incredible to watch. Through this expanded awareness comes empowerment, confidence, and satisfaction, all of which enhances their quality of life. I see the same transformation take place in many responsible cannabis users.

Enhanced Spiritual Practices

In indigenous cultures and throughout history, medicinal plants have been highly respected for their ability to support the mind, body, and spirit. Psychoactive plants are considered to possess what many call "plant spirits." The idea of plant spirits seems wildly "woo-woo" to many people in the West. In the jungles of the Amazon, and in tribes across the world, plants are revered for their ability to heal or open the mind and heart for a deeper connection to the Divine. To them it is not the plant itself that provides a beneficial effect but the spirit of the plant that does the healing.

As in all things, I believe intention matters. If you would like to enhance your spirituality, if you approach cannabis use with that intention, you will likely have the experience you desire.

Cannabis is used by many before prayer, meditation, yoga, tai chi, tribal ceremonies, and other spiritual practices to help individuals increase their senses, open their minds and hearts, and relax to receive the knowledge, guidance, or peace they seek. For some, the greatest benefit cannabis will bring is the ability to be still or quiet the mind. Others may find it interferes with their connection to spirit but serves them in other ways.

Euphoria

Warning: Rant Ahead!

I've lived my entire life thinking that euphoria (defined as "a feeling of elation or wellbeing" by Webster's Dictionary) is an incredible state of mind. It cracks me up that it is often listed as a "risk" of cannabis consumption. When did feeling good become bad? Do you ever feel you are at risk of experiencing euphoria?

Relaxing and feeling euphoric helps balance body chemistry after experiences of stress. EUPHORIA creates a chemical cascade in the body that can be very healing. It is likened to the feeling of being in love or triumphant. Can you hear your doctor saying, "Now Betty (or Bob) don't use cannabis; you might feel happy?" Euphoria heals. Euphoria gives us a break from cascades of chemicals our bodies make in response to stress and disease giving us space to create healing chemicals and hormones necessary for long-term health. No one ever died of euphoria. If that is ever a choice, sign me up. That is how I want to go!

I'll probably get a flood of letters from addiction counselors telling me all the reasons I am wrong. I get it. Euphoria is a deep sense of well-being that people get from certain life experience such as orgasm, love, and triumph. It is the same sense people chase with physically addictive drugs such as opiates. But I cannot see the euphoria caused by cannabis as a risk. [See "Why is Cannabis So Safe?", on page 113.] Rather, for those who are very sick or stressed, especially those with chronic or terminal illnesses, euphoria brought by cannabis is a huge benefit allowing laughter and enjoyment where otherwise there could only be suffering.

A large number of type-A personalities have told me cannabis is the only thing that helps them relax and recharge without fear of negative effects or addiction. Keep in mind that few people who use cannabis report becoming addicted, and withdrawal symptoms for those who decide to stop are minimal and carry no risk of death, unlike many street drugs and drugs prescribed by doctors.

Contraindications and Cautions – Who Should NOT Use Cannabis?

Here are two important cases in which cannabis medicines should NOT be used:

- Anyone who has an infection that requires a strong Th1 immune response such as Legionella. (Aggarwal 2013)
- If you have a family history of psychosis or are at high risk of developing psychosis. This is especially important for teenagers, as there is more risk of developing psychosis when the brain is not fully developed. (Aggarwal 2013)

The Frail and Elderly

Frail and elderly people, and others at risk of falling due to loss of balance or dizziness, should use cannabis with caution and take safety measures to protect themselves from falling. With that said, elderly people benefit from cannabis use to control depression, memory loss, and many chronic ailments.

Seniors in retirement communities, assisted living centers, and nursing homes all over the world are catching on to the fact that cannabis makes growing old much more comfortable and enjoyable. There is even a non-profit educational organization, *www.thesilvertour.org*, which teaches seniors about cannabis and encourages them to vote for the reform of cannabis laws. The cannabis lifestyle website *www.seniorstoner.com* is also a good resource.

Patients with Heart Conditions

Patients with heart conditions should be cautious not to over consume cannabis and be careful to avoid plant varieties with high THC levels that are not balanced with CBD or a THC moderating terpene. THC can elevate heart rate. Science indicates that THC is cardio-protective in ultra-low doses but high doses can be dangerous. (E. B. Russo 2015)

Teens and Children

Recreational use of highly psychoactive cannabis should probably be reserved for adults since the brain isn't fully developed until the mid-to-late twenties. Many experienced cannabis physicians say the older one starts smoking cannabis, the more likely one is to receive its therapeutic benefits. In my conversations with a variety of cannabis science experts, I have asked them if teen cannabis use is a concern to them. Unanimously, they agree that use is not a health concern. The concern is when a teen is using cannabis in a way that interferes with school performance, attendance, and healthy social behavior.

Neuroscientist and researcher Staci Gruber, PhD and her team at the Cognitive and Clinical Neuroimaging Core at McLean Hospital in Belmont, Massachusetts, a Harvard Medical School teaching hospital, conducted multiple studies that indicate early onset cannabis smokers (those who start before the age of sixteen) have a lower IQ and are slower at tasks. This research has made a big splash in the media and been promoted as evidence that cannabis lowers IQ and interferes with normal brain development. (S. Gupta 2013) But let's not get ahead of ourselves.

It is important to note that this research included subjects who were heavy cannabis smokers—although they never say what defines a "heavy smoker." The study subjects also consumed other drugs which, in my opinion, totally voids the efficacy of the findings. A missing piece of information this research does not include is the potency level of the cannabis smoked. I assume a 5 percent THC cannabis is going to impact the brain differently than a 20 percent sample. When I contacted Dr. Gruber's lab to inquire about potency levels used in the study, they said my questions were more "opinion questions in nature" and referred me to the Public Affairs office, which never responded.

Dr. Gruber's studies have been promoted by many as proof cannabis use lowers IQ. Yet correlation does not equal causation. Just because two things increase in the same direction does not mean one causes the other. For example, did you know that as the number of churches in a city goes up so does the crime rate? Now, we all know that churches don't cause crime; both numbers are the result of larger populations. Gruber's research only tells us that stressed out self-reporting teenagers who use large amounts of cannabis and other drugs illegally have a high rate of familial and social exclusions, which likely directly impacts brain development. It is reckless and unfounded to say flat out that cannabis use in teens lowers IQ based on this evidence.

It is legitimate to ask if the brain responds differently to chronic versus occasional cannabis use and how this may differ in teens versus adults. Is there a therapeutic dosage window for older teens that may help with focus and positivity, two things research indicates cannabis can do for adults? I have heard from countless people that cannabis made it possible for them to focus when they were teenagers. Without it, they say, they would not have made it through high school. I would never consider any of these individuals as having a low IQ. In fact, they are among some of the most brilliant people I know. That doesn't mean I think cannabis made them smart; maybe it just gave them the ability to focus and get through their later teen years more comfortably.

Dr. Gary Wenk makes a compelling argument that kids shouldn't use cannabis before age fifteen in his Psychology Today blog "Does It Matter When You Start Smoking Marijuana?" He cites what he considers to be a well-defined survey of teens below and above age fifteen who consume cannabis and their non-smoking counterparts. Results of the survey indicate that teens who use cannabis regularly before the age of fifteen show long-term impairment in executive cognitive functions including problem solving, the ability to plan, organize thoughts, and control reactions. This study also shows there are no real cognitive performance differences between those who used cannabis regularly after fifteen years of age and those who did not use cannabis. (G. Wenk 2011) Dr. Wenk concludes that the age difference seen here may be due to the fact that early teen years are a vulnerable time of brain development.

It makes sense that teens should not be regular recreational cannabis smokers/users if for no other reason than lack of maturity to do so responsibly. Brain maturity isn't reached until the mid-twenties, and until then, cognitive function is not fully developed. That is why one must be sixteen to get a driver's license and twenty-five to rent a car! The brain is not sufficiently developed to safely operate a motor vehicle. I believe, as more studies are done, we will find a big difference between heavy consumption and light to moderate consumption, between pure THC use versus THC consumption that is accompanied by 4 percent or more CBD, and a big difference between using and abusing. An occasional fast-food hamburger is not going to clog your arteries, but habitual consumption will wreak havoc on your system. Just ask the author of *Fast Food Nation*. Until there is more detailed information about how cannabis impacts the brains of teens and adolescents, I will argue for healthy young people to abstain from cannabis until adulthood.

Sick children are a completely different story. I love it when a cannabis- skeptical physician discourages the parent of a child with autism, cancer, or epilepsy, who has tried everything to help their child, by saying, "We simply don't have enough information on how cannabis might affect the brain development of your child. You shouldn't use cannabis. We just don't have enough information." The only thing true about that statement is that the offending doctor does not have enough information. That is the same professional who took an oath to "first do no harm," yet they are happy to prescribe an array of mind-altering drugs that are highly toxic and can cause long-term damage to organs and tissue. But, because they are approved by the FDA (which takes money from pharmaceutical companies), it is assumed they must be okay.

I argue that for many sick children cannabis is the thing they need most to help balance their ECS. And, yes, that includes THC for some kids. Could it be that, in the case of childhood and adolescent diseases, the use of cannabis actually protects the brain? Would it seem totally out of left field to believe that in some cases it could repair damage caused by the disease or pharmaceuticals used to treat it? Unfortunately, there is not much research on treating children with cannabis; to many people it is considered unethical. I argue it is unethical NOT to conduct that research. This is especially true when you consider that parents across the country with children who have epilepsy, cancer, and autism are treating their children with cannabis, and many are seeing drastic and immediate improvement.

How can cannabis products that stop or greatly reduce seizure activity be worse for the brain than multiple seizures a day? How can burying your child who lost their life to brain cancer be worse than trying to treat it with cannabis oil? How can treating your autistic child, who speaks his first words at twenty-five after you have treated him for one month with cannabis (true story), be worse than that young person being locked in their own brain experiencing who knows what from the frustration of autism and the chemical cocktail they have to endure? It is my strongly held belief that cannabis has a place in treating children and further consideration and research is needed to help so many of the children and families who suffer. Helping them helps us all. Pharmaceuticals with huge risks to the child are prescribed all day long, but the risk/benefit ratio is considered reasonable. Yet cannabis, which has a better safety profile than any modern medicine, cannot be considered because we don't have enough information. Can't we do better?

Pregnant or Trying to Conceive

It seems like a no brainer to think pregnant women should not use cannabis, right? Maybe, maybe not. If you think getting a research study approved to investigate the effects of cannabis on sick people is tough, can you imagine what it would take to get one approved to study cannabis on pregnant women and their babies? Many of the studies that have investigated this have been poorly designed and include subjects who are also using cigarettes, alcohol, and other drugs. This research would lead you to believe that cannabis causes retardation, prematurity, and congenital abnormalities. While it may be true that women with high-risk lifestyles who also smoke cannabis have a higher likelihood of having children with such abnormalities, there is no evidence showing that is also the case for cannabis smoking women with low risk lifestyles. (Park, McPartland and Glass 2004) We all know heavy use of alcohol and/or tobacco negatively impacts fetuses. As with the research on teens above, correlation does not equal causation. There is no evidence suggesting cannabis alone can cause fetal abnormalities.

While I do not advocate expectant mothers get stoned out of their minds everyday of their pregnancy, data does not indicate cannabis use presents a danger to the child's IQ or long-term development in any significant way. With that said, there really have not been any studies on exclusively cannabis using mothers that followed the children through adulthood, which is what we would need to show empirical proof.

A NIDA-funded longitudinal study lead by investigator Melanie C. Dreher, PhD came closer to doing this than any other study. Dr. Dreher followed thirty women who smoked daily and thirty non-smoking, socio-economic, and educational matches through the children's fifth year. Her original findings, which followed the children through the third month after birth, were published in the article "Prenatal Marijuana Exposure and Neonatal Outcome in Jamaica: An Ethnographic Study," in the highly respected journal *Pediatrics*, in February 1994. What is remarkable to me about this study is, unlike most other studies of pregnant cannabis users, the subjects did not drink nor use tobacco or other drugs in any measurable levels, and Dr. Dreher was able to track data about maternal cannabis use, dosages, and the family environment. Dr. Dreher and her colleagues tested the babies at one day, three days, and thirty days after birth in this first study. There were no measurable differences on day one and three between the different groups. On day thirty, the cannabis-exposed groups did better on every measured variable and did **significantly** better on measures of autonomic stability (heart rate, digestion, blood pressure) and reflexes.

Dr. Dreher and colleagues received additional funding to go back and interview and test the children again at age four before they started school and age five after they had been in school one year. The results showed no measurable differences between the performance of the children of cannabis consuming mothers and non-consuming mothers. In a presentation to the 2007 Patients Out of Time conference, Dr. Dreher commented that, "We cannot really conclude that there is not impact from maternal prenatal cannabis use. But what we can conclude is that the child who attends basic school with good attendance, is provided stimulating experiences at home, who is encouraged to show mature behaviors, has a profoundly better chance of performing well on the skills measured by the McCarthy Test (cognitive and verbal tests that Dr. Dreher used in her research) in the study, whether or not his mother used *ganga* [the word used for cannabis in Jamaica] or not." (Dreher 2007)

Dr. Dreher tried to get additional funding from NIDA to go back and research the offspring from the study again at age ten, but NIDA was only interested if she was willing to take on a specific pro-NIDA researcher as the co-lead. Unfortunately, the study languished.

The historic literature about gynecologic uses of cannabis shows it has been widely used around the world during childbirth to stimulate uterine contractions and to treat dysmenorrhea, gonorrhea, and post-partum hemorrhaging. (E. Russo 2002)

Today, cannabis is often quietly used by pregnant women suffering from morning sickness. In the case of hyperemesis gravidarum (HG), a severe form of morning sickness where the mother is unable to keep food down interfering with the healthy growth of the baby and even threatening its life, cannabis may be a lifesaver for mom and baby. (Curry 2002) It is estimated that 10 to 20 percent of expectant mothers use cannabis. (Park, McPartland and Glass 2004)

Hyperemesis Gravidarum

An excellent article on this subject is written by researcher and then doctoral candidate Wei-Ni Lin Curry who suffered from HG during her own pregnancy. Her article "Hyperemesis Gravidarum and Clinical Cannabis: To Eat or Not to Eat" is an important read for anyone wanting to learn more about this condition. You can find the article with a search of the title at *www.cannabis-med.org*.

Anyone wishing to conceive a child may want to reconsider using cannabis while trying to get pregnant. The science on this topic is not conclusive and is done predominantly in animals. However, fourfold higher levels of *anandamide* were observed in one study of women who experienced miscarriage versus women with normal gestation. This is an indication that cannabinoids exposure during pregnancy could contribute to miscarriage for certain parts of the population. (Park, McPartland and Glass 2004) While there could be other unknown contributing factors, it is wise to err on the side of caution when trying to conceive a child—especially if you have had a previous miscarriage. While there is little literature to support this concept, cannabis does have high anti-angiogenic properties and *could* have been a factor in those miscarriages. *Angiogenesis* is the formation of new blood vessels required for the fertilized egg to adhere to the uterine wall. New blood vessels are only created in the body when the fertilized egg adheres to the uterine wall, when the fetus is developing, when an injury occurs, and when tumors grow. In the case of tumor growth, cannabis has been highly effective at preventing growth of the new blood vessels the tumor needs to sustain itself. It's not a reach to hypothesize that components of the cannabis plant might prevent impregnation or cause an early miscarriage.

This is not a one size fits all scenario. I know women who smoked cannabis regularly, even heavily, when they were trying to conceive a child and several women who smoked regularly, and even heavily, while they were pregnant. Not one of those women had complications in their pregnancy, and they all have healthy, bright, well-adjusted children. Each of them used cannabis as a medicinal herb not a drug of abuse. As discussed earlier, lifestyle choices of the mother are the most important factor in pre-natal health.

The endocannabinoid system plays an important role in the health and function of the male and female reproductive systems, where a high density of *cannabinoid receptors* exists. Cannabinoid receptors have even been found in human sperm as well. (Park, McPartland and Glass 2004) In their paper "Cannabis, Cannabinoids and Reproduction," published in the scientific journal *Prostaglandins, Leukotrienes and Essential Fatty Acids,* Park et al. write: "The presence of cannabinoid receptors in sperm suggests the possibility of a natural role for cannabinoids in modulating sperm function during fertilization. However, it remains to be determined whether smoked cannabis or oral THC at doses achieved during recreational or medical use has a clinically significant effect on the fertilizing capacity of human sperm."

Cannabinoids and Sperm

It is important to note that THC has been the major focus of research surrounding reproduction at the exclusion of other cannabinoids. This begs the question: Does CBD, other cannabinoids, or other active components of cannabis have a positive or negative impact on sperm and the fertilized egg?

Before You Inhale or Ingest

If you are thinking about using cannabis for the first time, or are relatively new to using cannabis medicinally, consider the following beginner tips:

Step 1: Believe you can heal

Raphael Mechoulam called cannabis "… a treasure trove of healing." While the cannabis plant has much to offer mankind, we have to do our part, too. As is the case with any healing regimen, the one in search of healing has to *want to be healed* and believe it is possible. Valerie Corral, co-founder of Wo/Men's Alliance for Medical Marijuana (WAMM), has been working with patients for over twenty years. She shared with me that she has never seen a patient healed of cancer, or any other disease, who didn't believe healing was possible.

Our intentions and thoughts have a tremendous impact on our healing. No matter how badly you want something, if you don't believe it is possible, it is unlikely it is.

Step 2. Choose a safe set and setting

Psychedelic drugs such as cannabis impact the mind as well as the body. For this reason, it is important to consider "dose, set, and setting," a term popularized by psychedelic researcher Timothy Leary, PhD. Taking the right dose, in the right place, when in the right frame of mind (or with the right expectation) will directly impact the outcome of your experience. The same is true for the wrong dose, wrong place, or wrong frame of mind. Try cannabis at home or another safe place with a friend/loved one who is NOT partaking or someone who is experienced so you feel completely safe. Be prepared to stay at home and not be engaged in activity for the duration of the effect until you understand how the product affects your body.

Step 3. Let go of old ideas and generational stigmas

Many of us have been taught that cannabis is BAD and people who use it are, too. Since you have made it this far in the book, you know this is not true. Let go of associations you may have around fears, misinformation, and past negative assumptions and associations with cannabis use, and with the act of smoking as well, if you are choosing to smoke. Your highest good, healing, and relief are too important to waste on fears of what others may think.

Step 4. Embrace the experience—do not be afraid

Remember you are dealing with one of the safest therapeutic plants in our pharmacopoeia. There is no reason to be afraid if you are using it responsibly and cautiously. If you are fearful, or feel you are trying cannabis under duress, the likelihood of a negative experience increases exponentially. Learn about the possible negative and positive effects so you know what to do if these things occur. If you experience dizziness, headache, shortness of breath, or any other negative effect, remain calm and remind yourself that this will pass fairly quickly. Allow yourself to embrace the heightened sense of awareness that may come with the medicine. Be open to the possibility of a pleasant result. In fact, I hope you expect it!

Step 5. Don't be surprised if you don't feel much the first time

I thought I was the only one who didn't have much of an experience the first time I tried cannabis. Frankly, it was a bit disappointing. I couldn't understand what all the fuss was about. Dr. Sulak says this is fairly common. The first few times we use cannabis the body is stimulated to start creating more cannabinoid receptors and make the existing ones more receptive. If this is your experience, you may not feel much of an effect until the second or third time. Nonetheless, you are still receiving benefit because your ECS is being stimulated. Even if you don't feel much the first time, only consume a small amount.

Step 6. Start with a small dose

Regardless of your intake method, start slowly. Sometimes potent medicines come in super-small packages—especially those made with a concentrate. A small ginger snap cookie can hold up to four or more doses. When available, purchase products that list cannabinoid percentages and terpene levels so you can find your ideal dose and stick to it. Research, my personal experiences, and many stories from cannabis users suggest a small amount can provide a strong therapeutic impact—especially for the novice.

Step 7. Buy from reputable people

If you live in a state where you can purchase from a dispensary or licensed retail shop, do so. Otherwise, ask a trusted friend, your children, a college kid who can be discreet, or other people who have the same ailment you have. Do NOT answer an ad on the Internet or ask a minor. I repeat! **DO NOT answer an ad on the Internet or anywhere else for that matter. That is a great way to end up duped or in jail.** Disease support groups are a great way to meet people who can point you in the right direction. But remember the first rule of Fight Club: "Don't talk about Fight Club." Protect your sources once you have them. Should you have a problem with law enforcement, do not give up your source!

Step 8. Buy local if you can or U.S. grown only

Mexican cannabis comes at the high price of many innocent lives lost because it is controlled by violent criminal cartels. This may sound harsh, but if you are buying Mexican cannabis YOU are part of the problem. There are local growers everywhere. Generally speaking, people who grow cannabis care deeply about the quality of their medicine and its potency and take great pride in their product. The fact that cannabis is becoming more widely accepted does invite "Johnny-come-latelys" (who are in it only for the money) to the market. Ideally, you want to find someone who cares about you and can help you get the right cannabis for your needs. Just like nearly anything else in this life, relationships matter. Take time to develop them. Many of the most reputable growers treat their operation like any other commercial enterprise. Every grower I know has tried to acquire specific varieties to help customers whom they consider their patients. They care about customer satisfaction. Regardless of whether they are growing as a state-licensed operation or have an underground operation, they are doing so at incredible risk to themselves. They are generally highly motivated to help make people happy and better. If you are buying Mexican cannabis, you are supporting violent drug cartels that torture and kill thousands of people every year. When you buy American grown cannabis, you are usually supporting a small, local enterprise that puts food on the table for people just like you and me.

Step 9. Experiment with different intake methods and varieties

It will take a little while to understand what works best for you. The first variety and intake method combination may be exactly what you need, or you may discover some other combination of delivery methods and varieties are best. It's likely you will discover one variety and delivery method is better for daytime use while another is better for nighttime.

Step 10. Do your homework

Research the science behind this safe and powerful medicinal plant so you feel secure and at ease with your choice. [See "The Science of Cannabis", on page 33.] There are a lot of details in this book, but it is impossible to catalog ALL the cannabis research available for every ailment. See a list of resources previously listed in the "Diseases & Symptoms Benefited by Cannabis" section.

Step 11. Be clear about the outcome you desire

Information in this book can help you decide what to buy/grow, how to ingest it, and how to dose effectively for your unique heath strategy. [See "What is Your Health Strategy?", on page 137.]

Step 12. Know the laws in your state

Plan for the possibility of requiring legal representation. I don't mean to scare you, but many people are oblivious to the law, repercussions of possession, and what to do if questioned by police or arrested. Visit the Know Your Rights section of the Americans for Safe Access website and the legal section of this book.

Step 13. Be discreet

Regardless of where you live, be discreet. Unfortunately, not everyone you know and love will be on board with your well-considered choice, even if your use is legal in your state/country. While broad support for the legalization of cannabis has grown to 54 percent in the last twenty years, 46 percent of American's do not support legalization. (Pew Research Center 2011) **The old phrase "loose lips sink ships" is true. If you live in a state where there is no medical cannabis law, be especially discreet if you have underage children, and never smoke in front of** them—not because you should be ashamed (you should not) but because many people will not understand if they hear your kids talking about your medicine. One day we will be educated enough as a society that therapeutic use of cannabis will be accepted in the same way taking an aspirin is. Until then, be smart.

Step 14. Smoke shops are a great resource for medical cannabis users

You will find people there who can show you how to roll a cigarette, good books, and equipment (often referred to as *paraphernalia*) such as rolling papers, pipes, and vaporizers. Remember, these are legal businesses in most places—but not all. Where they are legal, there is no need to don a disguise and sneak around the shop. If you live in a state that does not have a medical cannabis law, make sure you know if such establishments are legal and if paraphernalia is legal. Do not blatantly use the words "cannabis" or "marijuana" (until you have a feel for the place). You will definitely get the brow and may be asked to leave. Feel free to ask for advice on using the words "tobacco" or "smoking herbs" as long as that advice is specific to what they have in the store. Remember, if you are in a state where cannabis is not yet legal, this is NOT the place to ask where to source "smoking herbs" unless you are asking about a legal smoking herb.

Step 15. Learn about Marinol®

Some people use Marinol® to provide cover for their cannabis use. It is probably not wise to ask your doctor about this unless you have a close relationship. In some states it is illegal for them to have this conversation with you.

Step 16. Be informed about drug testing

If you are going for urine testing, it is hard to say for sure how long you should abstain from cannabis use. It depends on frequency of use, weight, metabolism, amount used, your body chemistry, and many other factors. The type of test being done is also a factor. Regular users can test positive for cannabis use up to one hundred days in a urinalysis, two to seven days for blood, and months with a hair analysis and fingernail shavings. If this is a concern, read the California NORML Guide to Drug Testing available on-line for free. The general rule of thumb is that it will take at least thirty days to leave your system, but don't count on that. Please do your homework.

Don't Let Perfect Be the Enemy of Good

Forward thinking physician and cannabis expert Dr. Sunil K. Aggarwal, who kindly agreed to join me for my first official cannabis education webinar in 2013, thoughtfully reminded me after our live event that we should not let perfect be the enemy of good. I was advocating that people strive to get access to chemical testing for their cannabis medicine because it would make it possible to more effectively treat their ailments. While this is really good advice, it's not practical for everyone. Currently, a little more than a third of Americans live in states where it is possible to get cannabis medicine tested by a lab. Does that mean the rest of us should give up on cannabis? No way!

Dr. Aggarwal's comment to me drove home the point that cannabis is really safe and versatile. Many people are not using cannabis in the optimal way, or are not using optimal quality plant material, yet they still benefit tremendously from its therapeutic properties. Furthermore, the benefits most people get from cannabis make it a worthy addition to their self-care regime—even if they are not using the best cannabis in the best way.

Cannabis Testing in the Palm of Your Hand

What if it were that easy? The CannaDX™ is the first handheld device that tells you the cannabinoid and terpenoid content of your cannabis. Laboratory testing is likely to be more accurate, but at least this device will give you an idea of what you have. Visit *www.cdxlife.com* to learn more.

Using the Whole Plant: Making the Most of Your Medicine

As we learned in the "Science" section of this book, there is great synergy between the various natural chemicals in cannabis. The most well-known and studied are the cannabinoids and terpenoids. These, and all of the other chemicals that occur in the plant, when used together, provide a stronger therapeutic effect to the user. My viewpoint is that the more diverse the chemical profile in a particular plant, the more therapeutic the sample is likely to be.

Now, let's talk about how to tell the difference between the good stuff and the not-so-good stuff, and what parts of the plant you can use for different applications.

If you plan to inhale cannabis, you will find the flowers or "buds" provide the best possible experience. Most people prefer seedless cannabis flowers commonly known as *sinsemilla*. Cannabis with seeds is considered lower quality. If you are making an edible, you can use buds, leaves, *shake* (loose plant material that often collects at the bottom of a bag of cannabis), or a combination. Please keep in mind that using buds only will yield a more potent butter, oil, or tincture simply because there are more trichomes, and therefore more therapeutic compounds, in the flowers. You need not consume as much of edibles made with flowers to gain your desired relief.

Cannabis Plant Uses

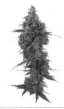

Green Plant
- Juice
- Tea
- Raw

Oil
- Internal
- Topical

Dry Bud
- Kif
- Smoking
- Vaping
- Butter
- Cooking Oil
- Concentrated Oil
- Tincture
- Shatter
- Hash
- Bubble Hash
- Dab
- Topicals
- Butter Wax
- Honey Oil
- Tea

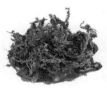

Dry Leaf
- Kif
- Butter
- Topical
- Tincture

Kif (sometimes spelled *keif* or *keef*)
- Pills
- Butter/Oil
- Vape
- Smoke

Spent Plant Material
- Butter
- Pill Caps (greenies)
- Topical Puck (for wound healing)

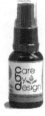

Tincture
- Straight
- Mix in food

Leaves and shake may be considered waste by some growers and are usually available for a much lower cost than flower buds. You can still derive excellent benefits from edibles made with leaves as long as you are using high-quality, potent plant material. If you have access to leaves, you can also use them to make your own hashish.

Oddly enough, the most potent butter I've tried was made with low-quality buds and shake. When talking with chemist Jeff Raber, PhD, it finally dawned on me, that the reason that particular butter was so potent was because it was cooked for over ten hours thus extracting a high quantity of cannabinoids from the material and fully decarboxylating the THCA into THC. Butters I had previously sampled were cooked only two to four hours. Even though these butters were made with significantly higher quality material, the therapeutic effect was not as powerful because the heating process was not long enough to fully decarboxylate the cannabinoids.

You will hear the term "whole plant" used to describe cannabis oils, tinctures, and other cannabis preparations. That means different things to different people. It can literally mean that the entire cannabis plant was used to make the preparation, or it could mean that buds and leaves were used to make the product or that buds only were used but that all the synergistic compounds in the bud are being extracted.

Varieties: Indica vs. Sativa

There is much confusion about how, why, and what to name various types of cannabis plants. The genus *Cannabis* is found worldwide and shares an ancient relationship with humans, who have used it for fiber, food, drugs and ritual purposes. Some more traditional botanists view cannabis variation worldwide as encompassed by a single species – *C. sativa*. More recent hypothesis propose that *C. sativa* only circumscribes European hemp, which is non-psychoactive, low in total cannabinoids and terpenoids, and definitely NOT the origin of medical cannabis. Other botanists accept a second and much more widespread species *C. indica*, which is native to the remainder of Eurasia and was introduced early on into India and Africa and eventually into the New World. *C. indica* varieties have been selected for centuries for high cannabinoid and terpenoid production, and they are the ultimate source of all drug cannabis used socially and medically.

C. indica can be further subdivided into several subspecies, two of which were the source of modern drug cannabis. Subspecies *indica* is the original medical cannabis first recognized by European physicians and the traditional source of the world's illicit marijuana. A second subspecies, *afghanica*, was introduced to the West from Afghanistan only in the 1960s and was traditionally used to make sieved hashish. Cannabis has male and female plants that easily interbreed via air-borne pollen. In North America and Europe, original, pre-1970s marijuana varieties were crossed with more recently introduced Afghan varieties, and modern hybrid *sinsemilla* medicinal varieties were born. Almost all medical cannabis available today shares its heritage with both the *indica* and *afghanica* gene pools.

Hybrid drug cannabis available today is characterized by its heritage but evaluated based on its effects. Two common terms are used today to describe drug cannabis varieties and their products, and although not based in science, they are certainly widely used and understood. The term "sativa" is used to describe the traditional narrow leaflet marijuana varieties, and the term "indica" is reserved for the wider leaflet hashish varieties from Afghanistan. Sativas are attributed with a certain suite of effects, and indicas with another. Recognizing that nearly all drug cannabis varieties are hybrids, what the terms really mean is that a certain variety has more sativa traits than indica traits or vice versa. However, users find it a useful system to categorize varietal differences for their own understanding. This is a great example of a botanically incorrect and clinically unproven taxonomy, which nonetheless is widely understood and is therefore of somewhat practical value for describing medical cannabis varieties. Most medical cannabis contains predominantly the cannabinoid THC, and only a small (but increasing) number contain the second most common cannabinoid CBD, and the other cannabinoids are rather rare. All cannabinoids are nearly odorless, and the subtle differences in the aromas and flavors of cannabis varieties are largely attributed to their aromatic essential oils that are rich in terpenoids. The aromatic compounds are chemically diverse, exhibit a wide range of physiological responses, and may account for differences in efficacy experienced in different cannabis varieties. In the future, we will likely describe cannabis varieties more by their aromas and associated effects rather than by their supposed heritage.

It will take a while for that nomenclature change to make it to the marketplace and everyone to get their head around the changes, which is why I have not discussed this earlier. It doesn't really matter what we call it. What matters is the active components of the plant and that it is in alignment with your needs.

Indica varieties are believed to cause drowsiness, which is why many prefer to take them at night. Indica is popular with people who are agitated due to medication, discomfort due to illness, or general life stresses. Popular indica varieties include: Blueberry, Gold Star, Northern Lights, Sensi Star, and White Berry. [See, "Terpenes", on page 53.]

Sativa varieties are widely believed to be more stimulating, and these varieties are often preferred for day use as they reportedly deliver a more energetic, cerebral, and creativity enhancing effect. Some say this effect is caused by the higher THC levels in sativas over indicas, but the differences more likely reside in the terpenes. It is commonly accepted that sativas make users feel optimistic and alert. Sativa varieties are thought to improve appetite and relieve depression, chronic pain, nausea, and migraines. (Erkelens and Hazekamp 2014) Popular sativa varieties include: Haze, Kali Mist, White Russian, K2, Kiwi Green, and Trainwreck.

Growers take pride in breeding their own plants and cross breeding different varieties. They sometimes make up names for their products like you would name a pet, car, or business. Don't rely on just the name when choosing your medicine. Your supplier should be able to tell you about the genetic background, cannabinoid content, terpenoid profile, and production method used. Not every grower or supplier is able to talk about the cannabinoid content or the terpene content—not everyone has access to lab testing— but they should be able to tell you about the general quality of the therapeutic experience. You will often hear people refer to the effect of a certain variety as an "indica high" or a "sativa high" referring to the commonly believed effects predominant in the variety.

There are so many different varieties of cannabis that it is hard to keep up with all the names. My all-time favorite name is Alaskan Thunder Fuck. The first time I heard that term, I couldn't help but think, "With a name like that, it must be good!" Maybe in the second edition of this book I will give a comprehensive overview of the majority of popular varieties. Until then, I am going to rely on *Leafly.com*, an on-line variety guide, to teach me more about this intriguingly named sativa. Leafly allows you to search by variety name, attributes, and therapeutic benefits, and you can even look up which dispensary has the medicine you seek. I like the way they allow users to leave reviews and share information about their experiences with different varieties. That said, the information available on line is highly subjective and each patient must develop their own set of criteria for effective medical relief.

> ### Cannabis Pharmacy by Michael Backes
>
> This is an excellent book complete with a variety guide and ailment specific information including data about varieties commonly used for specific conditions.

Leafly and other variety guides are good resources but not absolutely comprehensive. Often the name being used to market a plant sample does not match the true genetic profile of that variety. That is why it is important for all patients to have access to tested plant material. If you are in a legal state, be sure to buy cannabis that has been lab tested. You will then start to buy based on cannabinoid and terpene content not necessarily on just the name or sub-species.

New evidence suggests the therapeutic benefits and effectiveness of certain varieties are dictated as much by environment as genetics. This means two different plants of the same variety can have different therapeutic benefits and potency if grown in different conditions. Even medicine from different parts of the same plant can be significantly different, especially when it comes to terpene profiles. This is why lab testing is so important. If you know your medicine today has the same or a similar cannabinoid and terpene content as your medicine last week, you can be sure it will provide similar benefits and effects as it did last week, even if it goes by a different name.

Some people find using the same variety all the time can result in something called *strain drain* in which medicine that was beneficial at first ceases to be as effective when used over time. Friends report that using anywhere from three to ten varieties in rotation keeps their bodies responding optimally.

Potency and Quality

Even if you don't have access to laboratory tested medicine, it is still possible to have some sense of the quality of cannabis before you try it. Most quality flower buds are aromatic, *resinous* (thus sticky to the touch), and green (or sometimes red or purple).

> **Smell** – Most quality cannabis has a strong smell that can be described as sweet, floral, fruity, grassy, or "skunky." It is true some cannabis smells better than others. If a particular smell resonates with you, pay attention to that!

Your body and that sample are exchanging energy your body needs. There are a few varieties that do not smell as strong yet are still high in THC. Nevertheless, I strongly advocate using your sense of smell to find the sample best for you. The more aromatic the sample, the higher concentration of terpenes present and presumably the more therapeutic benefit the plant will have. Remember that terpenes provide an important synergistic effect when combined with cannabinoids. A strong terpene aroma also indicates freshness as well as maturity. [See, "Terpenes", on page 53.]

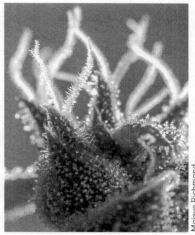

Trichomes

Mojave Richmond

Sight – If cannabis is brown or old looking, do not buy it. Look for varying shades of green, dark purple, and dark red. Many samples have what looks like colored hairs.

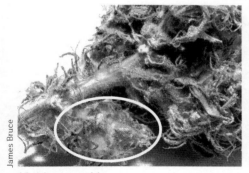

James Bruce

Moldy cannabis

That is both normal and desirable in many varieties. PLEASE look closely at what you are buying. Humidity greatly impacts the drying process. When there is too much, mold can occur more easily. It is important to buy mold-free cannabis. Some mold is not detectable with the eye. If you can see that a sample is moldy, do not buy it under ANY circumstance. Moldy cannabis can create an allergic reaction or make an already aggravated immune system weaker or more agitated. Additionally, do not buy ground plant material. Buy whole flower buds. I have heard of people grinding already vaporized cannabis and selling it as if it were fresh.

Touch – Cannabis flower buds that feel resinous or sticky have greater trichome density per square inch and therefore are more therapeutically potent. They may also be

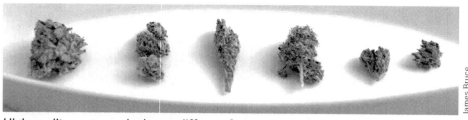

James Bruce

High quality nugs can look very different from one another.

fresher. Don't be afraid to ask to touch (with clean hands) before you buy, but don't mutilate it. Sticky is good!

Taste – Poor quality or old cannabis will taste bad no matter how you choose to use it. It may taste like dirty water from an ashtray, like dirty socks smell, or have an old musty taste. High quality cannabis will have a variety of different tastes when vaporized or eaten. You will likely find you prefer the taste or aftertaste of some types over others. This is completely subjective and different for everyone. I hypothesize that smells that are pleasing to us are an indication of how good of a match that particular plant material is for our needs. Of course, this is just something I wonder about not something I've seen in the literature.

Lab testing reveals that small leaves and trimmings are approximately 25 percent as potent as buds. This means you will need four times as much leaf or trim as you would flower buds to get the same level of potency. Remember that taste is important when making an edible. The smell will likely translate into the taste, so buy something that smells like it will taste good!

Regardless, buy high-quality cannabis. It will provide a much better experience all the way around. If you don't have access to a dispensary with lab tested medicine and knowledgeable folks behind the counter, you may need to take a leap of faith at first, and trust your instincts in deciding whether certain plant materials are worth buying. Use the tips mentioned above, and trust your body and your senses to let you know if it will benefit you therapeutically. In time, you will learn to easily distinguish between different qualities.

What to Buy?

In addition to outlining characteristics of the good, bad, and ugly, a few street terms might be helpful for those who cannot obtain medicine through a licensed provider.

What is the difference between good and bad?

- *Good Cannabis* is usually light green with a strong smell and lots of brightly colored red, orange, and sometimes blue or purple hairs. Much of the colors dissipate as the flowers are dried. Fresh flower buds will be sticky and slightly squishy to the touch, and there will be only a little **shake**—fine, dusty plant material collected at the bottom of the bag. Good cannabis is often referred to as "dank," "kind bud," or "chronic." Individual dried cannabis buds are often called "nugs." Nugs can be big or small, round or skinny, short or long depending on the variety.

- *Bad Cannabis* will be brown and likely have little smell. A bag of low quality street cannabis may have lots of shake collected at the bottom and a bad taste. It will often be overly dry and crumble easily. Who wants that? Bad cannabis is often called "schwag."

Is It SWAG or Schwag?

Lately, I have been hearing the term "schwag," that should be used to describe bad cannabis, as a word for giveaway items instead of the proper term SWAG—something we all get. It still makes me laugh aloud every time I hear "schwag" misused, especially when it is used by people of esteem in the community who would cringe if they knew what they were saying. On the other hand, can you imagine how surprised a group of college students would be to hear that they were getting a "schwag" bag? Several times I've had to explain to folks how it might be a good idea to use a different word. Thankfully they had a sense of humor.

What to Ask For

Bud is dried sinsemilla cannabis flower. It is the most expensive form of raw cannabis because it contains the highest concentration of therapeutic compounds. If you are inhaling your medicine, or making cannabis oil, bud is definitely the way to go.

Shake is the fine, dusty crumbs of plant material that break off the buds, leaves, and stems and collect in the bottom of a bag. If you are on a budget, consider making your butter and oil for cooking with quality shake instead of buds. You will still get a highly effective product but for far less money.

Leaves of the cannabis plant contain all the therapeutic properties of the bud but are not as high in active components. The closer to the bud, the more potent the leaf. Leaves have a fraction of the potency of the buds on the same plant. (Raber, 2013)

Kif (resin powder) sometimes spelled kief, is another misnomer and actually means marijuana or a mixture of marijuana and hashish in the Moroccan Arabic language. The brownish powder made solely of cannabis trichomes harvested from the buds, trim, shake, and leaves is more accurately called resin powder or by the Arabic word hashish. Resin powder is often much more potent than the plant material from which it was collected. After the leaves or buds have been dried and allowed to cure, they are put into a tumbler with a fine mesh screen or placed, along with dry ice, in a cloth bag with a fine mesh bottom and shaken to separate the trichomes from the plant matter. Hashish is usually a fine powder and high quality hashish powder can easily be pressed into a malleable shape. It can be mixed with lower-quality cannabis for smoking to increase therapeutic potency. It can also be used for cooking, decarboxylated and packed into a gel cap, used to make topicals, or sprinkled on top of cannabis flower and smoked. Kif is becoming increasingly popular, which can make getting cannabis leaves more difficult. If you want to vaporize kif, be sure to double check the directions for your vaporizer to make sure it will not clog.

Weights and Pricing

Cannabis is generally sold by the ounce, half ounce, quarter ounce, eighth ounce, or in grams. Begin by buying smaller quantities such as an eighth ounce until you figure out what kinds of cannabis you like and find therapeutic. An eighth ounce of high-quality cannabis is usually around $35-$60, though this differs from state to state. Lower quality cannabis will be cheaper. Prices will also be cheaper in states where cannabis is legally available. If you are buying underground, you can expect to pay up to $125 per quarter ounce for high quality cannabis, even higher for something considered boutique quality.

Mold, Bacteria, and Other Biologicals

A Word of Caution: It is important for medical users to buy from reputable people who know their products. Cannabis can contain bacteria, molds, pesticides, fungus, and other nasty things not visible to the naked eye. Consuming any of these can exacerbate whatever medical condition you are addressing. When the U.S. legalizes cannabis, it will be easy to obtain cannabis that is guaranteed free of bacteria, mold, fungus, and pesticides by a reputable testing lab. The Werc Shop says that, as an average, 20 percent of the cannabis samples they receive test positive for pesticide exposure and 25 percent test positive on the microbial screen, most often for mold. Other labs in California report even higher percentages of positive tests, especially for residual pesticides and plant growth regulators.

If you are buying cannabis illegally, it is good to make friends with cannabis nerds—also known as weed geeks. They are everywhere. These are the people who are passionate about growing excellent cannabis. They will know their medicine inside and out and can talk about it in the same way a wine or cheese expert can talk about the properties of their delicacies.

If you can see mold or fungus on cannabis, DO NOT consume it. If you get sick from smoking or ingesting any cannabis medicine, be suspicious of the material and take appropriate action. If you are unable to return it, destroy it carefully without dispersing the mold into your environment. Pain and stuffiness of the sinuses and sinus infection are key signs that you may have inhaled molded cannabis. If you have smoked moldy cannabis, try using a nasal saline spray to clear your sinuses.

Since cannabis is illegal, there are no certified organic standards for its cultivation, harvesting, storage, or distribution. This means there's no way to guarantee your cannabis is free of the most harmful pesticides. Even if someone is using a certified organic pesticide, it is unlikely it has been studied or tested for use on a combustible and inhaled product. Some organic pesticides are closer to nature than others. Without doing your homework, it's difficult to know which these are. This is another good reason to find a grower, dispensary, or distributor who is pro-organic and uses the most natural forms of pest control possible.

Storage

Cannabis needs to be cured for approximately three weeks before it is ready to consume for all non-juice or non-fresh applications. This will have been done before it gets to you. Store it in an airtight glass jar for optimal freshness and shelf life. Most people agree you should use cannabis within three to six months of harvest to get the most potent medicine. If it is older than that, it doesn't mean the cannabis isn't good; it probably is just not as good as it once was.

Research shows many of the most volatile terpenes are no longer present after one year of storage. Many people believe storing cannabis in the freezer helps it stay fresher longer. That is really only true if you plan not to keep taking the plant material in and out of the freezer and the freezer door is not often opened. Every time you open the freezer door, condensation will develop, and ice crystals will form on the plant matter reducing quality. That said, a freezer is the best option for long-term (more than a couple of months) storage. Be sure to seal the medicine in small amounts such as an eighth to a quarter of an ounce.

Keep in mind that oxygen and light degrade cannabis quality over time. That is why it is good to keep cannabis in an air tight container and either in a colored glass jar or in a dark place such as a cabinet. Do not let cannabis sit in your car in the summer heat. Your car will smell great when you get in, but the herb may lose much of its potency.

Antidotes

It is easy to consume too much cannabis if you are not careful, especially when ingesting edibles or oil. If this happens, remember that even though you may feel like you are dying, cannabis is not going to kill you. [See "No Lethal Dose Established", on page 114.] If you don't like the feeling, you will likely have to put up with it for six to nine hours. Antidotes such as pistachios, pine nuts, pine oil, lemon juice, and orange juice have been described in the traditional medicinal literature but not clinically tested. [See the "Risks and Harm Reduction" chart on page 149 for information about citicholine.]

While overconsumption of cannabis does not (as with alcohol) result in a hangover, it can produce an aftereffect that may include sedation, grogginess, and spaciness.

Intake Methods

While cannabis is commonly smoked, there are numerous ways to get its therapeutic benefits, and everyone needs to find their optimal treatment method. In figuring out what is best for you, consider the following:

- What is your primary cannabis care plan?
- Do you need immediate relief from symptoms?
- How long do you need or want the effects to last?
- Are you looking for relief that allows you to be present and function in a job or your daily life, or are you looking for something more sedating?
- What is available in your area?

As our understanding of medical cannabis grows, there will be an increased variety of cannabis medicines from which to choose. Here is a quick overview of the most common current intake methods:

Inhalation (smoking and vaporizing) of Dried Plant Material

Activation Time: Immediate: 0–5 minutes
Serving Sizes & Tips: Since relief can be provided in a single puff, it is wise to start with that. Should you need more, you can have more, but if you don't need more there is no reason to take another. Sometimes

a puff is enough. Someone else may need five or six. It just depends. **Notes:** Inhalation brings smoke or vapor directly into the Central Nervous System (CNS). Effects can be felt quickly, and sometimes increasingly so, for up 30 minutes before peaking. This is called *creeping.*

Special Medical Benefits: Inhalation is the best choice for rapid relief. It is important to note that while smoke inhalation is the most popular way to utilize cannabis, it is also considered by scientists to be the least effective medicinal intake method. Please note that vaporizing is a much healthier inhalation method than using a joint, bong, or pipe. [See, "Inhalation for Instant Relief", on page 186.]

Relief Period: 45 minutes–3 hours

Inhalation of Concentrates - (Dabs, Honey Oil, and other highly concentrated cannabis products)

Activation Time: Immediate: 0–90 seconds.

Serving Sizes & Tips: When trying any of these concentrated medicines, leave at least 15 minutes between inhales until you learn your optimal dose; it is easy to overdo! If you have access to a high CBD product, use it before you inhale a high THC product to help dampen possibly negative side effects of the THC and maximize its therapeutic potential.

Notes: Because these are highly concentrated, they are extremely strong, and it is possible to develop a tolerance to cannabis if they are used too often. These concentrates are useful for people with severe symptoms who require high doses of medicine to get relief such as people weaning off pain pumps and going through alcohol, opiate, or other drug withdrawal. Concentrates prepared with butane (and other non-food grade solvents) are not created equally, and may or may not be safe to consume. If you are dabbing for medical purposes, please make sure that your dab, oil, or hash is made by someone who uses quality herb, best practices, and makes a clean product. [See "Dabbing", on page 188.]

Relief Period: 45 minutes–3 hours

Edibles (food)

Activation Time: Slow: ½–2 hours

Serving Sizes & Tips: Begin with a bite! People who need sustained pain relief while being active will want to experiment to establish the ideal serving. It is smart to start small. Keep in mind that if you are using edibles for sustained pain relief, it is good to utilize CBD rich cannabis if you can find it.

Notes: Edibles go through the digestive tract. Therefore, it takes longer to feel relief, but it creates a longer lasting and more psychedelic affect (potentially 4x more psychoactive than if inhaled). [See "Dosing with Edibles", on page 220.]
Relief Period: 6–9 hours

Tea

Activation Time: Slow: ½–1½ hours
Serving Sizes & Tips: A normal serving is 1 cup or 6-8 ounces
Notes: Cannabis tea processes in the body similarly to edibles. While edibles are high in cannabinoids, cannabis tea will have more cannabinoids acids than cannabinoids. The effect, therefore, is much less psychoactive but still has the potential to be strong if you take too much. [See "Tea", on page 208.]
Relief Period: 6–9 hours

Tinctures

Activation Time: Moderate: 1–15 minutes & Slow: ½–1½ hour
Serving Sizes & Tips: This depends on the chemical makeup of the plant material, your chemistry, and the needs of your body. Some people take 2 drops under the tongue 3 times per day while another person may only take 2 drops before bedtime, while another will need 7-10 drops 5 times per day.
Notes: Can be taken either under the tongue or swallowed. Tinctures held under the tongue or between the cheek and gums provide relief quicker than swallowing the tincture but not quite as quickly as inhalation. Swallowing the tincture is similar to edibles in terms of activation time and relief period, as it has to pass through the liver to be metabolized. [See "Tinctures and Extractions", on page 204.]
Relief Period: 2–9 hours

Oils

Activation Time: Slow: 1–2 hours (for seizure control) & Gradual: 30-90 days (for cancers and treatment of some other conditions)
Serving Sizes & Tips: Cannabis oils are generally used in small doses daily for management of a seizure related condition such as epilepsy (CBD rich oil with low THC) and at high doses for 60-90 days for fighting cancer (high THC oil or combinations of high THC and high CBD oil). For cancer, pre-clinical and anecdotal evidence suggests starting slowly with very small doses for 30 days to allow for

tolerance. After tolerance is developed, a serving of up to 1g of oil a day is taken for 60–90 days.

Notes: Oils deliver high concentrations of THC, CBD, and other cannabinoids giving them the apparent potential to alter disease progression. There are no scientific studies on cannabis oil for the treatment of cancer or other diseases. This is purely anecdotal information and does NOT replace medical advice. Many people who advocate for the use of high concentration cannabis oil say that after the cancer is gone they suggest a small maintenance doses to ensure the environment that made it possible for the cancer to grow in the first place is not repeated. [See "Cannabis Oil", on page 196.]

Topical Applications

Activation Time: Immediate: 60–90 seconds, and Gradual

Serving Sizes & Tips: Using a topical properly depends so much on what is in it and what you want it to do for you. Some are rubbed directly into the skin for relief of muscle, bone, and joint pain, whereas it might be better to keep a skin growth covered with a bandage and a more liberal amount of topical to ensure it is constantly in contact with whatever you are trying to heal. Other topicals are rolled on and evaporate quickly.

Notes: Topical applications provide antioxidants directly to the skin and may prove a powerful medicine for skin cancer and other skin-related issues. They also provide relief to sore muscles and help heal wounds. I have seen cannabis topicals make pre-cancerous skin spots and pencil-eraser-sized growths (of unknown cell type) disappear from the top of the skin in 14 days. I also know people who use cannabis topicals to treat dry skin and eczema as well as bone, joint, muscle, and nerve pain. Cannabis topicals can also make great facial care products and have recently become popular as sexual lubricants/enhancers.

Relief Period: ½–3 hours

Kif Resin Powder Capsules

Activation Time: Slow: ½–2 hours

Serving Sizes & Tips: Finely ground plant material and plant trichome resin powders are both erroneously referred to as kif. Both can be baked for 20-30 minutes between 212-230° F, which decarboxylates and activates the medicine which is then measured and placed into empty gel caps.

Notes: A fat such as coconut or olive oil is required for maximum absorp-

tion. Some people eat a handful of fatty nuts or a spoonful of coconut oil or toast with butter when taking kif capsules. Others put the coconut oil directly into the kif capsule. [See "Cannabis Gel Caps", on page 209.]
Relief Period: 6–9 hours

Suppository

Activation Time: Within 15 minutes
Serving Sizes & Tips: A single suppository can provide a high dose of medicine that is more efficiently absorbed into the body than other cannabis intake methods. It is important NOT to use too high a dose nor insert the suppository too far into the rectum; otherwise, an extreme high may occur. Dosing size depends on your desired outcome and the patient. A therapeutic dose could be as small as 2.5 mgs of the needed cannabinoid then slowly increase the dose in small increments as necessary to control symptoms.
Notes: While this is considered to be one of the more efficient ways to deliver cannabis medicines, you may have already guessed it is not the most popular. Suppositories act fairly quickly because they do not have to pass the liver and are directly absorbed into the bloodstream and cross the blood brain barrier. This form of delivery is especially good for people who are bedridden and extremely sick, have limited lung capacity, cannot swallow, suffer from nausea and vomiting, have prostate issues, colon cancer, do not want to smoke or eat edibles, or are frail. [See "Suppositories", on page 210.]
Relief Period: Up to 12 hours

Raw Juice

Activation Time: Gradual
Serving Sizes & Tips: Raw cannabis juice works more like a dietary supplement to be taken daily or several times a day. Because the plant material is not heated, the cannabinoid acids are not converted to cannabinoids. Therefore, there is no direct effect on consciousness. Due to the legal status of cannabis, it is difficult to get access to a sufficient amount of plant material (2-6 large fresh buds/day) to use this intake method regularly.
Notes: Because of its high cannabinoid acid content and raw terpene content, fresh cannabis juice from buds may prove an excellent anti-inflammatory and antibiotic medicine that helps reset the immune system. Not enough is known about raw juicing to really tell how or why it works. For many people it has provided great health benefits. Dr. William Courtney is the most vocal proponent of using raw cannabis

juice for healing. Many of his colleagues take issue with the fact that they do not agree with his methodology or claims, but most agree that raw cannabis juice should be investigated using scientific method. [See "Raw Juice", on page 195.]
Relief Period: Benefits build over time. There is no psychoactivity.

Pharmaceuticals (Marinol® and Cesamet®)

Activation Time: Slow: 45–60 minutes
Serving Sizes & Tips: These are prescription medicines made from synthetic THC. Follow your doctor's instruction or that of the manufacturer for your specific condition. One of the major complaints about Dronabinol, (brand name Marinol®) is its psychoactivity and the fact that the patient cannot titrate their own dose. Once they have had too much, they are uncomfortable until it is out of their system.
Notes: Dronabinol is the isolated version of THC taken in pill form. It is prescribed to control nausea and vomiting in cancer patients and as an appetite stimulant in AIDS patients.
Relief Period: Dranabinol is generally taken 2-3 times per day.

Cannabis Based Medicines (Whole Plant)

Activation Time: Moderate: 10–15 minutes
Serving Sizes & Tips: Follow your doctor's prescription.
Notes: Sativex® is the only drug made from whole cannabis plant extracts. It is an oral-mucosal spray. Sativex® is currently in Phase III clinical trials in the U.S. for treatment of cancer pain. It is approved in the UK, Canada, and 26 other countries. It is effective in treating spasticity in M.S. patients and neuropathic pain in cancer patients. This drug is made with two plant varieties, one rich in THC and one rich in CBD, and seems to be well tolerated by many patients with a variety of ailments.
Relief Period: Sativex® 45 minutes–2 hours

Transdermal Applications

Activation Time: 0–15 minutes
Serving Sizes & Tips: Transdermal applications are usually standardized to a specific amount of cannabinoids and terpenes per patch, or pump. If you are using a commercially made product, simply follow the instructions or your doctor's recommendation.
Notes: Transdermal applications work quickly by absorbing directly into the bloodstream. Effects are felt almost immediately but may

take up to 15 minutes. This is a highly efficient intake method, and it comes without the smoke associated with inhalation, the waiting time of an edible, and is fairly easy to titrate. One of the great benefits of a transdermal patch is that some can be time released providing continuous relief for a longer period.
Relief Period: Up to 8–12 hours depending on one's metabolism.

Inhalation for Instant Relief

Smoking, dabbing, and vaping are especially useful intake methods for people who need immediate relief from nausea, vomiting, spasticity, and pain. Many people get relief with as little as one puff; others require more. I've never understood why nausea medicine comes in a pill. Have you ever watched someone who is vomiting try to keep down a pill?

Smoking

Smoking is the most widely used and accepted form of consuming cannabis but also one of the least efficient. While many people enjoy the immediate effect of smoked cannabis, the smoke itself can be an irritant to the throat and lungs—

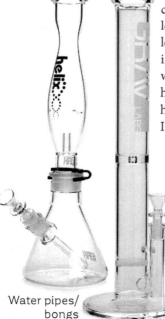

especially when smoking a paper rolled cigarette. Pipes create smoke but deliver a cleaner, cooler drag and are less irritating to some than smoking a joint. They waste less cannabis than joints. If you use a water bong, keep in mind that some of the cannabinoids will be lost in the water. Because of the design of the bong, the user has to hold their mouth in a way that allows for a deeper inhale. One hit is equivalent to several from a joint or pipe. I once asked someone, "How is a bong different from a

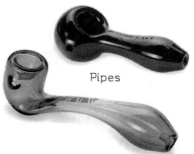

Pipes

Water pipes/ bongs

Photo Courtesy 420Science.com

joint?" He responded, "A joint is like drinking a beer while a bong is like taking a whiskey shot." He was not exaggerating.

Vaporization

Vaporizers are an alternative to smoking that provides immediate relief with inhalation. They deliver therapeutic compounds in smoke-free air with comparable benefits to joints, pipes, and bongs. A vaporizer heats plant material without combusting it thus releasing the cannabinoids and terpene rich essential oils into a smoke-free vapor that is inhaled. Many experts believe the temperature sweet spot is 210°C or 410°F. At this temperature, which is below the combustion point, terpenes are released and cannabinoid acids such as THCA and CBDA are decarboxylated and converted to cannabinoids at therapeutic levels. Vaporizers deliver the same amount of cannabinoids but measurably reduce the pyrolytic smoke and other non-desirable compounds generated when cannabis is combusted. (Gieringer, St. Laurent and Goodrich, 2004) Cannabis combusts at 230°C (446°F). It is for this reason the VolcanoMedic vaporizer does not exceed 210°C. Previously, Volcanoes, which are the gold standard in vaporizers, went to 230°C.

Vaporizers are widely considered a healthier option than smoking joints and pipes because they deliver therapeutic compounds at a much cooler temperature while providing a more pleasant user experience and reducing irritation to the lungs and throat. Additionally, vaporization makes more efficient use of the material because all the therapeutic compounds released go directly into the vapor. On the other hand, when you smoke many of these compounds

1: Volcano Classic, 2: Magic Flight Launch Box, 3: Pax 2, and 4: Donut KandyPen. Vaporizers 1-3 are specifically for dry herb. Number 4 is for concentrates.

Photo Courtesy 420Science.com

"go up in smoke," combusting before they reach your lungs. Also readily available are vaporizers that accommodate oil and concentrates for those who don't want to use flower.

Using a vaporizer aka vaporizing or vaping is by far the best way to go for anyone with a chronic ailment who needs immediate relief and chooses to inhale their medicine. Carcinogenic tars do exist in cannabis smoke when combusted in a pipe, bong, or joint but are reduced, if not totally eliminated, when cannabis is vaporized. While cannabis appears to be rich in therapeutic ingredients that counterbalance the negative impact of tars and carcinogens created by combustion, it makes sense to minimize exposure to potentially harmful compounds, especially when ill. [See "Cannabis vs. Tobacco", on page 129.]

Dabbing

Dabbing (aka dab, dabs) is a relatively new recreational phenomenon that converts a highly concentrated cannabinoid wax, shatter (shatter looks like a sheet of light amber glass instead of being viscous or sticky like its concentrate counterparts), honey oil, butane hash oil (BHO), CO_2 oil, cannabis oil, or resin to a vapor at high heat using a dab rig or a vape pen. Each of these concentrates mentioned delivers high amounts of cannabinoids and, depending on the production process, may also be high in terpenes. Each concentrate is different in how it was produced, its color, and its consistency. Availability of concentrates will have much to do with whether you live in a legal state or not.

Using a dab rig can be intimidating at first. The first time I saw one, I thought to myself, "Yikes! That looks like something used for crack or heroin intake." The concentrate is placed on what is called a nail. This is a flat surface that once heated (using a blow torch which is like a powerful butane lighter) is where

Photo Courtesy 420Science.com

Dab rigs, like all other cannabis paraphernalia, come in many designs. Pictured are Grav Labs glass dab rigs with quartz nails.

you place a small amount of concentrate. Nails are usually made from glass, quartz, ceramic, or titanium. One can use an e-nail where the nail is wrapped by a heating element connected to an external power source that keeps the nail hot without having to use a blow torch. As soon as the concentrate hits the surface it vaporizes. At the same time the concentrate is placed on the nail, the dabber will inhale drawing the vapor into their lungs. Some dab rigs have water chambers to cool the vapor but others will not.

For medical use, dabbing can be extremely helpful in relieving symptoms of opiate, alcohol, and other drug withdrawals. It can also be useful for helping people who are weaning themselves off heavy pain medications such as a pain pump. When pain is extreme and unbearable, dabs work instantly and provide great relief. Because of the high cannabinoid content in oil extracts, dabbing rapidly drops your blood pressure. Thus, it is wise to dab seated, or you will quickly find yourself sliding to the ground or nearest chair. In fact, that is what happened to my friend Larry who tried a dab at the first legal High Times Cannabis Cup in Denver. Larry has been consuming cannabis daily for fifty years. He was offered a dab by "some kid." When the young man offered the dab, he suggested that Larry take a seat. Larry declined thinking the "kid" didn't know with whom he was speaking. In a matter of seconds, Larry's blood pressure dropped, and he found himself seated on the floor. **Those with low blood pressure should take necessary precautions.** Exercise caution if you choose to use dabs, and please talk with a cannabis educated doctor. Yet, few physicians are knowledgeable about dabbing, as it is a recent phenomenon. You may find excellent "street research" and information on various cannabis and dabbing blogs.

Each concentrate uses a different process to extract a high amount of cannabinoids. Connoisseurs choose concentrates for purity of taste, their cannabinoid profile, and the strong high. Dabbing is especially pleasant for recreational users who have built up an extremely high tolerance. It makes it possible for them to get higher than they could with smoking or vaporizing alone. But, it also down regulates the endocannabinoid system and increases their tolerance level.

Because the cannabinoid content in concentrates is SO high—25 to 95 percent (usually THC in the form of THCA, although there are also concentrated CBD dabs on the market), their effect is immediate and intensely magnified. A single dab can be as powerful as a joint or an entire bowl from a small to medium size pipe, and in some cases more. Recreational dabbing should not be employed by novices or anyone who does not already have a tolerance to the effects of THC and should be done with someone with previous experience. It is wise to wait at least fifteen minutes before a second dab until you know how you respond.

The products in the concentrate market range from what I consider dirty and potentially harmful to fairly clean and safe. All the different extraction technologies (butane or other hydrocarbons, super critical CO_2, and ethanol) have trade-offs between safety, efficacy, cost, and yield. More important than the specific technique one is using to make concentrates is the knowledge of the process, use of safe and quality equipment, quality plant materials, clean solvents, and safe and reasonable production procedures. As an example, butane is toxic if consumed, but if clean butane is used in a process where it is all recovered then safety concerns are minimized. CO_2 is not flammable at room temperature, yet (unlike butane) it needs to be highly pressurized to perform a cannabis extraction. A pump failure with CO_2 could cause an explosion resulting in the release of the solvent gas, which is poisonous to humans.

Butane hash oil/wax/shatter, oils extracted with ethanol and CO_2 oil are probably the most popular or widely available concentrates for dabbing. Generally speaking, CO_2 products are made by larger companies because of the cost associated with the equipment whereas butane extraction methods can be done with homemade and/or more cost effective equipment.

Butane has a bad name in the medical cannabis community, yet it is widely popular on the market. As technology improves and standards are developed, the medical community may become less skeptical of butane extractions.

Part of the problem with butane (and other non-food grade solvents) is that it exists in varying grades of mixes with other solvents. An excellent example is lighter fluid, which is made from butane and varying amounts of other hydrocarbons all of which are neurotoxins according to Jeffrey Hergenrather, MD, head of the Society of Cannabis Clinicians. (California NORML 2013) Because there are no industry standards for any of the products in the concentrate market, some well-intentioned but not well informed people use butane of questionable quality, and they use processes that are unsafe for the operator and not efficient at fully evaporating the butane from the concentrate. For this reason, if you choose to use butane extracted concentrates, make sure you choose products from suppliers who are quality and safety oriented and have the lab tests to prove it!

Developments in technology continue to improve the quality of butane products on the market. The CEO of Tamisium Extractors, David McGhee, says, "... butane can be one of the safest and most cost effective extraction methods when used properly. The key is that the butane needs to be cleaned in advance of being used for extracting cannabinoids and terpenes." This is done through distillation. His company has a patent pending for this technology. There are different opinions among doctors and scientists about whether or not all the butane is actually boiled off in the finishing process, and if it is not, whether any remaining butane can cause health problems.

CO_2 has its own set of challenges but is considered one of the cleanest ways to extract highly concentrated cannabinoids. Liquid CO_2 under high pressure is used to wash cannabinoids and terpenoids from cannabis flowers or leaves. If done in one pass, the terpenes will be lost, but if CO_2 is applied twice at the right pressure for cannabinoids and terpenes to be extracted, then a CO_2 oil can be fairly complete. Currently, there are no standards regulating the use of butane, hexane, naptha, CO_2, and other solvents (except ethanol) for use in products for human consumption. This is likely to change as the industry matures.

A hot new trend in the DIY concentrate market is to make rosin by pressing dried cannabis bud with a flat iron used to straighten hair. This simple, solvent-free method requires good bud, parchment paper (to hold the bud and collect the oils), and a flat iron with an adjustable heating element. The ideal temperature for extraction is between 230-300° F. (Bienenstock 2015) Once your device is at the proper temperature, put a bud in a fold of parchment paper, place it in the flat iron, and press for three to five seconds. Once the resin cools, scrape it into a container. The article "How to Make Weed 'Dabs' at Home," posted on *www.motherboard.vice.com* is an excellent resource on this practical, easy, and relatively safe extraction method. This method may well become a favorite among concentrate users for its purity, smooth taste, ease of production, and delivery of high concentrations of cannabinoids and terpenes without solvents.

Each of the concentrates has pros and cons. What is most important is that the maker starts with clean, quality material; that they are using the proper process for a specific technique; and that they employ lab testing to ensure the safety of their product.

CAUTION: Dabbing high THC wax can lead to rapid tolerance to THC making it difficult, if not impossible, for the user to get high from anything but dabs. If you are a cannabis novice, and are not going through drug or alcohol withdrawals or suffering excruciating pain, please try other cannabis intake methods before dabbing.

Inhalation Tips

Breathing seems such a natural thing that it's funny how complicated it really can be. Novices tend to take much shallower breaths. They are often timid and don't inhale enough smoke or vapor leading to under consumption for treating their issues. Most adults are short breathers anyway. Have you ever noticed how when a baby sleeps their entire belly, chest, and ribcage move up and down as they breathe? Watch yourself breathe in the mirror, or observe another adult breathing. You will not see their belly move. As we get older, we begin to hold on to our stomach muscles and shorten our breath. Yoga, meditation, and Tai Chi are great for helping you become aware of your breath connecting mind, body, and soul. Proper breathing technique can greatly increase the quality of your inhalation, the amount of medicine pulled into your lungs, and the extra hold time making it possible for your plant material to go further.

The tips below may reduce your trial and error phase, but you still need to experiment with what is the best technique for you. You may notice that none of my tips or instructions mention joints or cannabis cigarettes. I'm not a fan. This is partly because I couldn't roll a joint if my life depended on it and partly because they are wasteful and lead to consuming more tars and toxins than other methods. If this is your chosen delivery method, the tips below still apply.

1. *Titration* (self-dosing) is easy with the inhalation method because you feel the effects quickly if not immediately. Take one drag at a time. Let a few minutes pass until you know how the cannabis affects you. If you need more, you will know in ten minutes. Effects of smoked cannabis can last anywhere from forty-five minutes to three hours depending on volume of intake, your body, your pain or discomfort level, and the variety of cannabis.

2. If you are using a pipe or bong, you will get a much better drag if you pack the herb tightly into the bowl. This provides a more efficient drag thus conserving your supply and reducing the amount of smoke generated.

3. Most adults only use the top third of their lungs when breathing, which minimizes their capacity to intake air, smoke, and vapor. For better inhalation, relax your throat and belly, allow your ribs to expand gently at their widest point (two or three inches under the arm pit), and breathe slowly and deeply from the base of your belly. Remember that one drag from a well-packed pipe or vaporizer may be all you need.

4. Pull the vapor into your lungs for an inhalation count of five to ten seconds, depending on your lung capacity, and then slowly exhale. Relief may be immediate. Holding vapor or smoke in the lungs longer than five seconds may lead to higher volumes of tar left in the lungs and can give a false sense of effectiveness due to the dizziness that comes when holding your breath too long. Holding your breath cuts off the oxygen supply to your brain; this is counterproductive. Don't do it!

5. Take a couple of deep inhalations after each drag to increase your oxygen supply and improve circulation.

6. Light your bowl quickly while inhaling. Don't keep the flame on the plant material. Once it is lit, quickly remove the flame. Most pipes will have a hole on the side of the bowl. This is called the *carburetor*. Keep your finger on it while you inhale. If you want the plant material to stay lit so you can take another drag or share, you need to keep your finger on the carburetor. There are many different types of pipes. If you are using a pipe that has to be filled after each inhalation or two, this is called a *one-hitter*. It will not have a carburetor. If you are using a pipe that allows the bowl to be filled for several puffs, you should get one with a carburetor. If you are using a water pipe, it will have a bowl but not a carburetor. Thus, the inhalation technique is slightly different. If using a bong, place the outside of your lips to the inside of the hole at the top of the neck. Light the herb in the bowl, and inhale at the same time. This will make the water bubble;

you will hear it. After three to five seconds of inhaling, pull the glass bowl out of the neck of the water pipe and continue to inhale. This pulls the vapor created and cooled in the neck of the bong into your lungs.

7. Do not constantly hold the flame to the plant material; that is a good way to "burn" through your cannabis wastefully. It degrades the therapeutic impact of the cannabinoids and terpenes and increases the likelihood of inhaling lighter fluid fumes. Even worse, cannabinoids and terpenes evaporate at too high a heat, so the less time the flame is touching the plant matter the more therapeutic compounds you receive. When starting a fresh bowl, it is better to light a small part of the green herb instead of the entire bowl face or a large amount of herb. This helps conserve the medicine, and for those who enjoy the taste, it will give a fresher tasting drag or hit.

8. If you are using a pipe or bong, the best quality drag will come from what experienced smokers call a *cherry*, referring to the glowing ball of embers that sticks around a few moments after you make the initial light. Once the initial flame has died, the plant material will burn slower at a lower temperature. It will have the same color of reddish-orange that charcoal gets when it's just right. Because the plant material is burning at a lower temperature in this form, you will get a smoother, cooler, and more therapeutic drag. You can continue to take drags off a pipe with a cherry, as long as it is glowing, without the need to relight. If you are passing a pipe with a cherry, immediately cover the carburetor to keep the cherry alive, or experienced smokers may give you the stink eye.

9. If you are sharing a pipe, joint, or vaporizer with another person, please make sure you **practice good hygiene**. This includes cleaning the apparatus frequently and NOT sharing with people who have a cold or virus. When using a water pipe, change the water frequently.

10. If you are using a vaporizer, be sure to read the instructions. Each vaporizer technology is different. While one vaporizer (i.e., the Volcano) is designed to hold the vapor in a chamber for a full drag on demand, others, such as the Magic Flight Launch Box, may require more of a sipping technique than a single, long drag for optimal performance. If you are in the market for a vaporizer, be sure to find out if the heating element is separate from the plant material. If not, the machine is actually combusting the medicine and leaving toxins in the smoke. **Make sure the material never comes in contact with the heating element.** Not to sound like a broken record, but be sure to read the instructions, specifications, and lots of on-line reviews before buying a vaporizer.

Is It Safe to Smoke If Your Lungs Are Sick?

Unlike one of our presidents, my mom did not inhale. She consumed cannabis edibles. We reasoned that smoking was not a good idea since she had lung cancer. In hindsight I have often wondered if she would have received more relief by utilizing a vaporizer in tandem with the edibles. Inhaled cannabis is known to kill lung pathogens (Tashkin 2008) and works as a bronchodilator, helping increase airflow into the lungs, which would have made it easier for my mother to breathe and improve her low oxygen levels. While it seems paradoxical for a patient with compromised lungs to inhale cannabis, I cannot help believing we should have used a vaporizer as part of her regimen. Is using a vaporizer any different from using an inhaler?

Ingestion for Lasting Relief

Ingesting cannabis does not provide immediate relief the way inhalation does. It does, however, provide sustained pain relief for six to nine hours (sometimes longer) depending on the volume and potency of the herb consumed and your own body. Compare that to the forty-five minutes to three hours of relief provided by inhalation!

Ingested cannabis passes through the gastrointestinal tract and cannabinoids are metabolized in the liver. For that reason, it takes thirty minutes to two hours to feel the effect. The time it takes for the cannabinoids to be metabolized and delivered to the blood depends on the contents of the stomach and the person's rate of liver metabolism. For that reason, it is important to start with a small dose of any edible—and I do mean small— such as a teaspoon or a single bite of a low potency preparation. Wait an hour and a half before consuming more. The cannabis-wise agree that if one does not get the desired effect after ninety minutes, **only consume half of what was initially consumed.**

When cannabis enters the stomach as an edible, concentrated oil, pill, tea, or tincture, the THC is processed in the liver and converted to the metabolite 11-hydroxy-THC, which *may* (or may not) pack a more psychoactive punch than THC in inhaled cannabis delivered directly to the blood via the lungs and then to the central nervous system. (Abrams and Guzman 2009) It has long been thought that 11-hydroxy-THC is much more psychoactive than THC. New pharmacokinetic studies examining blood levels call that theory into question. When the same amount of THC is consumed orally compared to inhaled, the reports of experimental subjects do not necessarily offer evidence of a magnified psychoactive effect of THC taken orally. (E. B. Russo 2015) This is a difficult subject to study scientifically since levels of THC in the blood do not necessarily correlate with levels in the brain. (E. B. Russo 2015) What accounts for the vast difference in effect or experience between edibles and inhalation? It likely boils down to actual cannabinoid intake and absorption. (E. B. Russo 2015) When one uses an oral intake method, much more of the cannabinoids may be absorbed into the bloodstream if the dose is large thus providing a stronger effect.

Usually, consuming a serving of cannabis that has one half teaspoon, or 2.5-10 mg THC, in a mild canna-butter or cannabis infused cooking oil (not highly concentrated cannabis flower oil extracts) is more than enough for the beginner. Depending on the potency of the plant material used and how long it was cooked, less than a teaspoon may be sufficient to provide relief. A cannabis-wise doctor will help advise you on what serving size will work best based on your symptoms, unique body chemistry, and the potency of the medicine. [See "Dosing with Edibles", on page 220.]

As you can see, dose titration is more difficult when ingesting cannabis than when smoking; however, people who dislike inhaling or need longer-term relief may find edibles a great therapeutic delivery system. Many of the therapeutic users interviewed for this book have told me that edibles help them get a good night's sleep. One of my favorite people on the planet swears cannabis edibles are the best medicine for her chronic hip pain. She says that when she has this kind of pain she usually cannot sleep, which makes the pain worse. Eating a cannabis edible dulls the pain and makes it possible for her to relax and sleep soundly. We all understand the importance of quality sleep to health and healing.

Raw Cannabis

Early anecdotal research suggests that consumption of raw cannabis juice may have many healing properties and may even reverse effects of certain conditions such as lupus, rheumatoid arthritis, and endometriosis (without making patients feel "high") and possibly eliminate the need for some, if not most, pharmaceutical medicines. While clinical research in this area is lacking, the anecdotal evidence is promising. Raw cannabis is high in *cannabinoid acids*, which do not alter consciousness and are believed to be strong anti-inflammatories, antibiotics, and immune system supporters. (Courtney 2010) The best source of cannabinoid acids are the buds not the leaves. Since we cannot feel the acids working in the body, it is hard to know how long the cannabinoid acids provide a therapeutic impact. There is little research in this area.

Kristen Peskuski's story of healing with cannabis is amazing. When she began juicing cannabis, she was taking over forty different medications for her lupus, rheumatoid arthritis, endometriosis, etc. Within six weeks of starting her juicing program, she stopped taking pain medication. Kristen spent most of her youth sick. Doctors thought she wouldn't see her thirtieth birthday and, due to her severe endometriosis, never thought she would have children. In her own words, she says they were "just trying to keep me comfortable." She is now a healthy mom with healthy children. All her conditions have remained in sustained remission. She directly attributes this result to flooding her body with cannabinoid acids. Hear her tell her story on the Cannabis International website at *www.CannabisInternational.org*. She and her doctor, William Courtney, MD, are now married and work together at Cannabis International to advance cannabinoid acid research.

Together, they deserve credit for popularizing the concept of juicing raw cannabis. However, many people in the cannabis science community are not as quick to jump on the band-wagon. Many take issues with how Courtney says raw cannabis works, the dosage he recommends, and that he suggests it is okay to use fan leaves in the juice. Martin Lee of Project CBD has written an interesting article titled "Is Juicing Raw Cannabis the Miracle Health Cure That Some of Its Proponents Believe It to Be?" It is the counterbalance to the Cannabis International mantra. You can find the article at *ProjectCBD.org*.

Having access to enough cannabis for juicing is unrealistic in most places. As we move away from prohibition, that is likely to change, but for now this will be a major barrier to access for most consumers.

Raw cannabis is an exciting part of the therapeutic cannabis revolution. I look forward to raw cannabis being more widely available and development in raw cannabis research on its therapeutic merits.

Cannabis Oil

Cannabis oil is also known as concentrated cannabis oil, Rick Simpson Oil (RSO), Phoenix Tears, or Milagro Oil. Cannabis oil is usually a dark (except in the case of an olive oil based high concentration cannabis oil), thick paste, or gel of highly concentrated cannabinoids made from the flowers (and sometimes leaves – but I don't recommend that) of seed-free female cannabis flowers. Making cannabis oil requires extraction of the cannabinoids from the dry plant matter with a solvent such as naptha (potential carcinogen), butane (potential carcinogen due to contaminants), hexane, isopropyl alcohol, food grade ethanol, olive oil, or CO_2. When using naptha, hexane, isopropyl alcohol, butane, or ethanol (grain alcohol such as Everclear), you must cook off any remaining solvent after extraction. There are some new systems on the market that recover 99.99 percent of the solvent in the first pass before performing an additional evaporation. **The use of butane, hexane, isopropyl alcohol, or naptha extraction is an industrial process that should NOT be done by the home user, without proper equipment and training, because of the risk of explosion and residual solvent left in the medicine.** See the "Dabbing" section for more information about butane. Unless you have the proper equipment and really know what you are doing, the safer alternative solvents for making cannabis oil at home are ethanol, and olive or coconut oil extraction. If you are purchasing oil from a commercial producer, it is wise to ask for lab results to ensure purity regardless of the method used to make the oil. Over the coming years, what is available in the marketplace will change significantly. It is my hope that, for the medical user, standardized and tested cannabis oil become readily available and affordable. Currently cannabis oil can be found on the black market and the legal market from as low as $30 per gram to over $100 per gram.

Is Hemp Oil the Same as Concentrated Cannabis Oil?

Some people call cannabis oil "hemp oil," "cannabis hemp oil," or "high CBD hemp oil," which has led to much confusion in the market place. Just to be clear, I want to stress that concentrated cannabis oil is very different from **hemp oil, or hemp seed oil,** a legal, food-grade product made from pressing oil from hemp seeds grown specifically for this purpose and containing negligible THC. Please see the "Hemp" section earlier in the book for more clarification. While hemp oil is a highly nutritious product that does indeed support a healthy endocannabinoid system, concentrated cannabis oil supports the ECS in a different way. In case you missed this in the "Cannabis Science" section, I want to reiterate that CBD rich hemp oil products are hitting the market with their trumpeters misinforming people that they are legal. It is important you know what you are getting. These products are made from hemp and may contain CBD, but they may also contain other things not conducive to healing such as heavy metals, pesticides, and mold. Like other products, some are better quality than others. Please be aware that, according to the Federal government, all products containing CBD are classified as a Schedule I drug (regardless of source) and are completely illegal. (Kubasak 2013) If you are skipping around in the book, please read the cannabidiol information in the "Cannabis Science" section for clarification about CBD-oil.

Medical cannabis plants and hemp plants are genetically similar. However, hemp plants are poor producers of cannabinoids and therefore generally have low levels of cannabinoids, especially THC. Keep in mind that cannabinoids reside predominantly in the trichomes, which are the small glands on the exterior of the cannabis flower and leaf, not within the seed or stalk. While medical cannabis plants are bred to increase trichome density and flower size, hemp plants are grown primarily for fiber, food, and seed oil, so they tend to be taller with smaller flowers. While each product has merits, whole plant concentrated cannabis oil, hemp seed oil, and high CBD industrial hemp oil are completely different products with different purposes.

How Is Concentrated Cannabis Oil Made?

The gold standard for extracting cannabinoids is super critical CO_2 extraction. Equipment for this is expensive and not likely to become commonplace for home use in the immediate future. Rather, it is used by companies making bulk quantities of cannabis oil. This is the method used by GW Pharmaceuticals to make their prescription drug Sativex®, which is a whole plant cannabis extract.

The most popular solvents used for home extraction are naptha (a carcinogen that is not a single entity—it means different things in different places—and should be avoided) or ethanol (food-grade alcohol). Arno Hazekamp, PhD of Leiden University in the Netherlands and Luigi L. Romano, PhD of the University of Siena, Italy have done an interesting study evaluating different home extraction methods for making concentrated cannabis flower oil comparing naptha; petroleum ether (ether is VERY dangerous as it can anesthetize the user, set him ablaze, or explode); ethanol; and olive oil extractions. Butane is another popular solvent sometimes used in making cannabis flower oil. Although it was not included in this study, for the sake of this conversation we consider it similar to naptha.

Researchers discovered that olive oil extraction is the safest, best choice for homemade concentrated oil. Medicine extracted with olive oil retains a higher percentage of cannabinoids and terpenoids and is affordable, widely available, totally non-toxic, and without fire danger during preparation unlike naptha, ethanol, ether, and other solvents, which are all flammable. It should be noted that the naptha used in the study was a heavy naptha not a pure, light naptha as suggested by Rick Simpson who has popularized concentrated cannabis oil. The only minor downside to olive oil extraction is that the resulting medicine is not quite as potent, and thus patients may have to take a little more to reach their desired effect. (Romano and Hazekamp 2013)

Proponents of using naptha, petroleum ether, and alcohol claim these solvents are burned off at the end. However, Drs. Romano and Hazekamp ran chemical analyses of the end products of these types of extractions and found residual solvent did remain in medicines produced using all three methods. Their results have been corroborated by The Werc Shop in California. They test many cannabis oil samples on a daily basis and regularly find residual solvents in oils extracted using these methods. It just doesn't make sense to use a carcinogenic product to make a healthy medicine (although I know this happens all the time with prepared foods, pharmaceuticals, and some supplements). While, for some people, the alcohol extraction method may work well, it is important to note that not all the alcohol will be evaporated, which is an important consideration for an alcoholic.

There are different processes for making cannabis oil. Although making cannabis oil with olive oil appears to be the safest and best method for making it at home, the ethanol method remains popular and is efficient. To see a video on how to make small batch cannabis oil with ethanol, search YouTube for "Cannabis Oil Recipe by Doctor Diane."

Cannabis Oil: Olive Oil Base

This recipe is adapted from the previous referenced paper by Hazekamp and Romano.

¼ lb. (4 oz.) ground dried cannabis flower
5 cups purified water for processing
2 cups purified water for rinsing
2 cups organic olive oil

Place the dried ground cannabis flower, water, and olive oil into a double boiler or a water bath and heat to 208°F for one hour. Using the water bath or the double boiler (with water in the bottom of the first boiler) prevents the mixture from getting so hot that the terpenes and cannabinoids evaporate. I disagree with the one hour and encourage you to move your mixture to a crock pot that has a low setting and cook 10 to 12 hours if your variety has no CBD and 20 to 24 hours if it does have CBD. Use a candy thermometer to monitor the temperature of the oil and water mixture.

Use a large French coffee press to separate the plant material from the mixture. Lift the press and pour 2 cups of boiling purified water over the material and press again pouring the extra water back into the mixture.

If you find you have residual material in your oil and water mixture, use a quart canning jar with a cheesecloth to remove the remaining debris.

Remove the lid from the quart jar. Cover the jar with a piece of cheesecloth that is at least a 4" x 4" swath. Place it over the mouth of the jar. Screw the ring over the cheesecloth with enough room for there to be some sag in the cheesecloth to facilitate filtering. Pour the mixture over the cloth slowly giving it ample time to filter. A piece of t-shirt cloth works as well.

Pour your finished product into a glass container (a casserole dish or serving bowl is ideal). Cover it with a lid or plastic wrap. Let it sit overnight in the refrigerator. The oil will harden on top and separate from the water. Remove from the refrigerator. Poke two small holes (the size of a chopstick) in the top, ½ inch apart, and near the side of the container. Drain the water from the oil. The oil is ready to use and store.

How to Use Cannabis Oil

This information is for educational purposes and should NOT be considered medical advice.

Cannabis oil is so powerful that it requires taking what is called a titration dose if taken orally. Patients who are taking the medication orally start with an extremely small dose—something less than the size of a poppy seed. This will be 1/25th (.04) of a gram. Any more than this on the first day will be extremely uncomfortable. From then on, the patient takes thirty to forty-five days to work up to a gram a day depending on their ability to develop tolerance to the medicine.

Mara Gordon at Aunt Zelda's (*http://azcannaoil.com*), one of the leading voices and most successful people in treating cancer with cannabis, shares that, for the vast majority of people treating cancer with cannabis oil, she thinks a gram dose is too much. She also asked me to share with you that the THC:CBD ratio is an important factor in treating disease with cannabis oil. In recent history, CBD has been overlooked and under considered by many in the treatment of cancer. Constance Finley, Mara Gordon, and Valerie Corral, pioneers in helping patients manage or cure their disease with cannabis medicine, say they are having increasing success with patients who are taking CBD with a high dose of THC for the treatment of cancer. Gordon and Corral have their patients take CBD separate from THC. Gordon explains, "In most cases we have patients use the THC two hours before the CBD. The reason we separate the THC and CBD is because THC is a CB_1 and CB_2 agonist, and CBD is an antagonist. They work synergistically, but we don't want them 'stepping on each other'. We believe that this allows us to keep the dose much lower." Certain cancers require higher CBD because of the ID-1 gene, and in those cases, the THC dose is able to be reduced." *ID-1* is an inhibitor of basic helix-loop-helix transcription factors, which has been shown to be a key regulator of the metastatic potential of breast and additional cancers. (Desprez, et al. 2007).

Gordon takes a clinical individual approach to working with her patients. She matches the cannabinoid and terpene profile with the needs of the patient's ailment. After thirty days she evaluates how the oil, extraction, or topical is working and adjust the cannabinoid/terpene profile as necessary. In keeping with her scientific approach, she has founded Zelda Therapeutics (*www.zeldatherapeutics.com*) to support the work of a leading cancer research laboratory at Cumplutense University in Spain and to conduct pre-clinical trials in several different disease states.

Cannabis Ratios – What Comes First?

When talking about cannabis ratios, put THC first. A 2:1 cannabis oil or tincture would have twice as much THC as CBD. It is important to make sure when looking at ratios, it is clear which cannabinoid is listed in which order.

Although the science does show components of cannabis can kill cancer cells, there is no double-blind study yet to prove cannabis oil, specifically, can change disease progression in humans, yet the anecdotal evidence is strong. **People who have successfully treated their own disease, or helped many others do so, agree it takes 1 gram a day of a high THC cannabis oil taken for two months to kill cancer.** Just to be clear, it is commonly said that killing cancer is a ninety day protocol. The first thirty days are usually dedicated to building tolerance so the patient can take a gram a day for the next sixty days. Many believe it is smart to continue taking some sort of maintenance dose after the initial round is completed. Constance Finley, CEO and founder of Constance Therapeutics, a leader in the cannabis oil industry, shares that her cancer patients are having success with a three gram per month dose divided across thirty days. She considers the maintenance dose to be a critical part of their aftercare and encourages all cancer patients to do a maintenance dose.

Cancer and seizure disorders are not the only conditions holding great promise for treatment with cannabis oil. Lyme disease and tuberculosis are two exciting areas for potential success along with arthritis, ALS, HIV-AIDS, and a variety of other hard-to-treat diseases including ankylosing spondolytis, which is what brought Finley to the cannabis space. After being virtually housebound for over ten years, Finely found that cannabis oil, while it didn't cure her disease, it made a dramatic positive impact on her health. Now she works ten to fourteen hours a day raising awareness about the healing potential of cannabis, building a science based cannabis oil company and facilitating cannabis research.

The Rise of Concentrated Cannabis Oil – The Rick Simpson Story

Canadian Rick Simpson (who calls cannabis oil "hemp oil" or "cannabis hemp oil") has led the way in raising awareness about cannabis oil as a curative medicine. After stumbling across research about the cancer killing properties of cannabis, he decided to experiment with the oil himself to treat skin cancer lesions on his face. He created highly concentrated cannabis oil (95 to 98 percent THC) that he reports worked! After his success, he started sharing the oil with friends, and friends of friends, who were suffering from a variety of different ailments. Word got out about the successes many people were having using the medicine to treat cancer and other serious and chronic health problems. Simpson was in the spotlight. Excited about the potential to help many people, Simpson hoped his oil would be embraced by federal health officials as an alternative to more toxic mainstream pharmaceuticals and cancer treatments. However, instead of wanting to know more about what he had learned, the Canadian government, according to Simpson, went on the offensive. After receiving public attention for helping people overcome different diseases with cannabis oil, it wasn't long before the Royal Canadian Mounted Police raided his farm. His farm has been raided four times confiscating large numbers of highly medicinal plants and clones. He was fined $2,000 and prohibited from owning a gun for ten years.

While traveling in Europe, Simpson received word he was being raided again, but this time charges would be filed, and he would be put in jail. Fearing being incarcerated and therefore separated from his medicine, he opted not to return. He continues to work from Europe to raise awareness for the oil and to educate people on how to make their own. He has made two movies about concentrated cannabis oil titled *Run from the Cure* and *Run 2 the Cure*. Simpson deserves tremendous credit for raising awareness about cannabis oil. However, I caution you from using naptha as your solvent, as it is a very dangerous. In fairness to Mr. Simpson, he is adamant that one use only **pure, light naptha.**

Is Concentrated Cannabis Oil Right for Me?

Anecdotal evidence suggests concentrated cannabis oil holds great therapeutic promise for treating and managing certain conditions such as various forms of cancer and seizure related disorders such as epilepsy, Alzheimer's disease, arthritis, diabetes, Parkinson's disease, and many more. **I want to reiterate that to date there have been no clinical studies on the effects of <u>concentrated</u> cannabis oil.**

To many, cannabis oil is seen as a miracle cure or a Godsend helping repair the body from illness. While I believe cannabis oil holds great promise and should be legal, I must stress that **concentrated cannabis oil is not a cure-all**. There are many factors at play that contribute to the effectiveness of cannabis oil including: the strength and quality of the oil being used, the mental and physical state of the person being treated, their willingness to put their wellness first by making beneficial lifestyle changes, the pathology and progression of the disease itself, finding the appropriate mix of cannabinoids for the individual and disease being treated, and the patient's desire to live.

Constance Therapeutics

Constance Therapeutics (CT) is one of the companies leading the way in individualized cannabis treatments for cancer. California cancer patients can have their oncologist send CT a sample of their tumor. CT will then split the tumor tissue into several Petri dishes and test different cannabis varieties against the tumor to see which is best for that particular patient. Because of our federal prohibition on cannabis, only California residents can benefit. Nonetheless, it is an exciting glimpse at what is to come in cannabis medicine! See *www.cbdfarm.org* for more information.

Since the science is lacking in the area of cannabis oil, there is considerable debate in the medical community around whether such oils should be used as a stand-alone treatment or as part of an integrative plan. Furthermore, little is known about optimal dosages for various diseases. Chat with your doctor about treatment options, and don't be afraid to go for repeat visits to get additional answers. If your doctor isn't providing the support and information you need, find another. Do your homework online, and explore what others in your situation have found helpful. There are some incredibly powerful testimonials out there.

In the end, I encourage you to listen to your instincts, and tap into your "intuition," "gut feel," or "inner-knowing." Some of you feel more comfortable with this than others. No matter what, you need to be part of deciding how to move forward with treatment. It is unlikely cannabis alone will cure whatever ails you (nutrition and lifestyle are important co-factors). This is especially true when treating a disease that has progressed to a late stage.

Consider using an integrative approach that addresses mind, body, and soul. I like the concept of functional medicine. This term means different things to different people. It is important to be clear about the approach you prefer so you can find the right professional and communicate your needs. Complimentary or integrative medicine is usually a combination of Eastern and Western medicine or a traditional treatment such as chemo and radiation combined with alternative treatments such as meditation, acupuncture, lymph massage, and counseling. Functional medicine is more about treating the cause and the whole body instead of just symptoms. A functional medicine approach may combine several different natural healing philosophies and regimens with a combination of Western and alternative medicine.

Everyone's ideal treatment program will differ based on belief system, body, ailment, and the relationship with one's doctor. You may find mainstream treatment plus cannabis and changes in diet are the right mix. Others may decide cannabis oil combined with acupuncture, herbs, and dietary cleansing is the right combination.

Regardless of how you proceed, consider cannabis oil a piece of your healing puzzle rather than the silver bullet. Remember: Whatever is ailing you didn't happen overnight. Give your mind, body, gut, and soul the time and support they need to integrate and heal.

After reading so many testimonials from people who claim to have "cured" their diseases using cannabis oil and other natural medicines (in the medical community, cancer is not considered cured until absent for five years and there are not too many of those folks around yet because of the relative newness of cannabis oil) I cannot help but wonder why more clinical research is not being done in this area.

Constance Finley, has been working with a respected oncologist who, in 2012, sent her twenty-eight stage four patients who, were battling their second cancer occurrence. (Finley 2016) According to that oncologist, twenty-six of the twenty-eight went into remission after using CT cannabis oil for three months. In 2015, he verified that 76 percent (twenty-one) of the original twenty-eight patients who took the Constance Therapeutics cannabis oil were still alive. (Finley 2016) In the spring of 2015, the referring oncologist shared these results at an Integrative Oncology conference in Reno and introduced Finley to the group. She continues to work with several hundred stage four cancer patients each year with impressive success. (Finley 2016)

People I know who are using cannabis oil to help patients heal and beat their diseases have all said they observe a higher success rate with cannabis oil for patients who have not used chemo or radiation, and the sooner in the treatment process the patient starts using cannabis oil the higher likelihood they have of success. **Please note that an observation, like the one just stated, does not equate to scientific fact.** It would be reckless not to encourage you to consider all treatment options. And it would be reckless not to encourage you to consider cannabis oil if you have already tried conventional treatment. The more you know, the better you can make choices for yourself.

It is important to take a long, hard look at treatment success rates with traditional cancer therapy. There are huge differences that may impact the treatment options you choose. For example, the conventional treatment success rate with *leukemia* (cancer of the blood) is significantly higher than that of *glioblastoma* (an aggressive and hard-to-treat form of brain cancer). According to MD Anderson Cancer Center, there are twelve to fourteen thousand new cases of glioblastoma multiforme diagnosed in the U.S. annually. Less than 10 percent are alive within five years. Treatment for this disease is generally focused on slowing disease progression and keeping individuals comfortable. To say the least, treatment success rates for this cancer are dismal, and the treatments available can greatly interfere with quality of life. On the other hand, MD Anderson says on their website that there are over 43,000 new cases of leukemia diagnosed annually in the U.S. Advances in treatment have been so significant that the five year survival rate is over 60 percent and even higher for certain types of leukemia. If I were diagnosed with any form of cancer, knowing this kind of information would be a critical component of how I would decide to approach my treatment.

As a final note on this subject, I cannot help wondering if a tiny amount of cannabis oil taken daily, or several times a week, would help give the body an immune boost and serve as a good preventative for all sorts of diseases. I look forward to seeing this question explored in future studies.

Tinctures and Extractions

Sublingual applications, tinctures, cannabis extractions, and oral mucosal sprays are becoming increasingly popular. They are smoke free, discreet, easy to carry and use, and can be made or purchased to contain specific cannabinoid, and sometimes terpene, profiles. They work great for children, adults, and the elderly alike by simplifying intake and dosing while maximizing results. GW Pharmaceuticals has proved the medical efficacy of this delivery method with their sublingual prescription product Sativex®.

Tinctures are made with distilled alcohol and technically called *ethanolic tinctures* (ET). *Glycerol extractions* (GE) are also becoming popular and are incorrectly, but commonly, called tinctures as well. The difference is that GEs are made with glycerin in a heat process whereas ETs are made with ethanol in a, room-temperature process. Super critical CO_2 extractions, such as Sativex®, are believed to be the strongest and cleanest cannabis tinctures available.

Alcohol has been used for hundreds of years to make herbal liquid preparations. (Bone 2003) Ethanolic tinctures are efficient at extracting cannabinoids and have the added benefit of killing many, if not most, biological contaminants that could be present in the plant material. (Raber 2015) Additionally, tinctures reflect the true chemical spectrum of the plant provided the alcohol has not been evaporated. (Bone 2003) ETs can be taken in two ways. The most common is *sublingually*, which means you spray or drop the tincture under the tongue or between the cheek and gum to allow it to absorb directly into the bloodstream. Delivery is both relatively fast acting and long lasting because the therapeutic compounds are absorbed immediately. Putting the tincture in a small amount of honey, water, olive oil, or MCT oil and then placing it under the tongue or on the gums is recommended to make it more palatable and to dilute the alcohol to prevent burning. (E. B. Russo 2015) Adding the tincture to warm water and swallowing it is another option. However, be careful not to add too much liquid to the tincture. Internationally renowned herbalist Kerry Bone suggests you not exceed a 2:1 ratio, meaning two drops of water, oil, or honey to one drop of cannabis tincture. (Bone 2003) If you swallow the tincture, it will take thirty to ninety minutes to take effect.

One of the great cannabis extraction myths is that you have to put the tincture in the freezer. Another is that they take a long time to make. Neither is true. You certainly can put the ET in the freezer, but it is unnecessary. The tincture will be ready less than twenty-four hours after mixing. (Raber 2015) When it sits for longer periods, chlorophyll will be extracted adding nothing but a bad taste and a dark green color. (Raber 2015)

Over the last several years, glycerin-based extractions have become popular. While they certainly taste better, they are less efficient at extracting cannabinoids. Ethanolic tinctures can be anywhere from two to ten times more efficient than a glycerin extraction. (Raber 2015) Another challenge with glycerin extractions is that cannabinoids tend to clump in the solution making it difficult to dose consistently for a homemade extraction. (Raber 2015) A laboratory homogenizer is required to ensure the cannabinoids stay evenly dispersed in the extraction. (Backes 2014) Even so, this may only last a short time, as the emulsions are often unstable. This equipment is likely to be cost prohibitive for the home extraction maker. With all that said, there are still those who argue that they prefer a glycerin extraction. Even though the GE may have lower cannabinoid content than the ET, it can still be therapeutic. As discussed throughout the book, sometimes the lowest dose is the most effective.

Ethanolic Extraction Recipe

Use food grade alcohol such as Everclear, 151 Rum, or organic alcohol from some-one such as *www.organicalcohol.com*. If you cannot get that, use the highest proof food grade alcohol you can get, preferably over 70 percent. Standard distilled spirits are around 40 percent ethanol. Be sure to buy alcohol that does not have a flavoring or sugar added. The higher the proof, the more efficiently the cannabinoids will be extracted. DO NOT USE RUBBING (Isopropyl) ALCOHOL.

½ to 1 ounce of dried cannabis flower
1 pint of alcohol

1. **Choose Potency:** Decide if you want to use ½ to 1 ounce cannabis flower. The more you use, the more potent the tincture will be. One ounce of bud to 1 pint of liquid is the general rule.

2. **Grind Herb:** Grind or chop the bud into small pieces. Use a clean coffee or spice grinder, blender, or food processor. You also can chop the bud with a knife, or rub the herb between your fingers to break it up into very small pieces.

3. **Decarboxylation:** Place your ground herb on an oven safe glass or Pyrex dish and bake at 220-240°F for 20 minutes. Remove from the oven and let cool.

4. **Herb Mixing:** Place the decarboxylated herb into a glass container. Quart canning jars work great! If you are looking for a tincture that delivers cannabinoid acids, there is no need to decarboxylate the cannabis. Although I have not heard of anyone doing this, it would make sense to decarboxylate ½ or ¾ of the herb, and put the rest into the mix undecarboxylated (or vice versa depending on what you are trying to achieve) to get the benefit of the cannabinoid acids.

5. **Mix Alcohol:** Add alcohol, shake, and seal.

6. **Extraction:** Let the mixture sit for 24 hours in dark or low light place shaking periodically.

7. **Strain:** Use a micron bag or cheesecloth. Be sure to squeeze the alcohol out of the herb.

8. **Storage:** Transfer your tincture to a dark (brown or blue) glass tincture bottle with a glass dropper. Seal tightly.

NOTE: Recovering alcoholics who choose to use an extraction should use GE or another extraction, such as olive oil or MCT oil, based in something other than alcohol. If you choose an ET, please check with your doctor to make sure the amount of alcohol in the ET will not interact with other medications you take.

[See "Vegetable Glycerin Tincture Recipe", on page 258.]

Dosing with Tinctures

A certain number of drops are commonly recommended for all liquid cannabis preparations. While I don't think "a drop" is necessarily a consistent way to dose, it is one of the easiest ways to take cannabis based preparations. Be aware that the viscosity of the preparation, and the size of the dropper mouth, will yield different sized drops delivering varying amounts of the active ingredient. If you are taking a large amount of tincture, you may find using measuring spoons allows you to dose more consistently.

Albeit repetitive, the definitive answer on how to dose with tinctures and all things cannabis is that it depends on you. You may find that you do better with more CBD and less THC, or vice versa, or with a 1:1 ratio. Many people realize big benefits from fairly small amounts of THC. Others must have larger amounts of THC to get the results they want. For example, CBD is generally effective at helping people with anxiety. As you know, one of the potential side effects of THC is increased anxiety. It seems counterintuitive to think THC might be helpful in addressing anxiety, but the truth is that, for some people, THC is not only required to address anxiety, but they need fairly high doses to boot.

You may find that a little more THC at night will help you sleep. There is no one-size-fits-all. Take a look at studies done on Sativex®. You will see a fairly wide range of dosing used by the trial subjects. Although a small number of participants found relief using a 1:1 ratio oral mucosal spray (one spritz three times a day), the average daily use was 7.7 sprays per day, which equaled19.79 mg of THC and 18.32 mg of CBD. (Notcutt, et al. 2012) Research on Sativex® shows that doses above twelve sprays a day are rarely more effective and definitively increase side effects. (E. B. Russo 2015)

If you can find a Constance Finley, Mara Gordon, Valerie Corral, Dr. Dustin Sulak, or Dr. Michelle Sexton in your area, this will go a long way in helping to discover the most appropriate therapeutic dose for you. As with all things cannabis, start with a small amount. Give it fifteen minutes to take effect before trying more. It may take a little more time and practice to establish your therapeutic doses with tinctures.

It is worth repeating that some cannabis medicine pioneers are finding success using THC and CBD separately. You may find that taking CBD first, two hours before the THC, has a beneficial effect on healing or managing disease and/or managing unwanted side-effects of THC. As mentioned earlier, there are also reasons to take THC first and CBD two hours later.

Visit with your doctor about starting with one to three drops. Wait fifteen minutes before the next one. It may take a week or so to establish your therapeutic dose. Before taking the tincture, swallow to remove saliva from your mouth so the medicine is not diluted before it is absorbed.

Tea

We know cannabis has been used to make tea around the world for thousands of years. This preparation method is particularly common in Jamaica. In fact, Jamaica's young and old alike consume cannabis tea regularly, and it is considered part of a healthy diet. (Hazekamp, et al. 2007) Arno Hazekamp reported, in an article in *Journal of Ethnopharmacology*, that to Jamaicans, "The tea is attributed various therapeutic and *prophylactic* (preventative) qualities and is used as a remedy for fever, cold, and stress."

Why it works as a tonic is not completely clear. The fact that small amounts of cannabinoid acids (which are usually converted to cannabinoids in other intake methods) and cannabinoids are present in the tea does contribute to the tonic effect. However, the amount of cannabinoids and their acids are so low in tea that there must be more to the story for us to yet discover. Cannabinoid acids are not well researched at this time; however, a recent study published in *Trends in Pharmacological Sciences* did report that THCA, the precursor to THC, provides anti-proliferative/pro-apoptotic (causing cell death) effects in human breast, colorectal, prostate, and gastric cancers as well as in numerous cancers in animals. (Izzo, Borrelli, et al. 2009) Another study finds that THCA has strong immune system-modulating and anti-inflammatory effects. (Verhoeckx, et al. 2006) These findings help us understand, in part, why many people use cannabis tea and claim benefits.

Dr. Hazekamp and his team conducted a study on cannabinoid contents in cannabis tea. (Hazekamp, et al. 2007) Tea used in the research was made from a cannabis sample with a combined content of approximately 17 percent THC and THCA. One cup (200 ml) of this tea yielded 2.0 mg of THC and 8.6 mg of THCA. This combination of cannabinoids and cannabinoid acids creates mild effects lasting for several hours, a very different experience from other cannabis ingestion methods.

Cannabis Tea Recipe

Cannabis tea is fairly easy to make. The Dutch Office of Medical Cannabis in The Netherlands encourages medical cannabis users to make tea as follows:

> Add 1.0 g of cannabis to 1.0 L of boiling water, and let simmer for 15 min. Filter out solid parts by using a common

tea-sieve. Tea can be consumed immediately or stored in a closed bottle in a refrigerator for up to 5 days. (Hazekamp, et al. 2007)

Start with one cup of this tea per day. Dr. Hazekamp suggests it is helpful to add coffee creamer (I prefer organic half and half or full fat canned coconut milk) to the tea for stability when storing it. Doing this may also increase the solubility of cannabinoids thus helping you consume more therapeutic compounds in your tea where otherwise they would stick to the side of the cup. (Hazekamp, et al. 2007)

Cannabis Gel Caps

If inhalation, oils, tinctures, and teas don't tickle your fancy, maybe cannabis gel caps will. Preparation of gel caps requires that the ground plant material, or kif, which is predominantly made up of glandular trichome powder, be decarboxylated in advance of packing the gel caps. That is if it is cannabinoids you are seeking. If you are looking for the therapeutic benefit of cannabinoid acids, do not decarboxylate the plant material or kif/resin powder.

Kif is more available in some places than others. If you are growing your own cannabis, or can get access to someone else's trim (leaves that are pruned during the growing process or trimmed from the flower at harvest), you can collect your own kif. If not, you can ask your supplier for it. Some people may also refer to it as powdered hashish or resin powder.

To collect your own kif, you need:
- a bubble bag or bubble bowl (may be more convenient for small batches; search the Internet to purchase one)
- a large, clean mirror or a flat, clean surface
- 1 to 2 lbs of dry ice and dry ice gloves
- plant leaves
- stainless steel baking scraper or a quality straight edge

Place the dry ice and plant material in the bubble bag and shake it over the surface in an up and down motion until no more yellowish powder falls through the sieve. When the resin glands are exhausted and the plant material begins to break up, the powder becomes greener. Using a large mirror for this makes it much easier to see and collect the kif.

Next the kif/plant material will need to be decarboxylated. If you are using plant material for the gel caps, please grind the material first. To decarboxylate the ground herb or kif:

1. Place the material in an oven safe glass dish

2. Cook at 240°F for 30 minutes
3. Let cool
4. Fill the gel caps with the desired serving

There is a range of temperatures and times on the Internet and in books, but after visiting with cannabis chemist Dr. Jeff Raber, I'm going with his suggestion of 240°F. Once the material has been decarboxylated and cooled, you can begin to pack your gel caps with the desired serving. Be sure to consume the gel cap with a fat. Cannabinoids need a fat to bind to for them to have the maximum effect. A couple of ways to consume a healthy fat include: eat something with butter consume a teaspoon of coconut, flax, hemp, or olive oil, or take your fish oil supplement at the same time. Check the dosing section for additional information.

One of my cannabis angels, Richard (who showed up in my life towards the end of writing this book and has helped considerably in contributing to the book's content), used this method to control his M.S. It has worked very well for him for over five years. He has also supported people going through opiate withdrawal to use kif gel caps and dabbing successfully. Kif gel caps can also be used with children who need the medicine. If swallowing a pill is a problem, kif or plant powder can be added to coconut oil and eaten by the spoonful, or added to a smoothie or yogurt. If you do that, make sure you are not using a fat-free yogurt but a whole milk product instead.

A parent of a self-harming autistic pre-teen reported to me that small amounts (as little as 0.04 grams or ¼ or less of a gel cap) of high THC decarboxylated kif taken in a capsule with coconut oil reduced her child's self- harming and reduced some of the child's other disruptive behaviors. Parents of autistic children, and the doctors who treat them, are experiencing similar results, yet there is little research being conducted in this area.

If you choose to try this route, please remember that this method has the same activation and effect time as edibles, which is usually thirty to ninety minutes. Be sure to visit with your doctor about the appropriate serving for you, or start low and gradually titrate your doses to find your ideal dose range. I've seen one gel cap knock someone out for sixteen hours and make them groggy and stoned for another eight yet the same volume gel cap not phase someone with a high tolerance. It cannot be said enough to start with a very small amount until you understand how that batch of medicine works in your body or that of the person for whom you are a caregiver.

Suppositories

You can imagine the funny looks I get when I mention cannabis suppositories. All jokes aside, it is a viable delivery mechanism for the medicine and should be given serious consideration for many patients. Rectal suppositories and sublingual administration are the best forms of administration for maximum bioavailability.

(Pertwee 2004) There is little science to share on this topic. We have to rely on anecdotal reports from top cannabis physicians, patients, and expert oil makers.

With a suppository, the effects are felt within ten to fifteen minutes. I've read many reports where people had no psychoactivity and other reports where they had never been higher. The reason for the wide range of experiences is not clear. It could be that little psychoactivity is attributable to the fact that when inserted just past the sphincter the oil will be absorbed into the bloodstream in a way similar to smoking or vaporizing and thus going first to the brain and taking the long way around the liver. Others believe the intense psychoactivity experienced by some is due to the suppository being inserted too far into the rectum where it is absorbed into the Superior (upper) hemorrhoidal vein, which goes immediately to the liver and therefore increases the psychoactivity of the experience. (Cannabis Digest 2014)

After lots of reading and conversations with oil makers, dispensary owners, and physicians Sunil Aggarwal, Jeffrey Hergenrather, and Ethan Russo, I've devised the hypothesis that the level of psychoactivity one experiences is likely due to their own rate of liver metabolism and, in part, their tolerance to cannabis. It just is not clear.

Oil maker Sean Beeman at Genesis Pharms (*http://www.genesispharms.com*) in Eugene, Oregon sees patients fighting cancer use suppositories with concentrated cannabis oil as a way to shorten the time it takes to get to a gram-a-day dose of THC. He says his customers can adjust to this dose within a few days if not immediately. Suppositories can be a useful delivery method for the very frail who require a high dose of cannabinoids, those suffering with nausea and vomiting, or someone who has difficulty swallowing.

The bioavailability of rectal administration is approximately double that of oral ingestion due to the higher absorption rate and the fact that it is generally not having to be processed in the liver first. (Huestes 2007) Thus, one can use lower doses than with the other intake methods to get the same therapeutic effect.

Dr. Ethan Russo, in his paper, "Cannabis Treatments in Obstetrics and Gynecology: A Historical Review," writes that the use of cannabis for women's issues probably dates back to Ancient Mesopotamia in the seventh century. Evidence of suppository use for anal and vaginal applications was noted in the Egyptian pharmacopoeia since pharaonic times. (E. Russo 2002) Unfortunately, it seems much of that knowledge has been lost. Nonetheless, we can still look at history to learn ways to broaden our use of cannabis."

There is almost no recent literature on the vaginal use of cannabis. However, I am aware of people using vaginal suppositories containing cannabinoids to treat HPV, herpes, yeast infections, and female reproductive related cancers. It makes sense that someone with a reproductive related cancer, virus, or infection could get relief from vaginal suppositories. With that said, I am unaware of any clinical evidence to address these issues.

Rhea Graham, owner of Albany's Canna Kitchen & Research LLC, (*www.cannakitchenandresearch.com*) makes custom suppositories for her customers. She prefers to break up the gram-a-day dose into three to five suppositories per day to minimize potential psychoactivity and ensure high levels of cannabinoids are constantly circulating in the body. Graham, shared with me the stories of two of her patients who have had success with suppositories. One is a twenty-seven year old male with prostate problems who was making six or seven trips a night to the bathroom. He reported sleeping six consecutive hours the first night of using cannabis suppositories, and within three weeks his problem was resolved. The other patient had prostate cancer. The suppositories didn't make him stoned but addressed his pain and made it possible for him to take care of his family more comfortably thus significantly improving his life. She reports her customers are also having success using suppositories for erectile dysfunction.

To make your own suppositories, you will need the following:

- A base – use coconut oil, cocoa butter, or a combination
- 2.25 ml suppository molds (buy online)
- Cannabis or cannabis oil
- An easy dose spoon dropper or a pipette (available at your pharmacy) to fill each mold
- Freezer bags for storing the suppositories

Establish how many suppositories you will make and how much of your base is needed.

- If you are dividing the gram per day dose of cannabis oil into three suppositories, assume 1.9 grams of coconut oil to .33 gram of cannabis oil.
- If you are making one suppository using the 2.25 ml mold, use 1.25 grams of coconut oil to 1 gram of cannabis oil.

While it is true coco butter will hold its form better than coconut oil, I believe coconut oil is a better choice for absorbability. If you choose coconut oil as your base, you will need to keep the suppositories frozen or refrigerated until time of use and insert quickly.

Directions
The following directions are for a thirty-day supply of three suppositories per day for a total of ninety suppositories:

1. Warm 172.5 grams of coconut oil or the base in a well cleaned double boiler, crockpot, or a Pyrex 2 to 4 cup measuring cup in a water bath over a low setting until it becomes liquid. Do not boil.
2. Remove from heat.
3. Add 30 grams of high concentration cannabis oil and mix until the cannabis oil is completely blended into the coconut oil.

4. Use your spoon, dropper, or pipette to fill the molds. Everyone will have to find their own way to fill the molds. Experiment with securing the molds in an upright position having someone hold them while you fill them, or hold them yourself. Regardless of your preferred method, you need quality light so you can see the fill line in the mold. It is easier to fill a sleeve of 9 to 12 molds at a time.

5. Once your sleeve of molds has been filled, place them upright in the freezer.

6. When they are frozen solid, place your 30-day supply in a tightly sealed freezer bag or a well-sealed container. You can leave them in the freezer or the refrigerator until time of use.

7. If travel is required, you want to seal the top of the mold to prevent contamination and loss if the suppositories return to room temperature. Suppository sealers are available, but they are expensive. If you need to seal the mold, wait until they are frozen solid then place the open mouth end of the sleeve of molds into the crease of a folded piece of parchment paper. Hold the molds in place. Gently run your iron, set for medium heat, over the open end of the suppository mold that sits in the crease of the parchment paper. Be careful not to touch any other part of the mold with the iron. Return the molds to the freezer or refrigerator.

When you are ready to use it, warm the individual suppository (in its mold) slightly in your hand. Then make a cut at the top, if sealed, and remove the outer barrier. Be careful not to get the suppository warm to the point that it is not firm enough to insert.

Use Gel Capsules to Make Smaller Suppositories

Albany's Canna Kitchen & Research LLC, uses 000 gel capsules (available on-line) and a gel cap machine (also on-line for under $20) to make suppositories. They use Virgin Organic Cocoa Butter as the base. When the capsule is filled with cannabis oil and base it weighs 1.3 grams. You can use the same basic method mentioned above. Decide on the amount of cannabis oil you want in each suppository and adjust the base accordingly. Gel capsules do not melt in the rectum. Be sure to take the gel capsule off of the suppository before inserting.

If you need a visual for how to properly insert a suppository, a quick search of the Internet will provide some detailed instruction. It is easiest to roll over on your side or roll the one you are caring for on their side. Lift the top knee towards the chest making access to the sphincter easier. You may choose to apply a small amount of lubricant to the surface for easier penetration. Once the suppository has passed the sphincter, clinching the buttocks will help hold the medicine in place.

It is important to ensure your hands are clean and your nails are trimmed and smooth before inserting. My final word of caution is to point out that in some cases the contents of the suppository may not absorb fully. A well-placed sanitary napkin may be in order. Always wash your hands, before and after, with soap and water.

Dosing and Titration Best Practices

Why is cannabis a medicine? Because it works! Precise dosing protocols alone do not make a medicine.

Many of us automatically approach any kind of medicine as prescription medicine and want to know how many milligrams we should take and how many times a day.

Old school cannabis users will tell you that for inducing sleep, controlling nausea, reducing pain, and reducing anxiety, a simple dosing regimen can start with a single drag of inhaled cannabis followed by waiting five to ten minutes. If you feel you need more relief, take another drag. This method has provided millions of people great relief for centuries and is a perfectly acceptable way of medicating. While this dosing method is valuable, a more focused protocol can support more efficient use of the medicine and better therapeutic results. Focused, regular dosing has been reported as especially effective in managing diseases such as M.S., Parkinson's, epilepsy, fibromyalgia, Tourette syndrome, and in changing disease progression as in Alzheimer's, diabetes, and cancer.

The historically popular "drag and wait" method is considered *casual dosing* by some physicians. Since no two drags are the same, it is argued by some that a "hit" is not a real dose. To better treat their patients, many doctors have been developing more *formal dosing* protocols that are based on milligrams of cannabinoids (generally THC and CBD) in a tincture, patch, oil, or other cannabis-based product. In this chapter are basic guidelines and best practices for both casual and formal dosing. This is written for those who want to use dried cannabis for inhalation, are going to make their own oil, edible, tincture, topical, or suppository; or plan to buy something available at their local dispensary. If you choose to go the route of one of the prescription THC drugs, simply follow directions and keep your doctor informed of your progress and any complications.

DISCLAIMER: The words "dosing," "dose," and "serving" are used throughout the book. These are NOT intended to be medical terms or medical advice. These words are used for informational purposes simply because of the lack of more suitable words. Please do not construe this information as medical advice. It is NOT.

The last forty-five years have brought about a much more comprehensive scientific understanding of how cannabis works in the body and the wide array of ways it can benefit health. Thanks to this expanding knowledge, we now know that:

- different cannabis preparations are better for different purposes.
- dosing protocols for changing disease progression are different from managing symptoms.
- there are big differences in how various cannabis chemical profiles work in the body.
- different intake methods work in different ways for different people.

Two important factors drive our quickly developing advancements in dosing protocols. The first is the availability of prescription synthetic cannabinoid drugs such as the THC-only drugs Marinol® and the not yet approved in the U.S. (but available in Europe) whole-plant cannabis extract drug Sativex®. Dosing protocols and documented patient results provide strong clinical data from which to base dosing guidelines. The second factor is the growing availability of cannabis chemical testing, which gives us access to cannabinoid and terpene profiles and makes it easier to treat people with consistent doses of specific ratios of cannabinoids and terpenes. As we learn more and more about specific doses for specific conditions, more doctors and medical professionals are starting to embrace cannabis as medicine.

Whole plant cannabis medicines have always posed a challenge to traditional dosing simply because it is difficult to grow standardized plants. The medicinal grower would have to: A) know which variable stimulates the expression of a certain cannabinoid/terpene/flavonoid, and B) control that expression and grow identical plants repeatedly. However, most medical cannabis is grown from asexually reproduced cuttings which are genetically identical, so variation results from different cultivation and processing techniques. This is the same with any plant-based medicine. Due to differences in growing conditions and genetics, there is always variability. Since cannabis is such a safe medicine, this variability is totally safe as well and may actually be beneficial by allowing patients the opportunity to select differently balanced medicines as they progress along their healing journey. In time, we will see more standardized products, such as Sativex®, that are created by extracting different cannabinoids and terpenes separately and then combining them to target specific ailments.

Those of you who live in medical cannabis states have access to medicines that list cannabinoid contents, and their ratios are easy to determine, which makes it possible for doctors to recommend, and patients to follow focused dosing protocols. Everyone else must make do with what is available—not letting perfect be the enemy of good. With a set of best practices and good judgment, anyone can use cannabis effectively whether they have access to cannabinoid ratios for focused dosing or they dose casually and trust their bodies to know the ideal. Remember that titration by casual dosing is much quicker and easier when cannabis is inhaled rather than ingested.

Finding the Ideal Therapeutic Dose Range

Before we jump off the cannabis dosing high dive, let's keep in mind that a dose of two aspirin, a tablespoon of cough medicine, or any prescription drug dose is a guideline to benefit the widest range of people at the lowest, safest dose. How many times have you followed specific dosing directions, but the medicine didn't work, or you found the side effects outweighed the benefit? You may have found taking a medicine with food was better for you even though the directions said to take it on an empty stomach, or perhaps the medicine didn't work as advertised by your doctor. The point is that ALL medicines have a therapeutic dose range, which varies from person to person and even from day to day.

When I asked cannabis activist and researcher Lester Grinspoon, MD about the concept of proper dosing, he shared that he thinks that as research evolves and develops clinical dosing standards will be created. He said it is important, for now, to get people comfortable with the idea of using cannabis and helping them understand its safety and versatility. One of the things he advocates is for people to share their stories of how they have successfully used cannabis. There is so much we can learn from the experiences of those who have traveled the road ahead of us. You can read many patient accounts on his website at *rxcannabis.com* or read additional stories in his popular book *Marihuana: The Forbidden Medicine* co-authored with James B. Bakalar.

Because each of us is biologically unique, we react differently to different medicines, foods, herbs, industrial chemicals, bacteria, molds, viruses, etc. Doesn't it make perfect sense that some people are going to need more or less of a medicine than the tested average and that individuals will react differently based on their unique chemistry? What works for me may not work for you. Part of the beauty of cannabis is that its excellent safety profile makes it possible for patients to safely experiment with all the different intake methods, quantities, and chemical profiles to find what is right for them. This kind of experimentation would be dangerous with potentially toxic and lethal medicines such as many conventional pharmaceuticals.

While little clinical data is available to assist us in finding a baseline for dosing with cannabis medicine, the data available on dronabinol (Marinol®), a synthetic THC pharmaceutical, can provide us with a jumping off point for THC dosing. Dronabinol is available in 2.5 mg, 5 mg, and 10 mg doses and is prescribed for adult and pediatric chemo-induced nausea and vomiting and for adult anorexia. The following is dosing information listed on the dronabinol website (copyright 2015):

Prescribed for:	Initial Dose	Subsequent Doses	Maximum daily dose
Adult & Pediatric Nausea/Vomiting, Chemo induced	5 mg 1-3 hours prior to chemo	5 mg every 2-4 hours after after chemo	4-6 doses
Anorexia prior to lunch and dinner	2.5 mg 1 hour before lunch	2.5 mg 1 hour before super	20 mg given in 4 doses

Please keep in mind that the difference between cannabis, prescription drugs, and over-the-counter-drugs is the VAST therapeutic range and low toxicity of cannabis. Additionally, most pharmaceuticals are made from a single chemical whereas cannabis therapeutics and cannabis have many chemical components working together to provide a broader therapeutic impact and, at the same time, addressing side effects that could be caused by a single agent within the preparation or herb. [See "Why is Cannabis So Safe?", on page 113.] **For this reason, patients who are using cannabis to manage or relieve symptoms can safely experiment to find the serving or use pattern best for them.** If you are lucky enough to find a cannabis-informed doctor, like the physicians quoted in this book, I encourage you to tap into their knowledge and expertise for guided dosing—especially if you are treating a chronic illness or trying to change the progression of disease. Otherwise, it is up to you to get informed and use your best judgment to discover what is best for you or your loved one.

Dosing is between you and your doctor. I am not a doctor, so please do not take anything in this book as medical advice. What I am sharing here is strictly for educational purposes.

Making Sense of Dosing with Dried Buds

Dried cannabis is the most widely used form of cannabis medicine. Buds typically contain 8 to 25 percent THC by weight while the leaves usually contain 0.3 to 4 percent THC. So, one gram of dried cannabis flower will contain 80 to 250 mg of THC. (Carter, Weydt, et al. 2004) The average cannabis cigarette is 0.5 to 1 gram in weight. Therefore, an ounce of flowers yields approximately twenty-eight to fifty-six cigarettes depending on the amount used.

A survey of smoked medical cannabis patients in Washington and California indicates consumption ranges between 10 to 20 grams of raw cannabis weekly, which translates to 1.42 to 2.86 grams of cannabis per day. Survey respondents reported using medicine with an average THC level of 15 percent resulting in a presumed absorption of 34 to 68 mg THC per day. (Carter, Weydt, et al. 2004) While it is likely some of these patients are over-medicating and some are under-medicating, these results provide a good comparison point for novices who are looking for effective and responsible dosage levels for THC.

In order to underscore the potentially enormous differences that are seen in the potency of dry plant material and the volume needed to achieve therapeutic effect, let's compare the amount of cannabis consumed by participants in the above survey to the amount consumed by patients in the U.S. Government's Investigational New Drug Program (IND) on smoked cannabis administered by the National Institute on Drug Abuse (NIDA). The four remaining patients in the study have been smoking cannabis from twenty-three to thirty-nine years for glaucoma, nail-patella syndrome, multiple congenital cartilaginous exostoses, and multiple sclerosis.

The cannabis cigarettes they receive from the government contain 2.75 percent to 3.8 percent THC. One patient consumes 7 grams daily (3.75 percent THC), another 8 grams (3.8 percent THC), and two patients consume 9 grams daily (with one smoking 2.75 percent THC medicine and the others smoking 3.5 percent THC medicine). (Russo, Mathre, et al. 2002) When you compare the usage of these IND patients to the usage levels of the surveyed medical patients from Washington and California mentioned above, you'll notice a large difference in the grams of cannabis smoked per day. We can all agree this is almost certainly because the IND patients receive very low potency cannabis and therefore have to smoke a great deal more.

Not only are the IND patients receiving low potency cannabis, their cannabis cigarettes contain stem and leaf as well as flower buds. Most people who inhale cannabis for medicinal purposes would never choose medicine containing stem and leaf matter. In fact, most people in the know about medical cannabis consider cannabis cigarettes with leaves and stems far inferior because these parts of the plant have much lower trichome density and therefore much less therapeutic power. They are fine for cooking but definitely not what you want for inhalation. The cannabis provided to IND patients is also old—sometimes several years old—which negatively impacts flavor and potency.

Inhalation is one of the least (if not the least) effective intake methods, yet it is also the most popular. Inhalation makes it easy for patients to titrate their dose and provides immediate relief. For these reasons, I anticipate it will remain popular. It is important to keep in mind that some of the active components will be lost in the initial lighting process and in *sidestream* (the smoke that does not make it into your lungs) and exhaled smoke. The amount of cannabinoids/terpenes absorbed into the body when smoking is also impacted by the depth and vigor of each inhalation, the temperature of the flame or heating element being used, and whether you are drawing from the beginning or the end of the cigarette. When all is said and done, at least 40 percent of the active components of cannabis are lost in sidestream smoke. Of the 60 percent remaining, up to 27 percent of the active ingredients are believed to be absorbed into the body. (Carter, Weydt, et al. 2004) "Up to" is the key phrase here because of the learning curve for beginners—especially for non-tobacco smoking beginners. Absorption levels tend to be lower (as low as 10 percent) until users learn how to inhale and gain confidence in using their pipe, cigarette, bong, or vaporizer.

Dr. Gregory Carter and his team published "Medical Cannabis: Rational Guidelines for Dosing" in 2004. They used data from the clinical trials for dronabinol and other studies to design the following dosing table:

% of THC in cannabis	Amount of cannabis required to obtain:			
	2.5 mg of THC	10 mg of THC	30 mg of THC	60 mg of THC
5% THC	0.60 g	1.24 g	3.70 g	7.40 g
10% THC	0.30 g	0.62 g	1.85 g	3.70 g
15% THC	0.16 g	0.41 g	1.23 g	2.46 g
20% THC	0.10 g	0.31 g	0.93 g	1.86 g
25% THC	0.08 g	0.25 g	0.75 g	1.50 g
30% THC	0.05 g	0.20 g	0.62 g	1.24 g

This chart is an excellent starting point from which to establish how much dried cannabis bud you need to get specific quantities of THC. Below are the long-form calculations used by Dr. Carter and his team in their patient surveys from California and Washington. Patients reported using 1.42 to 2.86 grams of dried bud per day containing an average of 15 percent THC. Adjusting for the amount of sidestream smoke lost (40 percent) and the average available absorption of therapeutic compounds (27 percent), it was concluded that surveyed patients were absorbing 34 to 68 mg of THC per day. The following calculation shows how we get from 1.42 grams of bud consumed to 34 mg of THC absorbed.

Inhalation Dosing Equation Example

1.42 grams of bud x 150 mg THC (15% THC/gram) = 213 mg THC

213 mg THC x 60% potential smoke ingested after sidestream loss = 127.8 mg THC

127.8 mg THC x 27% potential average THC absorption = 34.506 mg THC absorbed/day

You can use this same calculation for any cannabinoid and terpene by filling in the blanks:

__ grams of bud x __ mg of cannabinoid/terpene per gram = __ mg of cannabinoid/terpene or "A"

"A" mg of cannabinoid/terpene x 60% potential smoke ingested = __ mg of cannabinoid/terpene or "B"

"B" mg of cannabinoid/terpene x 27% potential absorption = __ mg of cannabinoid/terpene absorbed

Keep a log of the different medicines you try, levels of cannabinoids and terpenes you consume each time you medicate, and the relief you receive. This information will help establish your ideal dosages and be incredibly valuable to your doctor if they are interested in cannabis. It is quite possible you may find a particular THC/ CDB/Other cannabinoid/terpene ratio is better for daytime use, but another is better for nighttime. You may also discover you get the best relief by blending several varieties at once. Tracking milligrams of the different cannabinoids and terpenes you consume each time will empower you to buy, grow, or make the ideal medicine. Knowledge is power! If you don't have access to reliable cannabinoid/terpene profiles, you will have to do more guesswork.

Dosing with Edibles

Did you hear about the Michigan police officer and his wife who called 911 because they thought they were dying? No, this is not a joke. He and his wife ate too many cannabis brownies, which resulted in an experience so unpleasant that they called the police to come save them. As you can imagine, that man lost his job. While this story makes the experienced cannabis user chuckle, I assure you that having too much of an edible is not a laughing matter. It can result in the spins, nausea, lack of motor functions, and low blood pressure. This is why you MUST start slowly (with a tiny bite) every time you try a new edible regardless of whether it is homemade or professionally manufactured.

Just because your buddy needs four brownies for a therapeutic effect doesn't mean you need that much. In fact, half (or even a quarter) of the same brownie might be just right for you. NEVER base your serving size of edibles on how much another person consumes. That is a sure way to get in trouble, especially if they are a regular user. Consider what happens when a 150 pound casual drinker tries to keep up with a 300 pound individual who drinks a twelve-pack per evening.

Keep in mind that the potency of an edible depends on the plant material used and how long and to what temperature it was heated. The time it takes for the effect to kick in is dependent on your unique biology and the contents of your stomach at the time of consumption. Naturally, if you consume an edible on an empty stomach it will take effect quicker than after a big meal. For that reason, I encourage those new to cannabis to consume edibles after a snack. Wait at least two hours before consuming more. If you feel you need more relief, you can consume another portion half the size (or smaller) of your first portion.

Some edibles are so tasty it's hard to use a small amount. If you are eating a cannabis-infused food you find delicious, it's wise to have a non-medicated back up. Hopefully, this will help you not overdo it on the tasty medicated drink, honey straw, brownie, pesto, chicken pot pie, chocolate, etc.

Whether you decide to make your own cannabis infused foods, tinctures, or oils or choose to buy them, it is likely going to take a little time to find your ideal dose. Because of the legal status of cannabis, products made with it are only regulated in states that have medical or recreational cannabis laws. There are no universal industry standards for consistency, labeling, or food safety. This means there is huge variability in quality between different edibles and even between edibles sold at the same dispensary.

Dosing with Dispensary Edibles

A leader in the cannabis edibles industry is Bhang Chocolate (*http://gotbhang. com*). Their products are triple tested, meaning the raw plant material, concentrate, and final product are all laboratory tested. In addition, Bhang adheres to best practices for food manufacturing and safety. When I asked Bhang Chocolate owner Scott Van Rixel what we should look for when buying a cannabis-infused food product, he suggested:

- Accurate and honest ingredients list
- Nutritional panel
- Milligrams per serving of active ingredients

Do not buy products that don't list ingredients or list them in loosy-goosy language such as "made with a gram of kif." How are you to know the quantity of therapeutic compounds in a single serving with that kind of vague information? You cannot determine a reasonable dose based on that.

Seek out edibles that are lab tested for safety and quality, or make your own at home with quality medicine you trust. This will protect you from consuming edibles made with low-quality cannabis tainted with mold or dangerous pesticides.

Van Rixel stresses that the milligrams of active ingredients (cannabinoids and terpenes) per serving is the most important information when consuming edibles. As he says, "One can go from medicated to miserable very fast with edibles." When you know how much THC, CBD, etc. is in each serving, you can follow your doctor's guidelines (or your own) safely and consistently and avoid unpleasant overdoses.

Ancient Formula's for Health – Siddhi Tonics

The edibles market has exploded with innovative products. One of my favorite product lines is Siddhi Tonics (*siddhitonics.com*) out of Washington and Oregon. Their products are designed to deliver specific amounts of cannabininoids along with other important adaptogenic herbs. All their formulations are based on the ancient healing traditions of Ayurveda (from India) and Traditional Chinese Medicine.

Let's take a look at a couple of popular cannabis infused products that have been crowd favorites at various High Times Medical Cannabis Cups, an important industry contest for medical cannabis products. This table gives a good idea of standard THC doses for edibles that can help pinpoint your ideal dose:

Product/Brand	Total THC Mg	# Servings	Mg THC Serving	Price
Bhang Chocolate Bar Bhang Chocolate	120	4	30	$10-15
Blackberry Dark Chocolate Bar Kiva Confections	180	4	45	$20
Sweet Stone Gummy Bears Magnolia Wellness	100	2	50	$15
Strawberry Lemonade 16 oz. Buds & Roses The Venice Cookie Co.	72	2	36	$14
Hearts of Hemp Granola Bar Cool Calm Collective	125	2-4	62.5-31.25	$10
Sparkling Peach Elixir 8.5 oz. Dixie Elixir	40 & 75	1	40 & 75	$14

Dosing Homemade Edibles

The following are two primary factors that impact edible potency and efficacy:

- Decarboxylation – The potency of cannabis butter or cannabis cooking oil varies depending on the level of decarboxylation of the cannabinoid acids in the raw material. Preparations cooked low for ten to twenty-four hours are the most potent. [See "Decarboxylation - How to Activate Cannabis", on page 52.]
- Maintaining cannabinoid integrity – Be careful to not overcook cannabis butter or oil when using it in your chosen recipe. If you cook cannabis butters and oils at too high a heat, you evaporate the cannabinoids and terpenes and lose some of the therapeutic benefit. Only use cannabis cooking oils in recipes that keep the temperature under 350°F.

The following is for the home cook to help develop a consistent serving size across all forms of edibles. I use butter as an example, but this equation works for any cooking fat you choose.

1 cup butter = 16 Tbsp or 236.59 ml
2 cups butter = 32 Tbsp or 1 lb or 473.18 ml

1 Tbsp butter = 14.79 ml
1 oz of bud at 15% THC x 1 lb. butter = 4252.35 mg THC
(132.88 mg of THC/Tbsp butter)

Let's assume your brownie recipe calls for 7 tablespoons of butter and makes 16 two-inch brownies.

7 Tbsp butter x 132.88 mg THC = 930.16 mg THC for the total batch
Divided by 16 brownies = 58.13 mg/brownie
Divided by 32 brownies = 29.06 mg/brownie

No matter how you slice it, that's a potent edible for the average person. If you are looking for a less potent recipe, replace a few tablespoons of medicated butter with non-medicated butter and adjust your calculation accordingly, or divide into smaller portions.

Tolerance

When you start using cannabis, it is likely you will not need much plant material to experience therapeutic benefits. After using cannabis for a while, you may find you need to increase the amount of plant material you are using or upgrade to more potent medicine. Occasional users may never experience this, but regular users frequently develop some level of tolerance thus requiring an increase in potency, amount, or both.

Sensitizing and Re-Sensitizing the Endocannabinoid System

Dustin Sulak, D.O. (*http://healer.com*) is a doctor of osteopathy in Maine who specializes in integrative medicine and has seen thousands of patients who use cannabis. He advises patients who are inhaling their medicine to begin with a very small sub-therapeutic dose of one inhalation a day.

By taking one inhalation a day for two or three days, Dr. Sulak says the patient is priming their endocannabinoid system to create more cannabinoid receptors. (Sulak 2014) After a couple of days of sub-prime doses, you can begin to experiment and discover your ideal therapeutic dose.

So many cannabis patients I have talked to told me they didn't experience much the first time they tried cannabis. As already mentioned, that was my experience. Dr. Sulak says feeling nothing as a new user is a good sign, unless you have lots of doubts about the efficacy of cannabis. If you need to feel a strong effect to relieve your doubts, he suggests inhaling just enough cannabis that you feel a minimal effect for the first couple of days.

Dr. Sulak is the first person I have heard talk about the concept of a *threshold dosage*. This is the dose at which one can continue to use cannabis at an optimum therapeutic level without developing a tolerance. This threshold is different for everyone. Dr. Sulak explains that, "Patients who exceed their threshold dosage develop tolerance to cannabis, which means they need more of the herb to get the desired effect, and the optimal benefit of cannabis disappears. While cannabis may still be helpful, those who exceed their threshold never get the great results they once had. Certain exceptions to this rule do exist." (Integr8 Health, LLC 2012) Dr. Sulak tells me his patients who have been willing to sensitize their bodies with sub-threshold doses when beginning to use cannabis, and those who are mindful of not exceeding their threshold dose, are rewarded with a safe therapeutic experience and can make better use of less plant material. (Sulak 2014)

Re-sensitizing the Endocannabinoid System

The good news is that, even if you have exceeded your threshold dosage, re-sensitization is both possible and fairly simple. I think a large number of people who use cannabis for managing a disease are probably over medicating and would likely benefit more from using less. Just because a little is good doesn't always mean a lot is better. In fact, some studies of patients with chronic pain have shown pain is magnified at too large a dose of THC in some patients. (Aggarwal 2013)

Dr. Sulak and his patients worked together to find a way for cannabis users to re-sensitize their endocannabinoid system after periods of over-use. The following is the protocol he graciously shared with me:

Cannabinoid Resensitization Plan:

Step 1: Take a forty-eight hour break from cannabis use. (Heavy users may need much longer than this but never more than a month.)

Step 2: Using a pipe or a vaporizer, break your fast with a single puff. Wait three to five minutes.
- If you can feel a minimal effect, leave the cannabis and go about your day.
- If you feel no effect, take another puff and wait three to five minutes. Repeat until you feel a minimal effect.

Step 3: Repeat this procedure up to three times daily for three days total. During these three days, your sensitivity to cannabis will increase.

Step 4: On day four, use as much cannabis as needed to produce the desired medicinal effects.

- Remember to wait three to five minutes between puffs. Once you have the desired therapeutic effect, you have found your threshold dosage. For most patients, this is usually one to four puffs of high-quality cannabis one to four times daily.

> **Important Note from Dr. Sulak:** "If at any time you notice you are developing tolerance to cannabis, meaning you need a higher dose to get the same effect, then you have likely exceeded your personal threshold dosage. Simply return to using just below the threshold dosage you discovered on day four, or repeat the resensitization plan."

> "Many long-time cannabis users have been delighted by the effect of the resensitization plan. I often hear patients exclaiming, 'I did what you told me, and now two puffs does more for me than two joints used to do!'"

> At the time of publication, Dr. Sulak and his team were working on developing additional patient materials on this resensitization protocol. Visit *www.Healer.com* to learn more.

Cannabis Analysis

Let me begin this section with special thanks to chemist Dr. Jeff Raber, owner of The Werc Shop (*http://thewercshop.com*), one of our country's premier cannabis testing facilities, for his generosity in helping me understand cannabis testing so I can share what you need to know. In states with medical cannabis laws, or having legalized cannabis, you can buy cannabis that has been lab tested for bacteria, mold, pesticides, THC, and CBD content and, less commonly, other cannabinoid contents and terpene profiles. Testing confirms for the patient that they are buying a wholesome product. Lab testing medicines also allows doctors to recommend specific quantities of cannabinoids and terpenes for specific conditions and allows patients to purchase exactly the right medicine for their needs. For example, a patient with a heart condition who experiences rapid heartbeat when he uses high THC varieties can buy cannabis higher in CBD or with a balance of THC and CBD. He may be able to use cannabis without worrying about rapid heartbeat. This buyer can also choose a medicine with a specific terpene profile that further dampens the effects of THC that do not benefit him, that bolsters the positive effects of both THC and CBD, and that provides additional desirable therapeutic benefits such as sedation for better sleep.

Much of the spotlight on cannabis testing is placed on cannabinoids and terpene content profiling. I have to say that for medicinal users, most especially those with lung problems and severely compromised immune systems, testing for microbes (mold, bacteria, and other unwanted living organism), pesticides, and residual solvents in cannabis oils and other concentrates is equally, if not more, important than cannabinoid and terpene testing in terms of increasing access to safe medicine.

Unfortunately, due to current lack of regulation in most places, not all labs are created equally. Right now anyone can buy test equipment and set up shop as a testing lab. To illustrate, I'll share the experience of my pal Charleen Justice who was a grower in Oregon and the creator of the Cannabis Awareness Collection. She had her plants and her concentrated cannabis oil tested at what appeared to be a legitimate lab. The first red flag came up when the owner of the company told her the wrong temperature at which cannabis decarboxylates effectively. The lab owner didn't realize he was speaking to an educated and knowledge-thirsty grower with a keen interest in cannabis science.

The second red flag came when she got her test results. The analysis of plant samples had been switched by the lab. That could have been forgiven as a one-time mistake. However, she later found out the lab was marketing themselves as having a relationship with a better known, well-respected lab when, in fact, they had only discussed it with the lab. Making themselves out to be something they were not was in line with their flagrant use of a bunch of marketing mumbo-jumbo words such as "accredited" and "certified" to bolster their reputation. Those words mean nothing because at the time there was no accrediting or certifying body overseeing these labs (this is changing in many legal states). If that were not enough, the lab promoted their equipment as "state-of-the-art." While the equipment may have been state-of-the-art, a loosely defined term, how it is operated is the critical component, and their team did not appear fully up to the task of being professional scientists. In fact, the equipment they were promoting as being so wonderful is capable of testing for cannabinoids, but it isn't the most optimal and ideal tool for the job. This is why it is important to check out a testing facility before working with them.

Cannabis testing as an industry and process is in its infancy. The fact that cannabis remains a Schedule I drug hampers the development of industry standards for cannabinoids. Terpenes are unscheduled and have been studied for many years already, thus some basic testing protocols of this type already exists in the food industry. Cannabinoid standardization is different. The real problem is that industry wide testing standards for cannabis do not yet fully exist so that users can compare apples to apples and more easily discern what chemical profile best meets their personal needs and preferences providing them a baseline for dosing.

Take apples as an example. There are hundreds of different kinds. Supermarkets generally carry anywhere from three to twenty varieties at any given time. What makes those apples different? Just like cannabis, the difference lies in color, taste, smell, nutritional composition, texture, moisture content, and more. How one intends to use the apple dictates which apple they buy. If I want to enjoy the apple as it is, I prefer a Honey Crisp or a Fuji. For juicing I enjoy anything with a high degree of sweetness; the Red Delicious is usually the most abundant and thus affordable. For baking I need something that remains firm and is less sweet, so I might pick a Granny Smith. If I'm in the mood to make hard cider, I seek one of the less-common varieties of bitter apple. Just like with apples, simply knowing the characteristics of a cannabis sample goes a long way in the patient's selection process. One day cannabis testing will advance to the point that we have extensive information about every medicine available, including quantities of therapeutic compounds and possible contaminants, and we will be confident the test results we see are accurate making it possible to compare apples to apples.

In a perfect world, I'd like to buy from a dispensary that tells me the top two or three cannabinoids and five to ten terpenes present in each medicine and that provides data proving my cannabis is free of mold, bacteria, other microbes, pesticides and all other agricultural chemicals. In my perfect world, it would be affordable for growers and patients to have their cannabis tested. As it now stands, it is economical only for larger operations to have their cannabis tested regularly. Dispensaries often buy in half pound or pound increments. Testing becomes shamefully economical at this point. Don't let a dispensary tell you that they don't pay for testing because it is not economical. That is a cop out. State regulatory schemes will soon require testing to be mandatory, and that will make sure all cannabis provided to consumers will be assured of purity and provided to patients with cannabinoid and terpenoid concentrations reported on the package.

In 2011, *O'Shaughnessy's: The Journal of Cannabis in Clinical Practice* reported on the growing pains of the cannabis testing industry in the article "How Accurate is Potency Testing?" (Gieringer and Hazekamp 2011) Identical samples were presented to ten different labs to test for cannabinoid levels in dry samples and tinctures. This is called a *ring test* and is a standard procedure in analytical testing for external quality control. What they discovered was an unacceptably high degree of variability between the labs. At least three labs were far outside the ranges reported by other laboratories on the dry matter samples. While this highlighted the gross variations in testing procedures and results, it helped the participating labs evaluate themselves and refine their process.

It is important to keep in mind that there will likely always be some variations between labs. One contributing factor is the simple fact that there can be almost a 100 percent variation in cannabinoid content on different flowers from **the same plant!** The bottom flowers may test at 10 percent THC and the top flowers may test at 20 percent. Sampling protocols are critically important and may lead to batch homogenization efforts being required in the future. As we move forward with the development of industry best practices, we will begin seeing a narrowing in the testing discrepancies between facilities.

Soon after this ring test, a state association for cannabis testing companies in California was established. In November 2013, the Association of Commercial Cannabis Laboratories (ACCL) opened their membership to all cannabis labs in North America. At the time of writing, there were twenty companies across eight states in the organization's membership. The organization is dedicated to developing "... best practices and certifications for quality standards" for medical cannabis testing facilities. To become a member of ACCL, labs are required to "... demonstrate satisfactory scientific acumen and expertise." I like the fact that these labs participate in ring tests to validate their testing process, share information, and work together to establish best practices. I feel much more confident in the validity of lab tests that come from labs willing to measure the accuracy of their equipment and techniques against their peers.

> **Association of Commercial Cannabis Laboratories**
> This professional association for cannabis testing labs is dedicated to scientific acumen, legal responsibility and reliability in the testing community. Learn more about testing and their membership at *http://www.cacannabislabs.com*.

The best equipment for the most accurate cannabinoid testing is High Performance Liquid Chromatography (HPLC). This equipment operates at room temperature, which allows measurement of the volume of both **cannabinoid acids** and **decarboxylated cannabinoids**. Terpenes are tested by a Gas Chromatography (GC) machine. Some places use the GC for cannabinoid testing too, but they generally measure a lower percentage of cannabinoids than the HPLC. GC machines are second to HPLC machines for analyzing cannabinoids. The High Performance Thin Layer Chromatography (HPTLC) approach is sometimes used for cannabinoid testing. It is, however, the least accurate of the three methods.

Know Your Testing Lab

How can you have confidence that the lab you or your grower/dispensary is using knows what they are doing? Here are a few tips:

1. Look at the resumes of the people running the lab. Look for backgrounds in organic chemistry, analytical chemistry, or microbiology. How much experience do they have? Trust your instincts, and don't be afraid to make decisions based on subjective opinions. Your safety is the top priority.

2. Look for a team rather than an individual. The more eyes overlooking the quality process the better.

3. Ask if the lab has participated in a ring test. If they have not done so, ask if they are willing. Has the lab tested their results? If so, how? Have they had customers blind test them by taking the same sample to the lab on different days under different names?

4. Ask what type of equipment the lab uses. Different equipment provides best results for different tests. Check the list above to make sure the lab is using the best possible equipment.

Cannabis testing is in its infancy. As in the entire industry, the testing sector is like the Wild West! Having access to tested material improves safety for all users, which is one of many reasons for legalization. Over time, the collection of cannabis chemical profiles combined with patient experience surveys will yield an incredible database that could be mined for the benefit of the industry at every level and for the public good. While our advancement in cannabis science in the last twenty-five years has been both immense and impressive, much remains to be discovered.

Chapter Nine

Onward

A dvancements in cannabis science stand to greatly improve public health while at the same time positively stimulating our economy, reducing our criminal justice burden, and making our communities safer. Cannabis is the safest, most versatile plant on the planet. I believe it exists to benefit mankind in more ways than we can comprehend at this time.

The discovery of the endocannabinoid system is by far one of the most important medical advancements ever. Advancements in science and medicine that could take place through the study of cannabis and cannabis-based products, and how the dysregulation of the endocannabinoid system plays a role in every disease, could unlock untold ways of helping the sick and suffering find relief. Additionally, such research could lead to the prevention and cure of certain diseases.

While our knowledge of exact dosing protocols for the control of symptoms, disease prevention, and cure is not where any of us would like it to be, I argue it is reprehensible to use this as an excuse to deny people access to cannabis when the science clearly indicates the highest level of safety and the lowest level of toxicity.

What is covered in this book barely scratches the surface of this topic. I encourage you to learn what you can and ask questions. There is much more to know about this benevolent plant. When used properly, it has great potential to improve the human experience: mind, body, and soul. Please join me in advocating for legalization at a national level and reasonable policies that do more good than harm. This section is intended to give you tools to be an effective cannabis advocate.

The American War on People Who Use Drugs

The War on Drugs has turned out to be a war on American citizens who use drugs. Our nation has spent billions of dollars over the last forty-five years on this "war." To what end? Drug use and availability has not decreased, yet our arrest rates and prison populations have skyrocketed.

The FBI reports that in 2011 there were 663,031 arrests for simple cannabis possession (under one ounce) in the U.S. What is the cost of processing these simple possession cases? How does this impact our jails and criminal justice system? Who pays for that? We do! According to *http://www.mytexasdefenselawyer.com*, indigent defense costs rose in my home state of Texas to $91 million from 2001 to 2012.

When people are faced with jail time, taxpayers have to pay for an attorney if the defendant cannot afford one.

Once imprisoned, it costs approximately $38,000 to $50,000 per year to care for that person not to mention all of the associated costs of court and law enforcement. And what happens to a young person who gets thrown into jail for a joint or sent to a court mandated rehab facility and ends up with a felony on their record? They are labeled criminals and addicts and treated as such by society. The net impact is usually social scorn and chronic underemployment. Then what? You can see where this negative spiral is going. There is nothing good here for individuals or society.

Our current marijuana possession laws are antiquated, expensive, and have a long-term negative impact on society. Money currently spent on prosecuting simple possession charges could be spent instead to make communities safer, children smarter, food safer, and the economy more vibrant. Current drug laws do none of these things.

Let's take my pen pal Chris Williams for example. Chris is serving a five year sentence in a federal prison for growing medical cannabis in Montana under that state's medical marijuana laws. I discovered his story by watching the documentary *Code of the West*, which is about the fight to change Montana's medical cannabis laws. Before setting up his operation, Chris and his partners sought legal counsel to review their risks.

On October 19, 2009, U.S. Attorney General Eric Holder released a memo that said, "The guidelines make clear that the focus of federal resources should not be on individuals whose actions are in compliance with existing state laws, while underscoring that the Department will continue to prosecute people whose claims of compliance with state and local law conceal operations inconsistent with the terms, conditions, or purposes of those laws." (U.S. Department of Justice 2009) After reviewing this memo, Chris's lawyers advised that, as long as he was in compliance with Montana law, he should be safe. Chris operated to the letter of the law and even worked closely with his local law enforcement and legislators to educate them about cannabis. The DEA raided Chris's facility on March 14, 2011 destroying all his plants. He was indicted and was expected to spend eighty years to life in prison because of mandatory minimums associated with the charges brought against him. Public outcry at the trial was such that the Federal Government backed off and offered him a five year sentence if he promised not to appeal.

That Chris was operating his facility in accordance with Montana state law was not allowed into evidence. After posting on Facebook about my outrage over Chris's situation, one of my bright lawyer friends, Julie S., contacted me to explain that because of the way the Constitution is written, the federal government has supremacy over states, and therefore his compliance with state law was not admissible in federal court. That means no matter what the U.S. Attorney General says about how the government is going to allocate their resources or enforce cannabis laws, **no one in this country who grows, sells, dispenses, smokes, or is in anyway involved with cannabis is free from potential prosecution until our federal laws**

are changed. Even if you are operating in accordance with your state law, the feds can come after you. Ask Chris.

Not only will he have lost five years of his life sitting in prison, he lost his business, assets, and now his livelihood. He will be changed forever by this experience. His employees lost their jobs, and several hundred patients, grandmas and grandpas included, had to go elsewhere—possibly onto the black market—for their supply of medical cannabis. Now what is he going to do? It's not easy for a "felon" to get a job. This man could have been generating tax dollars for his state and federal government, providing quality jobs in his community, being a father to his teenage son, and supplying quality medicine to several hundred people. Instead, he is sitting in prison with people who've committed violent crimes and costing you and me $50,000+ a year. How is this justice? This conflict between state and federal law puts everyone in the cannabis business and patients at risk.

What about the kid who gets caught smoking pot in her dorm room? She is kicked out of school, loses her federal aid, has her driver license suspended, and is probably in hot water with her parents. There is no doubt she shouldn't have been doing something illegal on school property. She broke the rules, but breaking rules should not break the teenager or ruin her future.

What about the black teen who gets caught on campus or elsewhere with cannabis? **Black males are four times more likely to do jail time than white males for possession.** They are more often than not prosecuted to the fullest extent of the law, have difficult experiences in prison, and are released to face an equally difficult time getting a job and lack of access to funds for education and self-care. This can lead to cycles of criminal activity and arrest because law breaking becomes one of the few ways to make a decent amount of money.

Our national drug policies do not work. In fact, they do more harm than good to people and communities. They divert precious tax dollars from the more important work of fighting serious crime, and they clog the justice system. To drive home the points I'm making, I share the following staggering facts compiled by the Drug Policy Alliance (DPA), the nation's leading organization promoting drug policies grounded in science, compassion, health, and human rights:

- Amount spent annually in the U.S. on the war on drugs:
  More than $51,000,000,000
- Number of people arrested in 2012 in the U.S. on nonviolent
  drug charges: 1.55 million
- Number of people arrested for a marijuana law violation
  in 2014: 700,993
- Number of those charged with marijuana law violations who were
  arrested for possession only: 619,809 (88 percent)
- Estimated annual revenue that California would raise if it taxed and
  regulated the sale of marijuana: $1,400,000,000
- Number of people killed in Mexico's drug war since 2006: 70,000+

For more American Drug War statistics visit *www.drugpolicy.org/drug-war-statistic*. These statistics are eye opening. Many people are being hurt by these policies, and who is being helped? Clearly, current federal drug policy benefits law enforcement, often funding their budget shortfalls through property seizures. Other benefactors include drug cartels, the private prison industry, big pharma, drug treatment centers, and the alcohol and tobacco industries. And, last but not least, every politician who is supported by any of these lobby groups benefits tremendously from keeping the laws as they are.

Former President Jimmy Carter said, "Penalties against the use of a drug should not be more damaging to the individual than the use of the drug itself, and where they are it should be changed." Agreed! We must change our cannabis laws at the national level.

Your Voice Counts

Cannabis policy debate is happening all over the U.S. and the rest of the world. For far too long, most people have been too intimidated to speak up on this issue. I was one of them. As a result of my newfound knowledge about cannabis, I've discovered the power of one voice, the importance of talking about meaningful issues with the people we love, the importance of speaking truth to power, and the importance of exercising our rights no matter how difficult it may be. Regardless of the issue, your voice counts.

Current U.S. cannabis laws do not reflect the desire of the majority of our people. According to the Pew Research Foundation, as of April 14, 2015, 53 percent of Americans favor cannabis legalization. (Motel 2015) Why do elections and legislation so often fail to reflect the will of the people? My hypothesis is that it all boils down to the difference between apathy and action. The old adage the squeaky wheel gets the grease is true. Elections and legislation reflect the will of the entity with A) the loudest voices (read best organization and marketing skills) and B) the deepest pocketbooks. They are the squeaky wheels because they can make the most noise and the most trouble if they are ignored. You have to **find the courage to speak out.**

Maybe you are afraid of how you will be judged. What will be the repercussions of using your voice? Will you be persecuted actively or passively in some way? Will you be labeled? I was silent for a long time. Whom did that serve? Finding your voice and using it to speak out about your rights and needs is empowering. If you use your voice with conviction, and speak from a place of confidence and righteousness instead of fear, you will be heard. Conversely, if you are overly emotional or irrational in your delivery the conversation is over, and you have lost the chance to make your point and serve the greater good by broadening other people's perspectives.

Discussing our point of view calmly and compassionately is how we come to understand one another. Listening and seeking to understand other people's point of view is the only way we can find middle ground. You may not change minds over night, but at least you are planting the seeds of change regardless how long they take to flourish.

Each of us has an important story to tell. There is someone who needs to hear your story and who will resonate with what you have to say. They may be your doctor, another patient, a loved one, a neighbor, a legislator, or a complete stranger on the opposite side of the earth. Someone out there will benefit from the path you walk. When you share your experiences and beliefs about cannabis, be authentic. Speak from experience, and don't be attached to the outcome or how your listener feels about what you are saying. If a person doesn't respond positively, show compassion. They are coming from a place of fear that most likely has nothing to do with you. It can be difficult for people to change their minds about something that has been scary for them. It is hard to change your beliefs when you have hung on to them for so long. Be honest, direct, respectful, and authentic. I frequently say that you can say anything you want as long as you speak from a point of love, respect, or compassion—better yet, from all.

Three Simple Ways to Use Your Voice

1. **Talk to family and friends.** Start a conversation with your family and friends about cannabis with the intent to understand their position. Invite them to share their views on the situation, and ask good follow-up questions to gain a full understanding of their experience. When we understand what is important to people and where their fear originates, we can begin a meaningful discussion starting where they are instead of where we want them to be.

2. **Participate in a cannabis advocacy organization.** There are many well-organized groups (NORML, Americans for Safe Access, Patients Out of Time, International Association for Cannabinoid Medicines, Marijuana Policy Project, Drug Policy Alliance) that lead efforts at the local, state, and national levels to raise awareness about cannabis laws and cannabis science. Supporting these groups financially, signing their petitions, and sharing their newsletters and social media are easy things to do to help raise awareness and change laws. Attend their meetings and functions, and consider volunteering; you will learn a lot and feel good working directly to educate others, and you will meet like-minded people!

3. **Communicate with your elected officials.** Most elected officials want to hear from you. Go see them in person, meet with their aides, call them and state your position on certain issues, and ask for their support. Write them, and message them on social media! Good lawmakers track these things to discover what constituents want. They should be working for you. If they

don't hear from you, how can they effectively represent you? Politicians want to keep their jobs. Cannabis is something few mainstream people are willing to discuss openly for fear of the stigma that may be attached to them. Silence makes elected officials think this issue is important to only a small group of fringe people. They need to know this issue has broad support from their voting constituents. When they have confidence this is the case, they are going to be more likely to support pro-cannabis legislation.

Tips for Talking about Cannabis with Friends and Family

We all know it is easy to get emotional when speaking about a topic for which we have great passion. This often gets in the way of effective communication. If you can see each conversation as an exchange where you seek to share information and understand each person's position, you will find most people are willing to engage. Here are a few things I find help me engage people in discussions about cannabis and make them willing to listen:

1. **Be well informed.** When you have the facts straight, people naturally respect you. Vague or half-true information destroys credibility. If you are sharing anecdotal information, be sure to call it that. If you don't know the answer to a question, admit it. It is okay. This is an open door to follow up with the answer at a later date. Your observations and experiences count as being well informed when you are honest about exactly how much you know and how much you don't.

2. **Share personal stories.** Personal story makes you relatable. Use your experiences to find common ground with your audience. Invite them to imagine what it might be like to be you and struggle the way you have. When someone can put themself in your shoes, they will often hear what you have to say more openly. At this point, you have a higher likelihood of helping others understand your position and maybe adjust their own.

3. **It is okay to disagree, but don't be disagreeable.** Civility is critical to successful communication. We can attack a person's viewpoint without attacking them. Once you attack a person directly, they will become defensive and likely stop listening.

A couple of the most persuasive talking points about the benefits of medical cannabis I've discovered for effectively visiting with my friends, family, and anyone who will listen follow. I hope these serve you in developing your own talking points:

1. **Efficacy** – Chemicals in the cannabis plant mimic critical chemicals in our body that modulate or control every major function. They are designed to keep the body in balance. When unable to do that on their own, chemicals from cannabis are effective at helping bring the body back into balance. This is why cannabis is such an effective medicine for so many different problems. [See "The Science of Cannabis", on page 33.]

2. **Safety** – Cannabis is one of the safest and most versatile plants on the planet. No one has died from over consumption of cannabis because there are few cannabinoid receptors in the part of the brain that controls breathing and heartbeat. This is the part of the brain that is heavily affected by chemicals in opiate painkillers, which can lead to overdose death by depressing breathing and heartbeat. Additionally, cannabis has one of the lowest toxicity profiles in all of medicine and one of the widest therapeutic windows. Cannabis is safer than aspirin and has been tested and studied more thoroughly than 95 percent of FDA approved medicines. (Carter 2014) [See "Why is Cannabis So Safe?", on page 113.]

3. **Versatility** – Components of the cannabis plant work with the human body's innate harm reduction system, the endocannabinoid system, to maintain balance by reducing disease-causing cellular inflammation and building immunity. Inflammation and lowered immune system function are two root causes of a vast majority of diseases—especially those that are age-related. Because components of the cannabis plant help the body regulate these issues, they are effective at addressing a wide variety of symptoms, reducing inflammation and pain, managing nausea and vomiting, and stimulating appetite. This is just scratching the surface; components of the cannabis plant can also help change disease progression in epilepsy, cancer, Parkinson's, M.S., Alzheimer's, and more.

4. **Cannabinoid Patents** – The U.S. Government holds a patent on cannabinoids from the cannabis plant for its anti-inflammatory and neuroprotective qualities. The patent was written by a team of researchers that included a Nobel Prize winning scientist. It details not only how cannabinoids can help manage symptoms but also how they can change disease progression.

I could go on, but these are the highlights. It is easy to overwhelm people with information, so try to speak at the level of your audience, and don't assume that they have a cannabis vocabulary. Teach them from the beginning.

Dispelling Cannabis Propaganda

Once you start engaging people, you are going to be asked all kinds of questions about cannabis. Many will be based on fear and propaganda. I cannot tell you how many times someone has told me they support my work and think it is cool that I am writing this book. Then in the same breath that person will share with me some antagonistic propaganda driven sound bite about cannabis as if it is a fact. One day I was sharing with a colleague that I was writing this book. She was trying hard to not pass judgment and be supportive. She said, "Oh, well I support the use of cannabis for medical purposes for people who are dying or extreme pain, but because it is so addictive I think it is a dangerous gateway drug and should never be legalized for recreational purposes." I've come a long way in how I handle such responses. I used to respond more passionately. Time has taught me that the more gently and dispassionately I can deconstruct someone's misinformation, the more effective I am at opening their mind.

How people respond to my work on this book is a fascinating social observation. Responses range from wildly supportive to skeptical to everything in between including a few old pot smokers who feel I, as a newcomer, am somehow infringing on their territory.

About midway through the writing, I had a chance to catch up with a girlfriend whom I enjoy but don't get to see often. She inquired about what I was learning and seemed truly interested. As long as we were talking about cannabis as medicine for someone else, she was engaged. She listened intently and expressed support for my project. Several topics later she shared that an immediate family member was in the hospital, in a medical cannabis state, with a serious intestinal issue that was causing great pain. When I told her the different ways cannabis could help her suffering family member, she looked me in the eye and said, "Oh, no! We are not that kind of people."

While I didn't take her statement as a dig at me, I was struck by the fact that the D.A.R.E. program teachings were so profoundly embedded in her belief system that she was unable to embrace the potential relief this safe medicine can provide and how strong her judgment was against people who utilize it. As I look back, I'm grateful to have had that experience with someone I respect. It drove home that we have a long way to go in educating people. It also clarified for me that part of my role as an educator is to dissolve the cloud of shame, secrecy, and controversy around the use of cannabis and help the public see it as a safe, legitimate medicine.

People have all kinds of misinformation and misconceptions about cannabis. Here are a couple of the common myths I hear and how I respond:

1. **Cannabis is a gateway drug.** Many people support legalization of cannabis for medical purposes, but believe it is a gateway drug and therefore should not be legal for recreational use. In 2013, the National Survey of Drug Use and Health, the latest government report available, shows over 115 million

Americans reported having tried cannabis, yet only 24.6 million reported using it in the month prior to the survey. Additionally, the survey reports that 37 million Americans admit using cocaine, but only 1.5 million reported use in the prior month. Less than 5 million reported using heroin in their lifetime, and fewer than 300,000 American reported using it in the month prior. (Substance Abuse and Mental Health Administration 2014) If cannabis really were a gateway drug, wouldn't we have a much higher rate of hard drug use? I argue that the desire to use "harder," more dangerous drugs is more about family situations, natural propensity for addiction, social networks, neighborhood environment, access to steady and meaningful work, and the desire to alter one's consciousness in several different ways. People who want to experiment with multiple consciousness altering substances are likely to do so no matter what; there is no evidence that people tend to progress from using less dangerous drugs to more dangerous ones. In fact, many people with addiction to heroin, opiate painkillers, and pharmaceuticals find they can use cannabis to help STOP using dangerous substances for good. People who want to experiment with drugs are likely to try several in the same way someone who likes classical music will listen to multiple composers. The majority of people who try cannabis don't try harder drugs. (Martin 2015) In fact, the majority of people who use hard drugs are not addicted and lead normal productive lives. (Martin 2015) People who want to experiment with drugs are likely to do so no matter what.

Rx for U.S. Drug Policy: A New Paradigm

The James A. Baker III Institute for Public Policy, Rice University, published Rx for U.S. Drug Policy: A New Paradigm in June 2015, co-authored by their Director for Drug Policy, Dr. William Martin and Jerry Epstein This insightful report takes a fair look at how drug use and abuse is measured in the U.S., the absence of alcohol in the equation, that a drug-free America is not an achievable goal, how the War on Drugs has failed, why cannabis is NOT a gateway drug, and suggestions for sensible drug policy. This report is available at *www.bakerinstitute.org*.

2. **If cannabis becomes legal, how do we keep it out of the hands of children?** This supposition is ironic. The quickest way to obtain cannabis in any community is to go to the local high school or middle school and ask around. It is prevalent in all schools. By legalizing cannabis and bringing it into the fold of the legal marketplace, we increase the safety level for patients and communities and can limit access for minors. Plus, I cannot help believing that legalization will make cannabis lose some of its

rebellious allure to minors. Additionally, by having a more open cannabis marketplace, we also will have better education about cannabis including risks and harm reduction, which would almost certainly result in more responsible and informed use by all.

3 **If we legalize cannabis, won't it make it easier for people to get hard drugs?** No! (Oops, that's a bit passionate.) Have you ever been at a grocery or liquor store buying alcohol and been invited into the back to look at cocaine, heroin, or meth? I haven't either. Making cannabis more accessible through normal market channels takes cannabis buying out of back alleys and reduces the buyer's potential exposure to hard drugs. Hard drugs are frequently related to drug cartel activity. By moving cannabis into the open market, we take money and contact with cannabis consumers away from dangerous drug cartels and put it in the hands of local business owners and medical professionals.

4. **Doesn't pot make you a lazy stoner?** Some people fear cannabis legalization will result in society going crazy smoking pot and an epidemic of laziness will take hold. While it is true some cannabis varieties slow you down and make you lethargic or sedentary, the reality is that most people want to use cannabis in a way that increases quality of life— not to interfere with their productivity or lifestyle. The "stoner" stereotype does not accurately represent the profile of regular users. Most people would be surprised to find out who in their circle uses cannabis. The vast majority are highly productive, responsible people who pay taxes, participate in their communities, love their children, and have dreams and aspirations like normal people and not lazy, bleary-eyed couch potatoes who cannot string two sentences together, beginning every sentence with "dude," and constantly lose their cars.

Taking a position on cannabis can be scary at first, especially if you are afraid speaking out may harm you professionally or socially. Although it took me a year to work through this myself, I now realize if I don't stand up for what I believe who will?

Conclusion

Hopefully, by now you are convinced of the safety and efficacy of the medicinal qualities and potential benefits of cannabis and feel well informed to decide if it may improve your quality of life or that of a loved one. My desire is that you feel empowered to move forward with confidence and know where to start looking for answers to remaining questions. While there is much more for science to teach us about how cannabis can be used as medicine, we know enough to form a solid foundation for expanding how we view cannabis as an important and valid part of our culture, pharmacopeia, and economy.

Although society is rapidly shifting towards more open viewpoints about cannabis, I think it will take We the People to move our government to de-schedule cannabis and enact thoughtful policy. There are powerful forces at work to impede such progress. Through diligently sharing our knowledge with our social circles, medical professionals, and elected officials, I believe we will succeed. It will take all of us to help elected officials find the courage to vote for legalization. They need to know they have the support of their constituents. I am hopeful we can develop these policies from a base of science, maturity, and rational sensibility. Several hundred million Americans could benefit from such policy changes including those with chronic pain (100 million), diabetes (25.8 million), heart disease (16.3 million), cancer (11.9 million), PTSD (7.7 million), and stroke (7 million) to name a few.

How to Regulate Cannabis

Transform is a charitable think tank that campaigns for legalization of drugs in the UK and internationally. Read their book *How to Regulate Cannabis: A Practical Guide* online at *www.tpdf.org.uk*. This book offers sound ideas for implementing responsible drug policy.

Suffering does little to advance public good. The financial cost of illness can be crippling to families. Damage done to communities and the economy is immeasurable. While I have a great deal of respect for doctors and medical professionals, I find our medical system flawed, favoring perpetuation of sickness for economic gain.

The problem is, in part, the way doctors are educated. The rest of the problem is the system in which they work. Thankfully, many doctors are starting to look more critically at the therapeutic benefits of cannabis and are becoming increasingly convinced of its merits. Cannabis used appropriately may either be the answer or a critical puzzle piece for many people to help them get their health back and improve their quality of life. The bonus is cannabis is low risk, low toxicity, and low cost!

The responsible use of cannabis and the manipulation of the endocannabinoid system, collectively and independently, hold incredible promise for improving the way we treat and manage ALL illness and, in some cases, prevent it. This point cannot be overstated!

Call me idealistic, but I believe in a world where ALL people have the choice and chance to impact the world from their wellness instead of their sickness. Those cannabis converts who have done this serve as beacons of hope for others who choose to live and die better. I've had the honor of supporting several loved ones during the end of their lives including witnessing two people crossing to the other side. Because I see dying as a sacred process, it is important to me that anyone I love or care for be able to make that journey without pain. If cannabis can play a role in making dying more comfortable and peaceful, why would we not use it?

I get phone calls and emails almost daily from people who have contacted me on my website asking if I can help them. Their stories are gut wrenching. I can't tell you how many emails I get that end with, "Can you please help my baby?" or "Can you please help me? My life depends on it." I cry over every one of those emails. Just thinking about them makes my eyes tear and my heart ache—especially ones wherein parents beg me to help their sick child. I'm a helper by nature. Being unable to help someone who wants to help themself or their loved one is painful. In part, I cry for each person I cannot help because it feels inadequate to tell a desperate person that I can only offer them information and, in part, I cry because I have to tell a large number that the only real options for them are to move or break the law.

How is it okay that anyone should be forced to make a choice between their quality of life or that of a loved one and obeying the law? I'd much rather be alive and have broken the law than be dead and obeyed it. This kind of suffering is unnecessary and disgraceful. **We are supposed to be a civilized society, but there is nothing civil about our national cannabis policy. The time has come for us to do better by each other and to expect more from our government and the medical system. It is time to bring science to the forefront of our national conversation about cannabis and dissolve the cloud of shame, secrecy, and controversy around the use of this benevolent plant.**

When my mom thought I should be bolder in life, she would say to me, "Nishi, the world is full of wrens, be a red bird!" That was her way of encouraging me to live my best life, to be bold, and to step into the fullness of my mind, body, and spirit. It was her way of telling me to embrace my gifts, my voice, my body, my internal and external power, and to let my light shine—to not hold back for fear of what others might think. In a way, she was metaphorically coaching me on moving from surviving to thriving.

It takes courage to step outside one's comfort zone and move from surviving to thriving. It takes courage to be a catalyst for change be it for you, your family, community, or beyond. It takes gumption and confidence in your viewpoint to speak truth to power and to speak up about issues such as cannabis use and legalization. Courage (and often divine guidance) is required to step outside the confines of the law to make a choice that is in your best interest.

Each of us has to walk our own path and make our own decisions as to what is in the highest good for ourselves and our family. I hope this book expands your knowledge about cannabis and arms you with the data to benefit your health and society. Regardless of how you choose to use your voice, and whether you choose to use cannabis or not, I hope you will always find courage to follow your inner red bird and choose that which is in your highest good. So be it!

Acknowledgements

No one gets where they are going alone! During my writing journey, the right people have shown up at the right time to offer knowledge, inspiration, stories, experiences, connections, financial support, kindness, curiosity, wisdom, and expertise. Words are inadequate to express my gratitude and love for each person who supported me. This book would not have become a reality without Nadine Whiteley, James Whiteley, Shana Whiteley, Alex Jayne, Ethan B. Russo, Sunil K. Aggarwal, and Julie Ermisch.

All people should know the joy and comfort of a loving supportive family like mine. They have carried me when I couldn't carry myself. My mother, Nadine Whiteley, had an incredible life giving so much to so many. Without her I would not have had the inspiration, courage, nor fortitude to complete this project. My parents have always been my greatest support giving me the confidence to chase my dreams. My dad, James Whiteley, has provided unconditional and enthusiastic moral, financial, and emotional support—without that, I'm not sure I could have done this. My sister Shana has also been a great champion of this project by supporting me with her kind and funny pep talks, giving sound advice, encouragement, financial support, and sponsoring some much needed vacations. I'm also grateful to my sister for allowing me to be such a big part of my nephew's life. My nephew Wesley is the light of our lives. Time with him is food for the soul, keeping my heart nourished and my spirit grounded. Wesley, Shana, Dad, and Mom I love you!

To my beloved Chad Gouge, thank you for sharing your immense knowledge of cannabis botany, concentrates, and the healing potential of varieties. I'm grateful for your support and encouragement to put my best foot forward, that you are always the first one to promote me and brag about this project, and for dreaming with me.

Sensei – (a.k.a. Alex Jayne) has been an enormous support by teaching me in a matter of months what would have taken me a year or more to learn on my own. Thank you for all the ways you have been an integral part of this project! Your friendship is a great blessing.

My loyal, wildly competent, and ever-positive assistant Julie Ermisch has been involved in every step of bringing this book to life. I'm grateful for her wisdom, kind counsel, and unwavering support. With all the options open to her, I'm grateful Julie choses to work with me.

Early in my writing journey, I reached out to respected medical cannabis expert Sunil K. Aggarwal, MD, PhD. Surprisingly, he not only picked up the phone but agreed to serve as the medical editor for the book, made critical introductions, and allowed me to use his name to open doors for key interviews. By the time I was ready for the next round of medical editing, Dr. Aggarwal had accepted a position at the National Institute of Health, which precluded him from continuing to serve as medical editor. Nonetheless, he remained available to answer my questions. Sunil you have been a tremendous mentor and friend. Thank you!

When Ethan B. Russo, MD—our country's top medical cannabis expert—heard Dr. Aggarawal would not be able to continue as my medical editor, he generously offered to take over. In my world that is like Mick Jagger calling up a rock-n-roll unknown and asking to record an album together. Dr. Russo's body of work was critical to the creation of this book. In his role as the book's medical editor, he has offered clear and practical guidance. Thank you Ethan for your mentorship, friendship, and your belief in me and my ability to translate the science into laymen's terms.

Special thanks to chemist Jeff Raber, PhD for generously helping me understand how cannabis is tested, teaching me about decarboxylation, and for improving my understanding of terpenes.

Thank you to internationally renowned cannabis botanist Robert C. Clarke for clarity about the difference between hemp and medical cannabis, sativa, and indica, and the different varieties of cannabis.

To the experts who graciously spent time answering my emails, giving interviews, and sharing their knowledge, resources, and contacts – THANK YOU: Donald Abrams, MD; Michael Backus; Brad Burge; Gregory T. Carter, MD; Valarie Leveroni Corral; Mohamed ElSohly, PhD; Constance Finley; Fred Gardner; Mara Gordon; Lester Grinspoon, MD; Arno Hazekamp, PhD; Jeffrey Hergenrather, MD; Martin Lee; Mary Lynn Mathre, RN, MSN, CARN; Raphael Mechoulam, PhD; Robert Melamede, PhD; John M. McPartland, DO; Pal Pacher, MD PhD; Mimi Pleleg; Michelle Sexton, ND; Sue Sisley, MD; Dustin Sulak, DO; Scott Van Rixel; and Gary Wenk, PhD; Jokūbas Žiburkus, PhD. It is an honor to have had the chance to get to know you and share your brilliance with my readers.

To all researchers and experts around the world working to advance cannabis science, thank you for your brave contribution to the greater good! Thank you to Rhea Graham, David McGee, and Sean Beeman for helping me understand different methods of making cannabis oil and the pros and cons of using different solvents.

Sharing one's personal cannabis story with the world can be scary. Thank you for trusting me to tell it; Clif Devall, William from Pennsylvania, Edward, my dad James Whiteley, Charleen Justice, Christopher Williams and my friend Mellissa.

The production of this book was partially funded through a Rocket Hub campaign. I was deeply touched by each person who so generously gave. I was especially moved by the generosity of the following people: James Whiteley, Loy and Helen Sneary, Mary Wilson, Julie Smith, and Firooz Gidfar. The full list of generous supporters include: Lance Abney, Dianna Amorde, Adeline Arjad, Chad Ballard and Paul Parkinson, Chelsea Bartell, Brad and Stephanie Bogus, Emily Castleman, Allan Chase, Dan Day, Patti DeNucci, Brian and Colette Donnelly, Allison Ellis, Julie Ermisch, Niki Jackson Fletcher, Jo Hatchell, Heidi Hutcherson, Alex Jayne,

Stephanie and Tom Jayne, Ashley Jones, Myrna and David K. Langford, Mishell Kneeland, Andrea and Marc Kohler, Robin Kressback, Tiffany Landry, Grant Leeman, Kim Lumley, Cheri Mathews, Mike McManus, Laura Merritt, Fred Meyers, Sarah Mount, Mitzi Muirhead, Marisue Mullins, Sandra and Wylie Ponder, Julie Pomerantz, Johannes Poulard, Susan Poynor, Karen Renick, Kay and Troy Ross, Stephanie and Chad Simpson, Cindy and David Smith, Jerry Stevens, Liz Stotts, Deeana Tilly, Anne van den Avond, Thomas Welch, Shana Whiteley, Bob Whitson, and Kathy M. and Wesley Wilson. Thank you for believing in me and having the courage to publicly support this project. Thank you to Kate Doner for fundraising advice, and to the makers of The Magic Flight Launch box and their representatives Julie Chairiello and Beacon Nesbit for donating vaporizers to our largest financial supporters!

Thank you Hodgson Eckel, Teresa Cantwell, Alex Jayne, Shana Whiteley, Beki Morris, and Linda Ryan for your honesty, hard work, patience, time, and support in bringing the Rocket Hub Campaign to life through video.

Thank you to my dad, Sarah Mount, Julie Pomerantz, Loy Sneary, and my fellow cannabis advocates Ian Benouis, Dawn McDowell Brooks, and Mark Zugsmith for giving constructive feedback on this book.

Thank you to my design and editing team: Anne Tara Szostek and Kurt Wilson for making this book better and me a better writer, indexer Theresa Raymond for her eagle eye and thoroughness, and to my graphic designer Jeanette Poer Dickens for bringing my vision of the logo, book cover, and interior book design to life. Thank you to my friends Drew Rice, James Bruce, 420Science.com, Sarah Todd, and Mojave Richmond for their photography contributions. Many thanks to my extended network who contributed their support, encouragement, and knowledge along the way including my lifelong friends Kay and Troy Ross, Scott Ross, friends Bradley Sanchez Houseton, Leah Farnsworth, Alan Bodovsky, and Christy Coward, Lorie Woodward, early supporters Karli Duran and Jamie Balagia, my first writing accountability partner Rich Martindale, Mike Meadway for his support, Jax Finkel and Heather Fazzio for their leadership in Texas to change our state laws, Jeff Downs for tech support, Jim Bachus for CPA services, Dianna Amorde, Patti DeNucci and Michelle Scappace for the self-publishing advice, my high school English teachers Cynthia Sivek and Cynthia Bradley for your help and support then and now, Betty Robertson for help with InDesign, and to the healers in my life thank you for your loving guidance: Fran Bell, Ron Banuelos, and Rebecca Hamm.

I'm eternally grateful for the friendship and support of my 11:11-sister Chelsea Bartell. To my original BFF Andrea Bachus Kohler and our husband (wink) Marc Kohler, and Julie Smith thank you for your moral and financial support – I'm so blessed we are friends. Thank you to Mike McManus for always being on my side and playing devil's advocate. Thank you to my family members who so loved my mother and have been supportive of this book: Cathlene Cox, Toby Cox, Shirley Ressler, Suzan Rossi, Mindy Turns, Mary Wilson, and Bob Whitson.

And to you the reader, thank you for your open mind and helping bring the information in this book into mainstream. Blessings to you all!

Cookbook Extra

C ooking can be hard when you are sick or in pain, and cooking for someone else who is ill is a tremendous responsibility. The recipes included here are compiled with you in mind and are intended to help you incorporate cannabis into nutritious dishes that taste great, incorporate a variety of healing foods, and do not sap all of your energy to make. While I do include a few recipes with a long ingredient list, all are simple and scalable. Many of the recipes listed take longer to prepare than cook, as I place a high value on fresh, clean, simple, quality ingredients. Hopefully, these recipes will help you find your own happy place of easy to make, nutritious, and delicious foods.

Nutrition Is Key! Tips for Healing the Body with Food

The modern western diet is not good when it comes to helping people heal. The American diet is the worst of all: high in carbohydrates, refined sugars, and processed food and low in quality fats, minerals, and general nutrition. Facing a health scare often prompts people to make lifestyle and food changes and get in touch with or heal their spirit. Please consider that food is medicine. At the most basic level, food is designed to help our bodies be well or become well.

Recently, I saw a poster at Whole Foods that read, "Treat your body like it belonged to someone you love!" Remember that you are worthy of the best of all things to help you on your healing journey. Food is a critical part!

By using good sense and guidance from medical science, we can develop better eating habits that promote healing. As you utilize some of the recipes in this book, please keep in mind the principles below:

1. **When you are eating something that gives you pleasure or satisfaction, your body relaxes. The key is to find the nexus of taste, nutrient density, and relief.**

2. **Food is a pleasure center for most people.** We all dislike some things. If you cannot stand something, stop forcing yourself to eat it. Find something you enjoy that is equally nutritious. You have bigger battles to fight than convincing yourself to like liver. I am not one who believes you should eat a food just because it is good for you. Wheatgrass is considered

healthful, but I cannot force it past my lips. It makes me want to gag. Good for those of you who drink it or love it. It is supposedly great for you. My point is that it is important to enjoy food. If you or your loved one needs dietary changes, try focusing on healthier alternatives that are pleasing. It will make the transition easier and increase your potential for success.

3. **Reduce sugar intake.** Refined sugar is not your friend. It is especially bad for cancer patients, diabetics, and anyone with inflammation: it spikes insulin, contributes to inflammation, and feeds cancer cells. It is my opinion that natural sugars from fruits and veggies are better for the body than refined sweeteners. Agave nectar has been popular in recent years because it has a low glycemic index and thus is diabetic friendly. However, even over consumption of natural sweeteners such as agave nectar, honey, maple syrup, or high sugar fruits can be problematic. Remember that cancer cells love sugar. While naturally occurring sugars (in small amounts) are essential to good health, we don't need as much of it as we crave and consume.

4. **Raw food can be very healing. Increase the volume of fresh foods in the diet.** For some, it may be best to introduce raw foods in small amounts or lightly steamed instead of completely uncooked. I do not recommend switching to a raw foods diet overnight, especially for people who are very ill, as this can cause an extremely uncomfortable digestive reaction. Introducing fresh juices, as we explore in the tip below, is a great way to introduce raw food. As a general rule, I like to have at least one raw food item per meal. It adds nutrient density, fiber, and a nice crunch. Additionally, fresh fruits and veggies help alkalize the body which, according to recent nutritional literature, may help contribute to preventing disease or promoting healing. Pestos, salads, side dishes, picos, and salsas are a great way to eat raw food. Raw garlic is one of my favorite foods to add; it has powerful anti-viral properties. Evidence suggests it may also help fight heart disease and strengthen the immune system. (University of Maryland Medical Center 2011) Yet raw garlic is not well tolerated by everyone, so use with caution and moderation.

5. **Juice!** Juicing is a great way to pack nutrients into the diet in a manner that is easier for the body to absorb while leaving more energy for the body to heal itself. Be aware of sugar levels in fresh juice, especially when juicing apples, oranges, carrots, grapes, and beets. Green drinks and veggie juices are usually best for healing. If you are well enough to enjoy an occasional alcoholic beverage, mixing your favorite alcohol with fresh juice is a great way to enhance the nutritional value of the drink. Fresh juice is remarkable as a base for salad dressings, for making popsicles, and for making ice cubes to enhance the flavor and nutrition of sparkling drinks or water.

6. **Grass-fed is good.** Regardless of whether you are a meat eater or a vegetarian, increase your consumption of foods from grass-fed animals. (Vegans can ignore this section.) Dairy products, eggs, and meats from grass-fed animals have higher nutritional value overall. They are three to five times higher in conjugated linoleic acid (CLA), which has been shown to help fight certain cancers. They are four times higher in Vitamin E (associated with lower risks of heart disease and cancer), lower in saturated fats, and higher in Omega 3s [See "Essential Fatty Acids", on page 65.] CLA is a newly discovered good fat that is prominent in grass-fed foods and is also reported to help arthritis suffers by lubricating joints. Visit *www.eatwild.com* for more information about grass-fed foods and where to get them. (Smith n.d.)

7. **Reduce inflammation-causing stressors and foods.** Stress of any sort triggers an inflammation response. Meditation, practicing forgiveness, yoga, and weight bearing exercise are great ways to reduce stress-induced inflammation. From a food perspective, avoid anything that affects you in even the slightest negative way. Many people are unaware of their sensitivity to *gluten* (a binding protein found in high quantities in modern varieties of wheat, rye, and barley). Removing gluten from the diet pays huge dividends for many people. According to *www.celiac.com*, one in 133 Americans have Celiac Disease, which is a genetic intolerance to gluten products. This presents itself in a wide variety of ways—most commonly as diarrhea and unexplained pain—none of which are conducive to healing. If you do not have Celiac Disease, it may not be necessary to cut all gluten out of your diet, but reducing the quantities you consume by sticking to products made with other grains (spelt, amaranth, buckwheat, etc.) that have lower gluten content and higher levels of other nutrients is healthy for everyone. It is also good to figure out if you are sensitive to night shade plants, nuts, legumes, or dairy. These are some of the most common dietary offenders. Once or twice a year, I like to do a twenty-one day cleanse. In many ways it is like a reset button for my health. The concept is simple: For twenty-one days, eat a diet of fresh foods that excludes all major dietary offenders. When you are done, slowly and systematically add those items back into your diet. If something makes you feel badly, you will know it, and because you have added only one thing back at a time, you can easily tell what is causing a problem. I do the twenty-one days cleanse in tandem with cleansing herbs and nutritional supplements to help ensure that my body makes the most of those days. Although my goal is to boost immunity, I enjoy the added benefit of losing pounds. Should you have an interest in doing something like this, Google "21 day purification diet." As you know, cannabis has been scientifically proven to help reduce inflammation in many different parts of the body. (Nagarkatti, et al. 2009) Making dietary changes will give the endocannabinoids system some relief from inflammation and a general boost while helping your cannabis regimen be more effective.

8. **Eat enough protein.** Don't think this means eat as much meat as you can. While meat can be a valuable source of protein, especially when it is grass-fed beef or lamb, free-range pork or chicken, or wild-caught or U.S. farm raised fish, meat is not the only protein. How do you think vegetarians survive? Greek yogurt, cultured cottage cheese, eggs, nuts, and whey protein isolate (look for the word isolate, which indicates the proteins are easy to absorb), rice or pea protein powder, chia, and hemp seeds are all great sources of protein. So are quinoa and greens. Adding your favorite protein isolate to smoothies, sauces, and baked goods is a wonderful way to pack nutrients into foods that are easily digested and assimilated by the one healing. An extra benefit of eating whey protein is that it increases the production of important antioxidants.

9. **Buy more organic foods.** I come from a farming family and have been close to the organic vs. conventional debate for years in my work at the state department of agriculture. Some conventional crops are more chemical intensive than others. For that reason, I always buy organic for the most chemically intensive crops including **apples, berries, greens, potatoes, and stone fruit.** Broccoli and cabbage, on the other hand, are low-chemical crops, so I usually buy those from the conventional section of the grocery store to save money. People in the food industry continue to bicker about organic vs. conventional and whether there is a quality or nutritional difference between the two. While I find it difficult to afford all organic groceries, I do believe organic foods are safer and more nutritious. The reason is simple: plants absorb nutrients from the soil. Organic soil is likely to be more healthy and alive than conventional soil because organic pesticides kill fewer beneficial microorganisms in the soil than conventional pesticides. Plants use nutrients in the soil to grow, and these are passed on when we eat them. Additionally, chemicals applied on conventional foods do all the work of protecting plants from disease and pests whereas organic plants have to fend for themselves and therefore produce healthy chemicals in their own flesh and fruit. These chemicals are good for us, too! You can learn more on The Organic Center website at *www.organic-center.org*. Another good reason to choose organic foods is that they are less frequently genetically modified. Jo Robinson's book *Eating on the Wild Side: The Missing Link to Optimum Health* is an excellent resource for what varieties of fruits and vegetables are the most nutritious and therapeutic.

10. **Add "super foods" to your diet.** Get creative to figure out ways to incorporate the following foods with your old favorites, or use them to create new recipes:

   a) *Hemp, Flax, and Chia Seeds* can go into smoothies, salad dressings, eggs, oatmeal, chili, and so on. Chia seeds have a sack around them that will absorb ten or more times its weight in liquid. They help your body get plenty of fiber and stay hydrated because they take a long time for your body to process in the gut. Flax is my least favorite of these. Your intestinal tract cannot break down the outer layer of the flax seed, thus you must grind it. But don't buy ground flax seed; it will have oxidized and may be rancid. If you choose to use flax, be sure to buy as direct from the manufacturer as possible, store in a cool place out of light, and grind the flax at the time of use. Honestly, I think flax is more trouble than it is worth. Hemp tastes good and is relatively shelf stable. I enjoy the seed and the oil in my daily morning shake!

b) *Greek yogurt* is delicious with honey, your favorite jam, maple syrup, or used just as you would sour cream. Make sure you read the label. Not all Greek yogurts are created equal. A true Greek yogurt is strained to remove water. Because it is more condensed, it is often more expensive than Bulgarian or other type of yogurts with higher water content. Many companies make watery yogurt thick by using corn starch or xanthum gum, thus making a cheaper product that can be advertised as "Greek" or "Greek Style." Corn starch is an unnecessary ingredient that provides no nutritional value and is frequently highly genetically modified. My favorite brand of Greek yogurt is Fage Plain, which packs twenty grams of protein per cup! A true Greek yogurt will have a similar protein content. I use it in place of sour cream and sweeten it for breakfast and dessert. White Mountain Yogurt is my favorite Bulgarian Yogurt. It tastes great and has one of the highest *probiotic* (healthy bacteria) ratios available on the market. It gives your immune system a big boost. Any yogurt you consume should contain live, active bacteria to help support your immune system.

c) *Kimchee, sauerkraut, salt-fermented pickles* – fermented foods like these stimulate enzymes in the gut to aid digestion and are full of healthy bacteria that help our immune system. They are easy to make at home. Visit the Nourished Kitchen website at *http://nourished-kitchen.com/recipe-index/ferments-cultured-food/* for recipes. If you are buying fermented foods in the grocery store, read the label, and watch out for unwanted ingredients such as MSG. Pickles prepared with vinegar do not contain the high levels of probiotics found in pickles prepared with salt only. Sally Fallon's book, *Nourishing Traditions* also offers wonderful fermented food recipes.

d) *Quinoa* (pronounced KEEN-wah) – This ancient "grain" is a seed people call a grain (but really is not) and is a super food because of its protein content and digestibility. It has 14 percent protein, is low calorie, and is a good source of magnesium, iron, and fiber. You can use it like you would rice or barley. See the Ecuadorean Quinoa Stew recipe on page 276. Before using quinoa, remember to rinse it thoroughly, until all bubbles are gone, otherwise it will taste bitter due to a naturally occurring chemical called *saponin* that coats the seeds.

Kitchen Must Haves for Patients and Caregivers

Regardless of your skill level in the kitchen, there are a few things you should have to make life easier and cooking more pleasurable.

Cuisinart

I love this food processor. If you do not have one, get one! Don't be chintzy; get the eleven quart size or bigger.

Vita Mix

The Vita Mix remains on my wish list. This is a powerful blender that can liquefy or puree anything. If your budget allows, be sure to treat yourself, or put this at the top of your wish list.

Immersion Blender

Hand-held immersion blenders make it simple to make smoothies, sauces, soups, and desserts in no time with little clean up. Simply place whatever you want to puree into a stable cylindrical container, place the blade into the mix, press the "on" button, and move the blender up and down until your mixture is fully blended. It's so simple! My favorite is the KitchenAid brand, but there are many good ones from which to choose.

Jack LaLane Juicer

It is difficult to consume the "recommended" daily allowance of fruits and veggies if you are trying to eat all of them whole. The last time I tried it I nearly exhausted myself (and I am a fairly healthy eater). However, this juicer changes everything! I also hear good things about the Breville juicers.

There are certainly better juicers available, and if you want to get one, please do. However, I have seen people spend anywhere from $20 – $2,500 on juicers. No one I have ever talked to was as satisfied with another brand of juicer as I am with Jack LaLane's. It is the nexus of easy to use, easy to clean, functionality, and affordability. You can sometimes find a Jack LaLane juicer for as little as $75 brand new. Never pay more than $130. It has four easy to clean and reassemble parts. You will develop the most wonderfully flavored beverages and significantly increase your nutrient intake, which is critical to healing. You can use the leftover pulp for fiber in baked goods to make your treats more filling and nutritious as well. My dad used a Green Star juicer (excellent juicer) to make my mother two green drinks a day. We all believe that these green drinks helped my mom maintain her strength as long as she did.

Large French Press

The French press is a great tool for making cannabis butter, tea, tincture, or oil. It reduces the mess of separating plant material from the oil, butter, water, or glycerin. And, of course, you can easily make yourself a yummy cup of coffee or yerba mate in one.

Magical Butter Machine

The Magical Butter Machine *(magicalbutter.com)* is a great cooking tool for making tinctures, cannabis oil, and cannabis butter. The machine comes complete with a built in grinder, a variety of temperature settings, and many different recipes. I appreciate Garyn Angel, founder of the company, for being committed to helping empower people to take back their health through better eating and body care. I love my Magical Butter Machine!

Two Food Book Must-haves

There are two books that are kitchen must-haves for anyone interested in being healthy. They are *Eating on the Wild Side: The Missing Link to Optimal Health* by Jo Robinson and *Nourishing Traditions* by Sally Fallon. Both books separate diet facts from fiction helping make it easier to use food as medicine and enjoy eating a healthy diet.

How to Make Basics

Butter

Making canna butter is a relatively easy process. There are many ways to do it. Regardless of which you choose, the most important thing is to cook the butter low and slow. The easiest way to do this is with a crock pot that allows you to cook the butter on a low setting. This allows the active ingredients to be slowly released from the trichomes and bind to the fat. If the butter/oil is made at too high a temperature the cannabinoids will be vaporized, and you will have wasted considerable time and money. I've talked to people who claim to make their cannabis butter in forty minutes. Others say it takes four to six hours. Expert cannabis chemist Dr. Jeff Raber says the best decarboxylation results are generated when you cook the butter for twelve or more hours but is scale dependent, too. If you have a high CBD plant material, you should cook it low and slow for at least sixteen hours, but twenty-four is better. [See, "Cannabis Cooking Tips", on page 259.]

Use the table below to decide how much plant matter you need to make canna butter:

1 Pound Canna Butter

Strength	Buds/Flowers	Leaf Trim/ Shake
Aunt Sandy's 10X Maximum Strength Formula	1 ounce	4 ounces
High Strength Formula	¾ ounce	3 ounces
Elevated Strength Formula	½ ounces	2 ounces
Low Strength	¼ ounce	1 ounce

Source: *Aunt Sandy's Medical Marijuana Cookbook: Comfort Food for Mind and Body*

Recipe
1 pound of unsalted butter or ghee. (Don't use salted butter for this!)
4 cups filtered or reverse osmosis (RO) water. RO is preferred.
1-4 ounces of cannabis depending on if you are using bud, leaf, or shake. Use the table above to determine how much to use.

Instructions
1. Ensure your pots, pans, and utensils are clean and dry.
2. Weigh your plant material.
3. Grind the plant material. The easiest way is with a food processor using the metal blade.

4. In a crock pot or a double boiler, bring 4 cups of purified water to boil. Please don't use tap water; it will have chlorine in it.
5. Add the un-salted butter.
6. Once the butter is melted, reduce the heat and add the cannabis.
7. Simmer for 10-24 hours stirring every 10-15 minutes.
8. Take off heat.
9. Strain the plant material into another bowl or container. Use a sterile cheese cloth or a large French press (I prefer this method) to strain the mixture and remove the cannabis. Rinse the remaining plant material with purified hot water to get any remaining fat left in the plant material.
10. Squeeze the cheese cloth or French press until you have removed as much liquid as possible.
11. Store in the fridge overnight in a covered glass dish.
12. Loosen the butter from the sides of the glass dish, and allow the water to drain while straining it again to catch any butter solids that may have broken loose. I like to use a chopstick to poke two holes in the top layer of solid butter and one hole in the butter on the opposite side of the bowl to make it easy to drain the water.
13. Store your butter in a glass container and refrigerate. It will keep in the refrigerator for a month. If you are not going to use the butter in that time, store it in the freezer.

Cannabis butter can be made without the water, but you will have to watch it closely to ensure that the butter and cannabis do not burn or get too hot. If you are not using water, I strongly encourage you to use a crock pot with a low setting. If you are looking for a visual guide to this process, there are many videos available on YouTube that will walk you through step by step. For a method similar to the one here, see CannabisLifestyle TV's video at *youtu.be/9EwGmmqfab8*. For a similar but different method, view the High Times video at *youtu.be/b1QIAD--b38*.

Variations:
If you choose to use coconut oil, you can follow the same instructions as above. If you are using oil, such as olive oil, that is liquid at room temperature, repeat the same process as above without water. Olive, coconut, and grape seed make nice canna oils that can be used for cooking and topical application.

Vegetable Glycerin Tincture Recipe

In addition to the alcohol tincture presented earlier in the book, I am sharing a glycerin extraction recipe that is simple and has extra nutritional benefits.

This recipe comes from *magicalbutter.com*, the makers of the Magical Butter Machine, the unique machine used to make cannabis butters, tinctures, and oils. This recipe has been slightly modified for those who do not have access to the Magical Butter machine.

Here are a couple of important notes before we get started:

DO NOT ADD WATER to the recipe!

You can blanch your cannabis in advance to get rid of the chlorophyll taste, but don't add water to the recipe. Many people think blanching the cannabis first gives the tincture a better flavor. Simply soak the cannabis flower or leaf in boiling water for three to five minutes. Drain the water and repeat. Once the plant material has cooled, squeeze all the water out of the herb and place the herb in your crock pot or Magical Butter machine. For detailed instruction on how to do this, visit *www.yellowjuanacake.com* and search the word "glycerin." You can add a drop of peppermint oil into the tincture to improve the flavor if you like.

Use sunflower lecithin. It helps your infusions immensely. Sunflower lecithin is an emulsifier widely used in food to increase its smoothness. It is high in essential fatty acids including several which are reportedly good for memory recall, smooth muscle conditioning, and the nervous system. Sunflower lecithin is widely available, and you will likely find it at most health-food stores that carry vegetable glycerin. It is both a food ingredient and a nutritional supplement and, as an added bonus, sunflowers are rarely genetically modified.

Ingredients

10 grams botanical per cup of vegetable glycerin
1 cup of vegetable glycerin
1.5 Tbsp sunflower lecithin

Instructions

1. Grind your herb in a coffee or spice grinder or food processor (if not using a Magical Butter machine (MBM).
2. Place all of the ingredients in your crock pot or MBM and heat to 250°F. Depending on how much you want to make, it is certainly easy to scale this recipe for larger batches.
3. Once the temperature hits 250°F, turn the crock pot to low or warm and cook for 8-24 hours. If using an MBM, turn it to the desired setting.
4. Strain, cool, and use.

Keep your extraction in a well-sealed glass jar or a colored glass tincture bottle. Brown or blue glass is best to protect it from light. Light degrades the medicine.

Cannabis Cooking Tips!

When preparing canna butter or cannabis oil for edibles, it is important to remember that the longer the plant material is cooked, the more potent the butter or oil will become. **Cannabinoid acids begin to convert to cannabinoids at 100-105°C or 212°F. Cannabinoids decarboxylate over time at both low and high temperatures. When cooking, it is good to go with a low temperature.** Canna butter (and cooking oil) recipes are a dime a dozen. Everyone has their own way of doing it and often their own video showing how it's done. You will hear cooking times ranging from 3-4 hours to 8-10 hours or longer. Dr. Jeff Raber suggests that to get the most out of the plant material it should be **cooked low and slow for 10-12 hours. If you are using plant material that has a measurable amount of CBD, you will want to cook it twice as long to decarboxylate the CBDA into CBD effectively.**

You cannot bake the plant material directly into the dish to get the desired effect. While the heat will convert a small amount of the cannabinoid acids to cannabinoids, the conversion is inefficient resulting in minimal potency edibles. This is a waste of perfectly good cannabis unless you are seeking cannabinoid acids.

What if it's too strong? Simply cut the canna butter or oil with regular butter or oil to get the exact amount the recipe suggests. For example, if the recipe calls for 1 cup of canna butter and you want it to be less potent, use ½ cup of canna butter and ½ cup of regular (non-medicated) butter.

What if it's not strong enough? You can reheat the butter, add fresh plant material or kif, and continue to cook low and slow. Or you can add already decarboxylated kif to the mix.

If you can, test ½-1 teaspoon of your butter or oil after each preparation to know how it affects you. This will make it easier to create recipes that produce the desired effect. Choose a consistent measurement that you will use each time so you know how to modify your recipe.

After cooking and separating the plant material from the butter or oil, save the strained plant material (if it is seed and stem free) to add to a soup, meatloaf, muffins, or whatever you are cooking for increased nutritional value or save it to make a salve or poultice for bruises, burns, or joint pain.

Drinks

You can add cannabis tincture or cannabis olive oil to your favorite drink. You can also try cannabis tea [See "Tea", on page 208.] If you choose to use oil, use a whisk or an immersion blender or shaker to thoroughly mix the oil into the drink.

Green Drink

This drink packs lots of nutrition into a single glass. If you do not have a juicer, throw the ingredients into the blender and then strain with a French press, cheesecloth, or unused nylon stocking, or toss it all into a VitaMix and drink as is.

Ingredients
2 large leaves of fresh kale
1 large handful of baby spinach
5 large sprigs of parsley
1 cup broccoli sprouts or broccoli (sprouts are best as they are high in
   sulphoraphane, a super antioxidant/cancer fighter)
½ peeled cucumber
½ green organic apple
1 small clove garlic (optional – especially good for anyone with a virus
   Remember a little goes a long way)
1 serving of cannabis tincture or olive oil

Directions
Juice or blend all but the cannabis tincture/oil. Add in the cannabis tincture or oil. Whisk or shake well to make sure the medicine thoroughly mixes with the juice. Serves 1

Happy Apple Seed

This drink is even more refreshing when the fruits and vegetables have been chilled previously.

Ingredients
3 organic apples (green apples have less sugar)
1 inch piece of fresh ginger (good for circulation)
1 cucumber peeled (good for memory and movement)
1 serving cannabis tincture or olive oil

Directions
Juice apples, ginger, and then cucumber in that order. Shake or stir and divide into serving glasses. Add 1 teaspoon of tincture or oil per glass. Whisk or stir the cannabis tincture or oil into the drink. Serves 1-2

The Kiwi

I double dog dare you to try this. For several years I taught a three hour program each semester in an afterschool food discovery and health program for sixth graders. It never failed that they snarled their nose at this recipe (minus the cannabis of course) while we were making it, but 80 percent of them would come back for seconds. Every single time at least one child would ask to take some home so their parents could taste it. This juice is an excellent blood cleanser.

Ingredients
2 organic apples (green is good)
2 big leafs of kale or collard greens (kale yields a better flavor than collards)
2 lemons peeled
1 serving cannabis tincture or canna oil

Directions
Juice the above ingredients in order. Portion the juice and add your desired serving of tincture or oil to each glass. Serve chilled or over ice. Serves 1-2

Peppermint or Lavender Fizz

Peppermint and lavender essential oils have many wonderful therapeutic benefits. Peppermint is useful for nausea and vomiting. It is also taken for fevers and cooling the body. (Rose 1992)

Lavender is the most versatile essential oil. It is stimulating yet soothing, anti-spasmodic, decongestant for the respiratory system and sinuses, antiseptic and healing for skin wounds and burns. (Rose 1992)

When using essential oils, it is paramount to remember 1) a little goes a long way, 2) more is not better, 3) use therapeutic grade oil that has no other ingredients, 4) do not put any essential oil straight on the skin or tongue, and 5) make sure you do not buy essential oil diluted in a carrier oil. There is a big difference between oils that simply smells nice and oils that make you feel better. Look for products labeled "100% Essential Oil."

This recipe has saved many a friend from a horrible hangover and helped my mom manage some of her early chemo-related nausea before we discovered cannabis.

Ingredients
20-24 ounces of sparkling water or use Sierra Mist (made with sugar not high fructose corn syrup), Ginger Ale, Sprite, or 7Up
1 small drop of peppermint oil and/or lavender oil (you may want to stick a clean toothpick into the bottle and then whisk it into the base liquid to ensure that you are getting a very small amount—too much of either oil is unpleasant)
1 serving of cannabis tincture per 8 ounce glass
1 tsp Agave nectar (use only if you are using sparkling water)
Twist of lemon – optional

Directions

Mix ingredients, stir well and serve. Serves 2-3

Lemonade

This hydrating drink is excellent for someone who is suffering from physical exhaustion, has been in the heat, or has been vomiting. This recipe comes from a cooking class I took with Dr. Viajanti "Jay" Apte, a nationally regarded Ayurvedic practitioner. (*http://www.hnwellness.com*) She says the combination of sugar, salt, and lemon or lime juice and the pungent flavor of the cardamom make it a healthy well-balanced electrolyte beverage. This is a wonderful drink to enjoy with friends. Simply add a serving of cannabis tincture into the glass of lemonade for those who are medicating with cannabis. Adding the tincture to each drink after preparation insures an even distribution of medicine.

Ingredients

10 lemons (or limes) juiced
¾-1 cup sugar (or ⅓ cup agave nectar or xylitol)
5 cups of water
1 tsp cardamom
1 tsp Celtic or Himalayan salt
Canna tincture

Directions

Mix ingredients and adjust lemon, sugar, or salt to taste.
Don't feel like squeezing your own lemons? Use store-bought lemonade prepared with natural sweeteners instead. Fill an 8-10 ounce glass ¾ full, add a pinch of salt and a pinch of cardamom, top off with water and tincture, and enjoy! Serves 3-5

Tip: Cardamom can be expensive. Shop at an Indian or Pakistani store for significant savings. For example, there is an international food store near my house where I paid $2.50 for the same amount of spice that was $11 at my traditional grocery store.

Snickerdoodle Smoothie

This is both a great breakfast and a good snack to help someone get ample amount of easily digestible protein.

Ingredients

1 scoop unsweetened protein powder [See "8. Eat Enough Protein", on page 252.]
1 cup of sweetened or unsweetened vanilla almond milk (milk, rice milk, coconut milk will work) – the vanilla flavored makes a much better drink
1/3 frozen banana
1/2 tsp cinnamon
1 Tbs of hemp seed or hemp oil (optional)
1 serving of canna olive oil

Directions

Blend in your blender or use your hand-held immersion blender. Serves 1

Variations:

Add 1 Tbs hemp seeds/oil for more protein and essential fatty acids. To get more nutrients, add a handful of spinach. I call this variation the Green Goddess or Green Monster drink depending on my audience. Dark chocolate powder and/or a scoop of peanut butter are good additions, too. If you use unsweetened vanilla almond milk, consider using more frozen banana for sweetness. A nice addition is 2 Tbs of soaked or cooked oatmeal.

The Smooth Tropical

This smoothie makes a wonderful breakfast or snack. Play with the ingredients to figure out which blend is your favorite. Note that coconut milk contains medium chain fatty acids (MCFA) or "good fats" that the body can process and covert to energy immediately rather than storing as fat.

Ingredients

1 scoop unsweetened protein powder
1 ½ cup of sweetened coconut milk
½ frozen banana
1 frozen mango or 1 cup of cubed mango
1 Tbs of hemp seed (optional)
1 serving of canna coconut oil, olive oil, or tincture

Directions

Blend all ingredients in your blender or use your handheld immersion blender. Make sure the fats are thoroughly mixed. If you are using canna coconut oil, it will become solid when exposed to cold fruits. You may not be able to blend all the lumps in completely, but they will dissolve immediately in the mouth providing an interesting sensation. Serves 1-2

Breakfast

Hot Oatmeal

Oatmeal is a wonderful food. It is rich in fiber, aids in lowering cholesterol, and is relatively low in calories. I am generally disappointed with oatmeal that I don't make myself, as it is usually a flavorless gelatinous mess, but it doesn't have to be. May this recipe bring some life and taste to your morning routine.

Ingredients
1 ½ cup of water
¾ cup of steam rolled oats
2 Tbs organic raisins
Pinch of sea salt
¼ tsp cinnamon
1 tsp brown sugar, coconut sugar, or local honey, or for a sweeter flavor with
    fewer calories, try xylitol
1 serving of canna butter or canna coconut oil

Directions
Put raisins, water, and salt in a saucepan and bring to a boil. Reduce to medium heat. Add oats, stirring until you have the right consistency— creamy, not dry. If you overcook your oatmeal, simply add some more water. Add sweetener and butter (cannabis or plain) to taste. Remember, this should taste good and nourish your body! Serves 1

Variations:
Add ¼ of an organic apple, chopped, to the water when cooking for a sweeter apple pie taste. Bananas, berries, and nuts all make great additions. Some fresh shredded green apple for garnish is a nice touch!

Cold Oatmeal

This is a tasty summer treat for breakfast or a snack. It can even pass as a dessert!

Ingredients
¾ cup rolled (not instant) oats
1 Tbs chia seeds
3 Tbs organic raisins
½ tsp tincture (more if desired)
½ tsp cinnamon
1 cup of sweetened or unsweetened vanilla almond milk or coconut milk.
    Top off the jar with more liquid if there is room.

Directions
Fill a glass jar with the ingredients. Shake the ingredients and put your jar in the fridge. Stir or shake occasionally and let sit in the fridge for 2 hours up to 1

week. If you are looking to add more protein and hydration to the body, add ¼ cup of chia seeds and reduce the oatmeal to ½ cup. You may need to add more almond milk to get the desired consistency. This is also nice with fresh fruit instead of raisins. Serves 1-2

Quiche

Crust
½ cup (1 stick) chilled, unsalted canna butter
½ cup (1stick) chilled, unsalted non-medicated butter
3 cups flour (All-Purpose Gluten-Free Flour works well for the GF people in your life)
10 ounces chilled cream cheese
1 cup shredded cheddar cheese
1 tsp salt
¼ tsp white pepper, fresh ground is best
1 large egg

Directions
Pre-heat the oven to 375°F. Cut the butter into 16 small pieces. Place the butter and flour in the bowl of your food processor with the metal blade, and pulse until crumbly. Add the cream cheese, cheese, salt, and white pepper. Continue pulsing just until the dough forms a ball. Roll the dough out to make a large round for your pie shell or 8 individual portions. Lay the crust in the dish, poke holes in the bottom, and bake for 10 minutes. Remove from oven. Serves 6-8

Basic Filler Ingredients
3 Tbs canna butter melted
8 large eggs
3 cups half and half
¼ cup finely diced onions
¼ cup ground flax
2 Tbs hemp seed
1 tsp salt
1 tsp dried mustard
½ tsp cream of tartar
Additional ingredients: bacon, sausage, Gruyere, feta, cheddar, goat, or your favorite cheese, tomato, green chili, spinach, garlic, and anything else that sounds good.

Directions
Whisk the eggs until well beaten. Add the cooled melted butter then all remaining ingredients. Mix well, and add all the ingredients to the pie shell or ramekin. Bake for 60 minutes at 350°F. Let stand for 15 minutes before you cut and serve. For leftovers, reheat to 350°F for 30 minutes or until warm in the center. The quiche will be done when it is firm in the center.

The buttery crust is a wonderful delivery mechanism for cannabis oil or butter. However, a prepared pie crust will work just as well. If you are using a prepared crust and want to include cannabis, you have several options: brush the crust with butter, add more butter to the basic filler, or top off the quiche with tomatoes, garlic, and cilantro tossed in canna olive oil.

Variations:

Bacon Cheddar: Add 1 cup bacon (ham or sausage) + 1 cup shredded cheddar cheese to the basic filler recipe.

Spinach Gruyere: Add 1 cup raw or frozen spinach and 1 cup shredded Gruyere to the basic filler. If you are using frozen spinach, thaw and drain it before adding to the filler. If you are using raw spinach, give it a rough chop.

Tomato Feta: Add 1 cup diced tomatoes + 1 cup crumbled feta to the basic filler. You can also use sun dried tomatoes for a sweeter flavor. If you are using the dried version of sun dried tomatoes, rehydrate before using. If you are using a sun dried tomato from oil, use as is.

Two Minute Egg Tower

This is pretty tasty stuff—especially if you are looking for quick, easy, and substantial.

Using a microwave is not something I normally do. However, this particular recipe works well in the microwave if time is going to prevent you from having a healthy meal. It is based on using a 3 inch microwave-safe ramekin but can easily be scaled up if you are using a larger ramekin.

Ingredients
4 free-range eggs (they are higher in omegas)
⅛ tsp cream of tartar
¼ tsp dry mustard
¼ cup filtered water
½ tsp of canna butter per ramekin

Directions
Whisk all ingredients, except the canna butter, together using a fork or whisk. Line up 4 three inch ramekins, and place ½ tsp of canna butter in the bottom of each—unless you are microwaving the Egg Towers. Using your fingers, spread the butter evenly around the inside of the dishes. Divide the mixture evenly between the ramekins. Bake for 30-40 minutes at 325°F or microwave for 2 minutes on the medium setting. If you choose to use the microwave, add the butter at the end so you don't kill the cannabinoids. Serves 4

Variations:

I like to use a biscuit cutter to cut a corn tortilla piece to fit in the bottom of the ramekin. You can do the same with bread. Add to the mixture ½ cup of your favorite cheese and maybe ½ cup of sautéed onions or ⅛ cup of chopped spinach to each ramekin. Crumbled bacon or sausage is nice, too.

Top this wonderful food with your favorite salsa, fresh tomatoes, or chives. Salt and pepper to taste at the table.

Sautéed Apples

Do you like simple and wonderful? This large, single-serving breakfast or dessert takes less than 5 minutes to prepare. This is also a great dessert when topped with cream or served over ice cream. Leftovers can be added to a shake, turned into apple sauce, served with pork chops, or used for empanada filling. Or add dried fruits and nuts and use as a stuffing with your favorite meat.

Ingredients

1 organic apple cored and diced with skin on
2 Tbs organic raisins
1 tsp dark brown sugar, coconut sugar, or agave nectar
½-2 tsp unsalted canna butter or ghee
½ Tbs of un-medicated, unsalted butter
Pinch sea salt
Dash cinnamon
Dash nutmeg

Directions

Mix the ingredients in a bowl (or mug for microwave use). If you are using agave nectar or honey, wait to add it until after the apples are soft. Sauté on the stove top with desired amount of canna butter and specified amount of non-medicated butter. Continue to stir until the apples reach the desired softness, 5-10 minutes.

To cook in the microwave, place the apple mixture in a serving dish and microwave for 35-50 seconds. Add canna butter, stir, and enjoy. Do NOT nuke canna butter, and be careful not to overcook the apples. Serves 1

Condiments

Pesto

Oh how I love pesto! This flavorful sauce is a great way to deliver nutrition and medicine. The basic pesto recipe starts with an herb, an oil, and garlic. From there you can do all sorts of great things. Below are two of my favorite recipes and several of my favorite versions of each.

Ingredients
2 bunches cleaned organic cilantro or basil
½ cup canna olive oil
2-4 large cloves garlic (depending on your love of garlic)
Salt to taste

Directions
Add the herbs, garlic, salt, and ¼ cup canna olive oil to the food processor and puree. Slowly drizzle more olive oil into the food processor until the pesto is creamy and well blended. Pesto will keep in the fridge for 2-3 weeks and longer in the freezer. When I have leftover fresh pesto, I put the extra in ice cube trays and freeze. Then I can pull out just a few pesto ice cubes at a time rather than thawing the whole batch. Makes ¾ cups

Variations:
Add any one, or a combination, of the following to mix up the pesto flavor: toasted nuts, almonds, walnuts, pine nuts, macadamias, or pecans. Adding cheese to the mix is also a great way to change up the flavor. Parmesan and other dry cheeses (pecorino, asiago, etc.) work best.

Lemon Edamame Spread

Ingredients
2 cups organic shelled frozen edamame beans (soybeans) heated per directions on the package
Juice of 2 lemons
1 large garlic clove
½ cup canna olive oil
1 tsp sea salt

Directions
Put all ingredients in the food processor and puree until smooth. This spread tastes great on dense bread served as a tea snack, on a sandwich with leafy greens and sprouts, or as a dip for chips and veggies. I was amazed at how many of the 6th graders in the healthy snack programs I taught in my local school district not only ate this but asked for more— canna free of course. Serves 4

Croutons

Put 1-2 tsp of canna butter on both sides of a slice of your favorite bread. Dust with garlic powder, sea salt, and possibly your favorite herbs. Cut the bread into small bite sized pieces, place them on a cookie tray, and toast at 300°F until the bread turns a light golden brown and the bread is crispy. This will take 7-10 minutes Serves 1

Dressings

Garlic Lemon Dressing

Ingredients
2 cloves fresh garlic
⅛ cup canna oil
¼ tsp lemon zest
1 lemon juiced
Salt and pepper to taste
Squirt of honey to cut acidity

Directions
Blend all ingredients in a small food processor or with your immersion blender. This basic dressing is delicious on salads, grilled/sautéed vegetables, grilled/baked chicken, fish, and roasted potatoes. Serves 4

Variations:
- Add ¼ cup cream and 1 Tbs of butter to make a cream sauce for pasta, chicken, fish, or pork.
- Add 1 tsp sugar or honey and ⅛ cup of white wine or champagne, and you have a slightly sweeter dressing that is wonderful on salad. Add a big strawberry for an even sweeter dressing.

Dijon Dressing

Ingredients
1 Tbs balsamic vinegar
3 Tbs Dijon mustard
3 Tbs local honey
2 cloves garlic
2 small minced shallots
¼ tsp sea salt
¼ tsp pepper
1 cup canna olive oil
1 Tbs hemp seeds

Directions
Puree all ingredients in a blender or emersion blender and serve. This dressing is great on salads and is also a good addition atop white fish before or after it is grilled. You can also toss baby greens with this dressing, and add them to a turkey or veggie wrap for extra flavor. Serves 8

Blueberry Balsamic

Ingredients

3 Tbs balsamic vinegar
1 Tbs apple cider vinegar
1 cup blueberries fresh or frozen
8-10 cherry tomatoes
2 clove garlic chopped
3 Tbs regular olive oil
1 cup canna olive oil
1 tsp fresh lemon juice
Sea salt to taste

Directions

Sautee balsamic vinegar, blueberries, tomato, garlic, and half the olive oil over medium heat. Once the berries and tomatoes are fully cooked and the mixture has been reduced, approximately 3-5 minutes, remove from heat and let cool. Add the apple cider vinegar, lemon juice, remaining olive oil, and canna oil, and puree all ingredients. I know tomatoes and blueberries sound like a weird combo, but I promise it works. Use this dressing to top off a pork chop or fish fillet or toss over mixed field greens with a variety of your favorite veggies, feta, and some toasted pecans. Serves 8-10

Appetizers and Basics

Cheese Bread

For all my talk about healthy eating and the importance of nutritional density, this is where I go off track. This bread is a delicious treat of epic proportions that few people can resist. When my family or friends find out this is on the menu, they go nuts.

This recipe is easy to modify if you are cooking for a mix of people who are medicating and those who are not. Simply make the recipe with regular butter and add 1 tsp of canna butter to the pieces of bread for those medicating. If you are planning on each person eating two pieces of bread, use ½ tsp of cannabis butter per piece. If you are gluten free, try Udi brand French bread. It will blow your mind!

Ingredients
4 large cloves garlic (more if you like) finely chopped
2 cups shredded mozzarella or an Italian cheese blend
1 cup shredded parmesan
½ cup canna butter, melted
½ cup mayonnaise
½ tsp garlic powder
Salt and pepper to taste
Small loaf of French bread

Directions
If you are using gluten free sandwich bread instead of gluten free French bread,, before you add the spread, toast the side that will hold the cheese spread. Then apply the spread to the toasted side. Otherwise, slice regular bread or rolls in half, or cut into individual pieces. Mix the cheese, garlic, butter, mayo, salt, and pepper. Mix well, and spread over the cut side of the bread. Bake face up at 350°F until the tops are browned to your liking—generally 7-9 minutes. While this recipe may not be so good for your waistline, it is good for your soul!

Enjoy as an appetizer or with spaghetti, lasagna, or your favorite dish. Serves 8

Soda Bread (Gluten Free)

This recipe comes from the wonderful cookbook *Healthy Gluten-Free Cooking* by Darina Allen with Rosemary Kearney. (Allen and Kearney 2005) No one will know this is gluten free. It is especially wonderful with soups, stews, and Italian food. It was the first bread I made successfully after I went gluten free. It was a big deal to me because I was desperately missing the texture of bread. When it came out of the oven, I nearly cried.

Ingredients
2 ¼ cups rice flour
1 cup (4 oz.) tapioca flour

½ cup (2 oz.) dried milk
1 scant tsp baking soda
1 heaped tsp gluten free baking powder
1 tsp salt
1 heaped tsp xanthum gum
2 Tbs superfine sugar
1 egg lightly beaten
1¼-1½ (10-12 oz.) buttermilk

Directions

Note: If you are using all-purpose gluten free flour with xanthan gum, simply use 3 ¼ cups of the four in place of the rice/tapioca/xanthan gum. If your all-purpose mix does not have xanthan gum, be sure to include it, or your bread will fall apart. If you want to use regular wheat flour, use 3 ¼ cups and do not add xanthan gum. FYI, xanthan gum is what holds together gluten free breads.

Pre-heat the oven to 450°F degrees. Sift all dry ingredients together in a large bowl. Mix well by lifting the dry ingredients up in your hands and then letting them fall back into the bowl through your fingers. This adds more air, and therefore more lightness, to your finished bread. Lightly whisk the egg and buttermilk together. Make a well in the center and pour in most of the egg and buttermilk at once. Using one hand, with your fingers stiff and out stretched like a claw, stir in a full circular movement from the center to the outside of the bowl in ever-increasing circles adding a little more buttermilk if necessary. The dough should be soft but not sticky. Mix as quickly and gently as possible to keep the bread light and airy. The key is not to over mix the dough. When the dough is fully mixed, turn it out onto a rice floured surface.

Wash and dry your hands. With rice floured fingers, roll lightly for a few seconds—just enough to tidy it. Pat the dough into a round about 2 inches in height.

Place in the oven for 5 minutes, then reduce the temperature to 350°F for a further 25-30 minutes or until done. If in doubt, tap the bottom of the bread; if it is cooked, it will sound hollow. Cool on a wire rack.

Serve warm with your favorite version of canna butter or a dipping sauce made with canna oil. Yummy! Serves 8

Hummus

Ingredients

2 14 oz. cans of garbanzo beans drained or 4 cups of cooked garbanzo beans
2 lemons juiced and seeds strained
½-1 cup canna olive oil
⅓-½ cup tahini – available at most grocery stores with a health or
    international section
2 medium cloves of garlic
1 tsp sea salt – add more if needed
¼ tsp cumin

Directions

In a food processor add garbanzo, tahini, garlic, salt, cumin, juice of 1 lemon, and ½ cup of canna olive oil. Puree. Taste. Add the additional lemon gradually to taste. If the mixture is too thick, add olive oil 1 Tbs at a time until you have the desired texture. Serve with chips, crackers, pita bread, or veggies. Serves 4

Variations: Add a small can of chipotle pepper without the sauce to increase the heat, or add 1-2 roasted red bell peppers for a different flavor. This makes a great snack, appetizer, side, or sandwich spread.

Soups

Sweet Potato Soup with Cilantro Cream

Ingredients
3 large sweet potatoes peeled and cut in 1" chunks
4 cups low sodium chicken stock
1 large onion cut in quarters
1 tsp sea salt
1 seeded jalapeño (optional)
1 tsp cracked pepper
1 cup Greek or Bulgarian plain yogurt
3-4 Tbs canna oil (you can use ½ oil, ½ butter for a great flavor)
1 clove garlic
½ bunch cilantro

Directions
Add salt, peeled and diced sweet potatoes, onion, and jalapeño to the chicken stock. Bring to a boil and then cook at a simmer until the potatoes are very soft. You can take the jalapeño out at this time for a milder spice, or leave it in for a spicier flavor. Use a blender or an immersion blender to puree the soup until smooth. Add salt and pepper.

In a separate container, puree the yogurt, garlic, cilantro, canna oil, and a pinch of sea salt. Put the mixture in a squeeze bottle for easy dispensing.

Fill each bowl ¾ of the way with soup. Add approximately 1½ Tbs of yogurt cilantro cream from the squeeze bottle; it is fun to make nice decorations on top of the bowl. Add a few sprigs of cilantro and serve. It's delicious with salad and hot bread. Serves 6-8

Beef and Barley Soup

Ingredients
1 lb ground beef (pork, turkey, chicken, or tofu)
1½ cups chopped onion
4 cups cooked pearled barley
2 large cloves garlic
4 tsp canna oil
1 cup chopped red bell pepper
3 cups sliced or quartered mushrooms
2 tsp Better Than Bullion paste
1 cup water
1 box or 2½ cups organic beef or vegetable broth
2 cups large cut carrots
2 large potatoes cubed
1 yellow onion chopped

1 cup cut green beans

1 cup anything else you want to throw in: corn, cooked soybeans, cooked kidney beans, spinach, etc.

Directions

In a skillet, sauté ½ cup onions and the mushrooms in 1 tsp canna oil over medium heat for 1-2 minutes. Add water and bullion. Once the bullion is fully dissolved, use a hand blender or food processor to puree. Hold back a portion of mushrooms to add later. This is the mushroom gravy. Pour into a dish and set aside.

Add the remaining 2 tsp of oil, garlic, and onion to the hot skillet and sauté 2 minutes. Once translucent, add the beef until it is browned—approximately 5-7 minutes. Add the cooked barley, mushroom gravy, and raw red bell pepper. Add broth or stock and all ingredients (except carrots) in a soup pot and cook until the potatoes are ready to eat, which will take approximately 25 minutes. Add carrots 15 minutes before serving.

If you wish to add more cannabis, make cannabis croutons to top the soup. [See, "Croutons", on page 268.] Serves 6-8

Lentil Soup

Ingredients

2-3 Tbs of canna coconut oil (or other canna fat)

1 cup finely diced yellow onion

2 cloves garlic, finely diced

2 cups dried lentils

2 ½ cups vegetable or chicken stock

1 can (14 ounces) coconut milk

Salt and pepper to taste

Directions

Sauté onions and garlic in the canna coconut oil over medium heat until translucent (2 minutes). Add remaining ingredients. Bring to a simmer then reduce to medium-low heat. Simmer for 2-3 hours until lentils are soft. Use an immersion blender to make the soup creamier. Either cream completely or give it a few pulses. If you don't have an immersion blender, put 2 cups of soup into the blender or food processor, puree, and add back to the soup. To make this more nutritious, top the soup with 2-4 tablespoons of hemp seeds before serving. Serves 6-8

Ecuadorean Quinoa Stew

Don't curl up your nose at this dish until you've tried it. My friend Dianna made it for lunch one day. Admittedly, I was not too excited when she described it, but it would have been rude to express my skepticism. So I tried it, and it is scrumptious! After my mom died, Dianna was supportive at times when others had moved on. She has also been supportive of my book and my education efforts. It seemed fitting to include her awesome recipe in the book. Besides, it is so good it would be wrong not to share it.

Quinoa is an ancient seed (most people refer to it as a grain) from South America. It is an excellent source of essential amino acids and calcium and has more protein than any grain. Because its carbohydrates are processed slowly, it does not cause a spike in blood sugar. I usually serve this as a main dish. It keeps well for several days in the refrigerator.

Ingredients
½ cup dry quinoa
2 Tbs canna olive oil
1 Tbs canna butter
2 cups chopped onion
1 tsp sea salt
1 cup diced potatoes
1 cup chopped red or green bell peppers
1 tsp ground coriander
1 tsp ground cumin
1 tsp dried oregano
½ tsp ground black pepper
3 cups water or vegetable stock
1½ cups chopped fresh tomatoes or a 14.5 oz. can of chopped tomatoes, un-drained
1 cup diced zucchini or yellow squash
1 Tbs fresh lemon juice

Optional Additions: Chopped scallion, chopped fresh cilantro, crumbled tortilla chips, grated Cheddar or Monterey Jack cheese.

Directions
Rinse quinoa in a fine mesh strainer under cold running water until it stops making bubbles. Set aside to drain. If you do not rinse the quinoa your dish will taste soapy.

Warm oil and butter in a non-reactive soup pot, add the onions and salt, and cover and cook on medium heat for 5 minutes stirring occasionally. Add drained quinoa, potatoes, bell peppers, coriander, cumin, oregano, black pepper, water or stock, and tomatoes. Cover and bring to a boil over high heat. Reduce heat and simmer 15-20 minutes or until all veggies are tender. Remove from heat.

Stir in the lemon juice. If desired, serve with a sprinkling of scallions, tortilla chips, and grated cheese. A dollop of Greek yogurt on top is delicious and will add protein. Additional butter or oil can be used for a more potent dish. Serves 6-8

Variation:
Meat lovers can add pieces of rotisserie chicken.

Main Dishes

Cilantro Beef

Ingredients

½ lb thinly sliced grass-fed sirloin or rump roast shaved to a #1 slice on a deli slicer if possible

3 Tbs basic cilantro pesto [See "Pesto", on page 268.]

1 small onion sliced thinly leaving the slices in 1" long pieces and 1 red bell pepper sliced in rounds or spears

Directions

Add 2 Tbs of cilantro pesto to a warming pan over medium heat. Add onion and cook 2 minutes or until translucent. Add meat and peppers together. Cook meat approximately 2-4 minutes until medium. Turn off heat, add 1 more tablespoon of pesto, and stir. Serve alone or over rice, quinoa, or mashed organic potatoes, and top with fresh cilantro. Serves 2

Variation:

For a vegetarian version, use sliced portabella and shitake mushroom in place of beef.

Chicken Pot Pie

I adapted this delicious recipe from the cookbook *The Pastry Queen: Royally Good Recipes* by Rebecca Rather. You can use canna butter in any combination of the filling, cream sauce, or crust. DO NOT let the ingredients list scare you; this is a simple and relatively quick recipe that takes only 60-90 minutes to make. Your taste buds, belly, and soul will thank you!

Filling

3 Tbs unsalted butter (canna butter or not)

1 medium yellow onion, chopped

1 large russet potato, peeled and diced

3 cloves garlic, minced

1 red bell pepper, diced

8 oz button mushrooms, sliced

Salt and fresh ground black pepper

1 cooked rotisserie chicken or a whole stewed chicken cooled, skin and bones removed, meat cut into cubes

8 oz fresh green beans cut into pieces and blanched

1 (8 oz) package frozen peas

Directions

Add butter, onions, and garlic to a pan over medium heat. Sauté 3-5 minutes, add all other ingredients, and cook 10-15 minutes. I like to add carrots, spinach, and peas at the end after the mix has been taken off the heat. To blanch the green beans, simply let them cook in salted boiling water for 2 minutes. Pull out of the water and place them into a bowl of ice water to cool. They are ready to add to the mixture. Serves 8

Cream Sauce
½ cup (1 stick) unsalted butter (canna or not)

1 cup all-purpose flour (for gluten-free, try ⅔ cup gluten free flour with xanthan already added + 1 Tbs organic corn starch or use ½ cup of arrow root)

2½ cups chicken stock, preferably homemade (otherwise choose a low sodium stock)

½ cup heavy whipping cream (or 1⅓ cup whole milk if using the gluten free flour)

1 tsp garlic powder

1 tsp salt

Dash nutmeg

Dash white pepper

Fresh ground pepper to taste

Dash Tabasco sauce

In a separate pot from the sautéing veggie mix, melt butter over medium heat, add flour (or cornstarch/arrowroot), and whisk. Once smooth, add chicken stock and all other ingredients steadily whisking all the while. Cook over medium heat while the mixture thickens to the consistency of cream soup. If it gets too thick, add more stock, milk, or cream until you have the desired consistency.

Remove from heat. Mix sauce with the chicken and veggie mixture.

Crust
1 cup (2 sticks) chilled, unsalted canna butter or use half canna butter and half non-medicated butter.

3 cups flour (all purpose gluten free flour works well)

10 oz chilled cream cheese

1 tsp of salt

¼ tsp of white pepper, fresh ground is best

1 large egg

Directions
Pre-heat the oven to 375°F. Cut the butter into small pieces. Place the butter and flour in the bowl of a food processor with a metal blade and pulse until the butter and flour are crumbly. Add the cream cheese, salt, and white pepper. Continue pulsing until the dough forms a ball.

Set the dough on a flat surface dusted with flour/arrowroot. Use a floured rolling pin to roll out to ¼ inch thickness. Measure the diameter of the pot, pie bowl, or casserole dish you will use. Cut the dough 1½ inches larger than the diameter. Lay the dough rounds on top of the pie or pies making sure dough hangs evenly over each bowl. Whisk egg in a small bowl. Brush dough lightly with beaten egg. Bake 20-25 minutes until golden brown. Serve immediately. This dish keeps well. You can also make individual portions and freeze for future use.

Variations: What do you like in pot pie? Carrots, chopped spinach, asparagus, and corn are good additions or substitutes for anything on the list.

If you want to make this dish non-medicated but wish to serve it to someone who needs the medicine, simply use non-medicated butter throughout the recipe. At the time of serving, add ½-1 tsp of canna butter to the patient's portion while it is hot.

Veggie Beef Turnovers

My good friend Chelsea made these for my family the week before my mom passed. They were so comforting. We added a teaspoon and a half of canna butter to my mom's serving. She really enjoyed these, and I hope you do, too!

Chelsea lost her mother Gloria to lung cancer a little more than a year before my mother died. Chelsea has often remarked how she wishes her mother would have been open to trying cannabis for her pain. She is convinced that if her mom would have been willing to try it she would have not suffered as she did.

Chelsea recommends the VIP brand mini pie crusts because they are so buttery, but any crust will do including mini homemade crusts like Elaine's Pastry Crust in the "Dessert", on page 291.

Ingredients
8 Mini frozen pie crusts
1 lb ground beef (chicken or turkey)
1½ cups potato, sliced into small cubes
1 small carrot, shredded
2 sticks celery, chopped
Salt and pepper to taste
½ tsp onion powder
1 tsp garlic powder

Directions
Preheat oven to 375°F. In a large sauce pan, sauté beef on medium heat until cooked thoroughly; season to taste with salt and pepper. Should take 5-7 minutes. Add raw potatoes, carrots, and celery. Add enough water to just cover beef and veggie mixture. Let simmer until potatoes are tender and the mixture has thickened. You can add 1 tsp corn starch, flour, or arrowroot if a thicker "gravy" is desired.

Keep 4 crusts in their foil tins, and fill them heaping full with the mixture. Remove the other 4 crusts from their tins. Place pie crusts mouth down atop each filled pie. Place in oven for approximately 25 minutes or until the top crust is slightly browned. Enjoy! Serves 4

Tuna Noodle Casserole

This recipe always seemed like poverty food to me, so I used to look down my nose when Mom made it. I probably even gave her an eye roll when she told me we'd be having this for dinner. After leaving home for college, I forgot about this meal. One day in my early thirties, I found myself craving it. It's packed with lots of flavor, protein, and some fiber. There is something warming and soulful about it. Every time I make it, I cannot help but chuckle and wish my mother could taste my version of her tuna noodle casserole. I think she would like it! The only difference between our recipes is that I add garlic, onion, and green peas.

Ingredients

2 cups egg noodles or gluten free noodles
5 cups salted water – use 2 tsp of salt
2 (5 oz) cans tuna
3 cloves garlic, chopped
1 small onion, finely diced
3 Tbs canna butter or oil (do not use coconut oil; it will not taste good)
1 12 oz can low sodium cream of mushroom soup. If you require a gluten free soup, try Pacific Brand.
1-2 cups sliced mushrooms—any mushroom but those boring button mushrooms, which have no real nutritional value. Try shitake or cremini mushrooms instead
1 cup frozen green peas
Fresh ground black pepper
Sea salt

Directions

Boil noodles in salted water until done. The package will tell you how long. Strain noodles reserving 1 cup of water. Rinse noodles with cool water and set aside in the colander. Add butter, ⅔ of the garlic, and all the onion and mushrooms to the pot you cooked the pasta in and cook for 3 minutes on medium heat until garlic and onions are translucent. Add tuna, mushroom soup, and ½ cup of reserve water from the pasta or milk. Stir over medium heat until the condensed soup mixture becomes creamy and smooth. Add the noodles and frozen peas. Cook another 3 minutes or until the peas are warmed through. If you want the mushroom sauce to be thinner, add 1 Tbs at a time of the reserved water or milk until the sauce reaches your desired consistency. Add the rest of the raw garlic, add salt and pepper to taste, and enjoy.

This is wonderful served alone as a one dish meal or served on a bed of mashed potatoes or quinoa with a side salad. Serves 4 to 6

Green Chicken Enchiladas

When I tell people I am making this recipe, they nearly invite themselves over for dinner. It is an excellent way to sneak in veggies for picky eaters.

Ingredients

2 cups shredded cooked chicken or turkey (use leftover baked or rotisserie chicken if you have it). Portabella mushrooms are a good substitute if you are vegetarian, but they need to be cooked and drained first.
1½ cups shredded zucchini or chopped spinach (These ingredients add nutrients, fiber, flavor, and moisture. My preference is to use zucchini.)

2 cups shredded mozzarella, Monterrey jack, or your favorite mild cheese

12-18 corn tortillas, the fresher and bigger the better. If you have a tortillaria nearby, they will have the best tortillias

4 cups of your favorite green salsa

2 large avocados

2-4 cloves garlic (depending on how much you love it)

1½ cups Greek yogurt – my favorite brand is Fage

½ bunch cilantro, stems and all (approximately 1 cup)

2 Tbs water

1 tsp salt

5-12 Tbs of canna butter –depending on strength desired

Directions

This recipe doesn't need much cooking once it's assembled and is a quick and easy way to get a hearty no-fuss meal on the table. It will take longer to read this and pull out the ingredients than it will to put it together. It is easy to make for the whole family and ensures that only those who need it receive the medicine. Simply prepare two pans, one with canna butter and one without. If you don't want to use two pans, make the recipe without canna butter. When the enchiladas are done, give them 10 minutes to rest. Remove the portion for the one medicating and add ½-1 tsp of canna butter to their portion while it is hot.

Pre-heat oven to 350°F.

Make the green sauce: Mix 4 cups of salsa with the garlic, 2 large avocados, 1½-2 cups of yogurt, cilantro, and salt in a blender or food processor, or mix with an immersion blender. Pour a few tablespoons of sauce into the bottom of the casserole dish. Add 2 Tbsp of water to the mixture and spread evenly on the bottom. Reserve the rest.

Soften tortillas with a tortilla steamer or warm them for 20 seconds per side over an open flame on your stove top. Doing this is more time consuming but does enhance the flavor. Wrap tortillas in a dishcloth to keep them pliable until you are ready to fill them.

Assemble each enchilada: spread ¼ teaspoon of canna butter or regular butter on a tortilla, lay it flat, and place some filling in a line down the center. Start with adding cheese – 1-2 Tbs or a healthy pinch, several pieces of shredded chicken (2 Tbs), then add a pinch (1-2 Tbs) of zucchini or spinach. You may have to adjust the volume for filling the tortilla depending on its size. Wrap the tortilla tightly and place in the pan. Repeat until the pan is full.

Pack the enchiladas so they fit into the dish tightly. Cover completely with the green sauce. Bake for 20-30 minutes at 350°F or until enchiladas are hot in the center and the sides are bubbling. About10 minutes before the enchiladas are ready to be removed from the oven, add more cheese to the top if you like. Let sit for 10 minutes before serving.

Toppings include fresh chopped cilantro, the cilantro pesto in this recipe book and Greek yogurt. Serve with a side salad or the Herbed Rice listed page 287 and some black beans, and you have a delicious, well-balanced meal. Serves 4-6

Sautéed Cabbage and Sausage

Cabbage is an underappreciated food. It is tasty and good for you. I'm still amazed that I'm able to get my nephew, who is ten, to eat this. He loves it—sans the cannabis of course!

Ingredients

4 cups cabbage cut into pieces the length and width of an average index finger
½ lb. ground pork sausage
1-2 Tbs of canna oil or butter or a combo of half of each for a great flavor
3 cloves garlic, chopped
2 green onions, sliced thinly (including the tops)
1 Tbs Braggs Amino Acids (or quality low sodium Tamari sauce)

Directions

Brown the sausage. If you need to add oil for browning, do not add canna oil. Use olive or another type of oil, and be careful the oil does not get so hot it smokes. Once browned, either rinse the sausage or use a paper towel to dab off the grease.

Add ⅔ of the garlic and all the canna oil to the pan, and cook on low heat for 2 minutes. Add the pork sausage back to the pan and brown it further by increasing the heat to medium. Once the meat is completely browned, add shredded cabbage and cook for 2-3 minutes. Be careful not to overcook the cabbage, and do not get the canna oil or butter too hot. Turn off the heat and finish by adding the remaining garlic, green onions, and Braggs Amino Acids. Serves 2 (meal)-4 (side dish)

Parmesan and Herb Pasta

This recipe is so easy!

Ingredients

1 Tbs canna butter
1 Tbs canna oil
1½ cup pasta – elbow macaroni, spirals, spaghetti, or bow tie. For those who are gluten free, try this recipe with Tikayada or King Soba brand noodles
4 minced cloves garlic
¼ cup shredded parmesan cheese
2 Tbs chopped fresh basil
1 cup diced cherry tomatoes

Directions

Boil pasta until it is al dente. Drain well. Leave pasta in the strainer; add oil, butter, and garlic to the pasta pot and sauté for 2-3 minutes over medium heat. Add pasta back into the pot with the parmesan, tomatoes, salt, and crushed black pepper. Add basil at the end and serve. This is great with baked or grilled chicken or with a simple side salad. If more medication is desired, add it to the warm pasta at the end. This is nice hot or cold. Serves 2

Herb Spring Rolls

This is an excellent, easy, and light dish that can be served with or without meat.

Ingredients
12 rice paper wrappers
12 pieces leafy green lettuce
1 cucumber, peeled and sliced in ½ rounds
6 pieces boiled or grilled shrimp cut in half or 6 strips of chicken the length and thickness of your index finger
1 cup shredded carrots
1 cup broccoli sprouts
1 Tbs fresh grated ginger
6 tsp cilantro or basil pesto [See "Pesto", on page 268.]

Directions
Fill a large dinner plate with water. Place rice paper in the water until it is completely soft and pliable. Remove it from the water to another plate. Assemble the spring rolls using 2 rice paper sheets per wrap for optimum chewiness: position 2 pieces of shrimp or 1 piece of chicken in the middle, top with layers of lettuce, cucumber wedges, carrots, and sprouts. Add 1 tsp pesto down the middle of the roll, tuck rice paper in on each end, then roll and enjoy! Serves 6

Black Gold Chili

One day I was craving chili but wanted something really healthy. I challenged myself to make a chili that is both super delicious and packed with nutrients. I call this sneaky food! It is true some of the ingredients may seem a little weird, but they are worth studying and figuring out how to incorporate into your regular diet.

Ingredients
3 cups cooked black beans (homemade or canned)
3 cups beef stock (homemade is best or choose low sodium)
1 lb grass fed ground beef (or turkey)
2 medium onions chopped + ½ cup chopped onion if cooking the black beans at home.
4 cloves garlic
4 Tbs canna oil or butter (add up to 8 total depending on how potent you want it)
3 large bay leaves
1 cup black rice
1 Tbs black lava salt (or other quality salt)
1 cup quinoa
½ cup Chia seed
½ cup ground flax
Toppings: Greek yogurt, chopped green onion, shredded cheese, chopped cilantro

Directions

If you choose to cook the black beans yourself, begin by boiling 4 cups of water. Take off the heat. Add 2 cups of dried beans and let sit for 2-4 hours. Bring to a boil then reduce to medium-low heat and let simmer for an hour or more. Add 2 teaspoons sea salt (black salt if you can get it), 3 bay leaves, and ½ cup chopped onion (this is in addition to what is already listed in the recipe) to the mix. Once the beans are soft, they are ready to use. Scoop out 3 cups of beans. It is okay to use some of the juice, but make sure you have mostly beans in your 3 cups. Reserve the bean juice for later in case you need to add moisture to the chili. If this sounds like too much trouble, open several cans of black beans.

In your stock or soup pot, brown the ground beef with 2 tablespoons of canna butter or oil, half of the chopped garlic, half of the onion, and ½ teaspoon of black salt. If you wish to enhance the potency of this dish, add 1 Tbs of decarboxylated finely ground cannabis bud or leaf powder to the ground beef. Allow ingredients to simmer 15-20 minutes before adding the other ingredients so the fats can help further release THC and CBD from the powder.

Add liquids and all other ingredients except the ground flax seed. The rice, quinoa, and chia seed will double in size. Be sure to stir every 10-15 minutes, and monitor the liquid level. It will take about an hour for everything to cook. If the chili gets too dry, simply add more beef stock, bean juice, or water as needed. Add the freshly ground flax seed 15 minutes before you are ready to serve. Lower the heat to the lowest setting, and continue to simmer lightly. Eat alone or with any combination of the toppings mentioned. Enjoy! Serves 6-8

Sides and Salads

Squash Ribbon Salad

Ingredients

3-4 medium squash medley with ends removed–a mix of yellow and zucchini
makes a prettier dish
1 lemon
¼ cup canna oil
Sea salt to taste

Directions

Use a potato or carrot peeler to shave the squash into ribbons. Hold the peeler
at the top of the squash and slice downward repeatedly until the entire squash
is in paper thin ribbons. Squeeze the fresh lemon over the squash ribbons, and
add canna oil, a pinch of salt, and some fresh cracked pepper. Toss and serve.
Serves 4

Variations:

Add one of the pestos in place of the canna oil. Fresh grated parmesan is nice,
too!

This dish is especially nice with grilled meats in the summer. It makes a nice
nest for grilled or baked fish.

Quinoa Tabouli

This is the tabouli solution for gluten-sensitive folks, but regardless whether
you are gluten free or not, give it a try! It is full of protein and easily digestible.

Ingredients

3 cups cooked quinoa
2 cups chopped fresh parsley
½ cup chopped mint
1 large juiced lemon
1 bunch green onions chopped
1 cucumber diced
4 diced ripe Roma tomatoes
½-¾cup canna olive oil
Salt and pepper to taste

Directions

First, you must rinse your quinoa to remove saponin, which is a natural
coating on the grain; otherwise, it will have a soapy flavor. Rinse quinoa until
it stops producing bubbles. Dr. Russo tells me heating it in a dry skillet also
works. Cook 1 cup of grain in two cups of water just like you cook rice; you can
even use a rice cooker. One cup of dried quinoa yields 3 cups of cooked quinoa.
Toss the ingredients, chill, and serve.

This is a great salad to keep in the fridge all the time. It is packed with flavor, protein, raw veggies, and herbs. It is highly alkalizing and easy to digest. Parsley is good for helping cleanse the blood. Serves 4

Broccoli Slaw

My sister introduced me to this concoction. It is wildly delicious and nutritious. It is great with grilled foods, summer meals, sandwiches, tacos, quesadillas, and all things Mexican. It's also yummy on a grilled pork chop (or fish) taco in a corn tortilla—heaven!

Ingredients
3-4 cups of pre-packaged broccoli slaw or finely shredded cabbage
1 large avocado
½ cup chopped cilantro
2 limes
4 Tbs canna olive oil
2 Tbs mayonnaise
Sea salt and pepper to taste

Directions
Mix the broccoli slaw (or cabbage) and cilantro in a salad bowl. Add the juice of both limes, the mayo, and the canna oil. Cut your avocado into chunky square pieces, add to the slaw, and stir until the avocado is well blended throughout. Salt and pepper to taste. Serves 4

Herbed Rice

Ingredients
2 cups cooked white or brown rice (I use ½ and ½)
2-4 Tbs of cilantro or basil pesto [See "Pesto", on page 268.]

Directions
Combine rice and pesto and enjoy. This simple side dish is a great compliment to grilled and baked meats and fish. Serves 4

Variation:
Add chopped tomato for flavor and color—especially when they are in season. Use quinoa instead of rice, or use a combination of rice and quinoa.

Stir Fried Rice

Ingredients
2 cups white or brown rice or quinoa (or try using half rice, half quinoa)
1 small diced onion
3 cloves of garlic
1 tsp fresh grated ginger

2 Tbs canna oil
1 tsp toasted sesame oil
½ cup frozen green peas or edamame
½ cup frozen or canned organic corn
½ cup shredded carrots
1 tsp Braggs Amino Acids–add more to taste if you prefer a saltier stir fry.

Directions

Sauté the onions and two thirds of your garlic (reserve the rest) in the canna oil. Once translucent, add the sesame oil and rice and stir well until all the rice is coated with oil. Allow the rice 1 minute between each stir for the rice to brown somewhat. Then add all the veggies. Cook for 3 minutes. Add the remaining garlic, fresh ginger, and Braggs Amino Acids or a quality shoyu or tamari sauce. You can also add left over cubes of pork, chicken, or tofu to make this a hearty meal. Serves 2-4

Robin Hood Corn

Ingredients

2 Tbs canna butter
½ cup yellow onion
½ block (5 oz) cream cheese cut into small cubes
2 cups organic sweet corn, fresh or frozen
1 cup diced red bell pepper

Directions

Sauté butter, onion, garlic, and corn on low to medium heat. Be careful of overheating. Allow corn to lightly caramelize for 5 minutes. Add cubes of cream cheese. Allow cream cheese to melt slowly on low heat. Stir until melted completely. Cook 15-20 minutes and serve. Add crushed black pepper and salt to taste. If you want to spice this up, try adding a fresh jalapeño. Serves 4

Baked Broccoli with Lemon Garlic Sauce

Ingredients

1 small head broccoli
1 large clove garlic
¼ tsp organic lemon zest. When using zest, I suggest organic lemons; the oil in the skin is a powerful therapeutic, and we want it to be as clean and chemical free as possible.
1 lemon juiced
⅛ cup canna olive oil or butter or a mix of both for great flavor. For an Asian twist, use canna coconut oil instead.
Pinch of salt

Directions

Bake or grill the broccoli to your liking. If you are baking the broccoli, it takes 5-7 minutes under the broiler or a similar time on the grill. If grilling, place the broccoli to the side of the flame for the first 4 minutes and then over a soft flame for 2-3 minutes—turning it once during that time. Be careful not to overcook and deplete the nutrients. Puree or whisk together the olive oil and garlic and slowly add lemon juice, then zest. Salt to taste. Once the broccoli is ready, pour the mixture over the broccoli and serve. This is great with a white fish or other mild fish. You can add (or substitute) Brussels sprouts, steamed spinach, steamed kale, green beans, and cauliflower. Serves 2

Spaghetti Squash

Ingredients

1 medium spaghetti squash
1 clove garlic diced
2 Tbs canna butter
½ tsp nutmeg
½ tsp salt
½ tsp cracked black pepper

Directions

Cut squash in half lengthwise. Bake in a casserole dish cut side down with an inch of water in it for 50 minutes. In a skillet, sauté the garlic, oil, and spices together over medium heat. Once the squash is soft, scoop out the insides and toss in the skillet with the other ingredients. Once completely blended, cook over medium heat for another 2 minutes. Serves 4

Fiery Mashed Sweet Potato

Ingredients

2 large sweet potatoes peeled and cut in rounds
1 cup chicken broth/stock
1 tsp salt
1 ripe banana
1 small jalapeño seeded and finely diced
1-2 Tbs honey or maple syrup to taste
¼ cup canna butter

Directions

Place peeled and cubed potatoes in a large sauce pan. Add 1 cup chicken stock and salt, and then cover potatoes with water. Boil potatoes until soft. Remove from liquid. Place on a cookie sheet and bake in the oven for 10 minutes at 300°F to reduce moisture.

Remove potatoes from oven, and mix all ingredients in a bowl with a hand masher or a hand blender. Whip until smooth and enjoy! Serves 4

Sautéed Kale with Balsamic Reduction

Kale is a healthy food that doesn't get enough respect. It is high in fiber, vitamins K and C, calcium, and produces sulphoraphane, which has strong anti-cancer properties. Boiling reduces the level of sulphoraphane, but stir frying, steaming, and sautéing do not. When kale is cooked briefly, the body is better able to take up all the good nutrition in the leaf.

Ingredients

5-6 cups chopped fresh kale
1 cup balsamic vinegar
½ cup golden organic raisins
3 cloves garlic, minced
1 small onion chopped (approx. ½ cup)
1 Tbs canna butter or oil
½ tsp of salt

Directions

Place balsamic vinegar in a sauce pan and simmer on medium for 15 minutes. This concentrates the vinegar. Add half the garlic, all the onions, and golden raisins and simmer another 5 minutes. The balsamic should reduce to ¼ to ½ cup.

Cut kale into bite-sized strips. Add kale and canna butter to the balsamic mix and cook until just tender—2-3 minutes max. Serve and enjoy! Serves 4

Dessert

Elaine's Pastry Crust

Our family friend Elaine makes some of the best pies you will ever sink your teeth into. While the fillings in her banana cream and chocolate pies are truly out of this world, it is her crust that send her pies over the top! Elaine suffers from the painful condition of Interstitial Cystitis, which is a hardening of the bladder and urinary tract, and the medications her doctor prescribes seem to cause more harm than good most of the time. Cannabis has been proven to greatly benefit people with this condition. She wants to try cannabis but does not because it is illegal and because she has to get blood tested often to make sure the medication is not damaging her liver. She is fearful of losing her insurance if it is discovered she tried cannabis. When making this crust, please say a prayer that we pass national cannabis legalization or that Texas passes a medical cannabis law soon so Elaine can get some Chronic Relief.

This is an excellent flaky all-purpose crust for your favorite pie or empanada. This makes enough for 2 regular sized pies. Dough can be refrigerated for 3 weeks or frozen for 2 months.

Ingredients

2 cups regular or all-purpose gluten free flour
1 tsp salt
½ cup cold canna butter
6-7 Tbs of 7Up. Yep! You read that correctly.

Directions

Tip: The less you work the ingredients, the flakier the crust!

Stir flour and salt together. Break butter into many small pieces. Cut in the softened butter in small increments. Use a fork, a pastry tool, or your food processor with a metal blade. If using a food processor, pulse a few times. Once the mixture looks like cornmeal, add the 7Up 1 Tbs at a time until the dough sticks together. Roll into a ball. Cut in half. Wrap each half in plastic wrap and chill for 1 hour. Then roll the dough out on a floured surface to ¼ inch or less thickness.

For pie, quiche, or tarts: Roll out to the desired size or cut in rounds and lift and drop evenly into a pie pan. You can mold the sides of the crust to the pie pan with your fingers to make it attractive, or press the prongs of a fork into the crust around the edge.

For empanadas and turnovers: Cut the crust into desired size rounds. I like to use the rim of a glass or an empty food can for my cutting tool. Place filling on one half of the circle and fold over the dough. Use your fingers or a fork to fasten the edges to ensure the filling is secure. Whisk one egg with 1 Tbs of water to make an "egg wash," and brush this over the outside of the crust to help it brown.

Apple Crumble Pie

Who doesn't LOVE apple pie? This recipe can be for a full pie, which can be frozen whole or in slices, or you can make individual servings using mini pie shells or small soufflé dishes.

Ingredients

8 small (4 large) organic apples, peeled and sliced
2 cups flour (gluten free works fine)
½ cup white sugar
1 cup brown sugar
1 lemon, juiced
1½ tsp salt
2 tbs cinnamon
½ cup +3 tsp canna butter, softened

Directions

Prepare crust using either Elaine's Pie Crust on page 291 or or a pre-made pie shell.

Toss cut apples with all the lemon juice, ¼ cup white sugar, ½ cup brown sugar, and ½ teaspoon of salt. Mix well until apples are completely coated.
Preheat oven to 350°F.

Mix softened butter, flour, remaining salt, cinnamon, and sugar in a large mixing bowl with a fork or your hands until crumbles form. This is the crumble topping. Put one 1" layer of apples in the crust, and sprinkle with about 2 Tbs of the crumb mixture. Add a few extra small pieces of canna or regular butter like you would pepperoni on a pizza. Add an inch of apples then another layer of crumbles and canna butter. When the pie crust is almost full, layer on the remaining apples, and spread the remaining teaspoon of canna butter evenly in small pieces across the top of the pie. Add all remaining crumbles on top.

Cover a cookie sheet with aluminum foil where the pie will sit. This will make cleanup much easier, as the pie will likely bubble over a bit. Cook for 30-40 minutes at 350 F. For the first 25 minutes of baking, cover with foil to prevent over-browning on top. It will be done when you can easily stick a knife through the center of the pie. You don't want to overcook the pie; a little firmness is a good thing. Serves 6-8

Oatmeal Chocolate Cookies

This recipe is strangely delicious and full of fiber. Dark chocolate is packed with antioxidants and minerals. Oats are well known for their cholesterol lowering ability. This is a relatively guilt free treat—especially if you reduce the amount of sugar.

Ingredients

2 cups sugar
1 tsp salt
6-8 tablespoon of 60-70% cocoa—use the good stuff!

⅓ cup canna butter (not oil)
⅓ cup milk
3 cups dried rolled oats

Directions

In a saucepan, melt butter over low heat, stirring until butter melts. Add sugar and cook 1 minute. Add cocoa and salt. Turn to medium-low heat and cook until the mixture touching the edges of the pan starts to bubble. Test for doneness by dropping some of the mixture in a cup of ice cold water. When it forms a soft, workable ball, remove the mixture from the heat.

Add 1-2 tsp vanilla and stir in 3 cups oats (uncooked).

Immediately, before the chocolate solidifies, drop teaspoon sized balls of dough onto waxed paper. Servings 16-24

Notes

You can cut the sugar to as little as half cup if you prefer less sweet.

Foster Styled Bananas

Ingredients

2 ripe bananas
2 Tbs canna butter or a mix of canna butter and canna coconut oil
1 Tbs brown sugar
¼ cup of dark rum (optional)

Directions

Over medium heat, add butter, brown sugar (or coconut sugar), and rum. Stir to mix until bubbly (4-6 minutes). Add a pinch of salt and fresh bananas. Cook 1 minute. Do not overcook! Serve as is, over ice cream, or over another dessert. Serves 2 to 4

Mexican Chocolate Sauce

Warning: Several years ago I wanted to make birthday cake for two of my best friends, Andrea and Julie S., who were having a joint birthday party. I ended up baking these Bundt cakes in an effort to get two perfect cakes for display and serving. I made the mistake of leaving the six cakes unattended only to find two other friends, Julie P. and Stephanie, with spoons in hand eating the icing (this recipe) from the center of the four not-so-perfect Bundt cakes. This icing makes people do strange things. Fortunately, it was un-medicated. Otherwise, they would have been in for a big surprise!

Ingredients

1 cup pecans
½ cup unsalted canna butter
¼ cup whole milk
½ cup high-quality dark cocoa powder such as Scharffen Berger
2 cups sifted powdered sugar (sifted then measured)

1 Tbs vanilla extract (I prefer Mexican vanilla)
¼ tsp salt

Directions

Preheat oven to 350°F.

Arrange pecans on a baking sheet in a single layer, and toast them in a 350° oven for 7 to 9 minutes until golden brown and aromatic. Chop the pecans.

Melt butter over low heat in a medium saucepan. Add cocoa and powdered sugar and whisk until glossy. Remove saucepan from the heat, and whisk in the vanilla, salt, and pecans.

Served hot or cold, this makes a wonderful sauce over fresh berries. It is a fantastic icing for any chocolate cake, cake balls, or torte and is pretty darn fine by itself on a spoon, too. Serves 10-14

Variation:

If you want truffles, add 1 ounce of chopped 60+% cacao to the cocoa powder and sugar, and mix until melted. Let cool in a bowl, then scoop and form the chocolate into tablespoon sized balls, refrigerate, and serve.

Chocolate Torte

Ingredients

4 oz semisweet chocolate, chopped (Valrohna is preferred)
½ cup butter
¾ cup white sugar
½ cup Ghirardelli cocoa or other quality dark cocoa
3 eggs beaten
1 tsp vanilla extract (use Mexican vanilla for best flavor)

Preheat the oven to 300°F. Grease an 8" rounded spring form pan, and dust with cocoa powder. You can also use a cake ball mold to make bite-sized treats that I call Happy Cake Balls.

In the top of a double boiler over lightly simmering water, melt chocolate and butter. Remove from heat and stir in sugar, cocoa powder, eggs, and vanilla. Pour into prepared pan.

Bake in preheated oven for 30 minutes (12 minutes if using a cake ball mold). Let cool in the pan for 10 minutes then turn out onto a wire rack and cool completely. Slices can also be reheated for 20-30 seconds in the microwave before serving. If you are making cake balls, allow them to sit 5 minutes before removing from the molds. Place them on wax paper and allow to cool if you are not serving them warm.

This gluten free recipe is a favorite among chocolate lovers and gluten and gluten-free eaters alike. Two Happy Cake Balls, or a slice of cake with a dollop of the above mentioned Mexican Chocolate Sauce and fresh berries, is a grand dessert. It is even better when you add a small scoop of ice cream.

Thank you to my friend Carolyn who brought this dish to our family corn harvest party. It was the first summer after I went gluten free. The dessert table was packed full of beautiful desserts I couldn't eat. When she told me it was gluten free, I stopped what I was doing, cut a huge slice, and promptly hid it! Is that wrong? Serves 6-10

Gluten Free Brownie

I guess this wouldn't be a cannabis cookbook without a brownie recipe, but since cannabis brownie recipes are a dime a dozen on the Internet, I thought I'd include something unique. This is one of my all-time favorite brownie recipes. It uses no flour of any kind, is more nutritious than traditional recipes, and is naturally gluten free. These brownies are chewy and full of flavor.

This recipe has been modified from *Healthy Gluten-Free Cooking* by Darina Allen with Rosemary Kearney, one of my favorite gluten free cookbooks.

Ingredients
2 oz best quality gluten-free dark semisweet chocolate, 70%
7 tablespoons (3 ½ oz) canna butter
2 eggs, whisked
½ tsp pure vanilla extract
¾ cup (3 oz) ground almonds
½ tsp gluten-free baking powder
Pinch of salt
1 cup (4 oz) chopped walnuts
8 in square pan, lined with silicone paper

Directions
Preheat oven to 325°F.

Melt chocolate in a double boiler or a heatproof bowl suspended in a water bath on low-medium heat. Cream the butter and sugar together with a fork or in a standing mixer until pale, soft, and light then beat in the lightly whisked eggs, vanilla, and melted chocolate. Lastly, stir in ground almonds, gluten-free baking powder, salt, and chopped nuts. Spread mixture in the pan, and bake for 40-45 minutes. Leave to cool then cut into 1" or 2" squares. Enjoy! Serves 16

Appendix

Email to Friends - Moving Nadine Forward

The following email was sent to family members and friends three weeks before my mother died. I encourage others to do something similar when faced with the same situation. This email let our support network know what was going on, what we needed from them, and it politely set our boundaries so we could make the time we had left as delicious and comforting as possible for my mother and our family.

Hello Friends and Family,

We hope you are well.

Sadly, Nadine has been encouraged by her oncologist not to pursue more treatment. Hospice came Thursday to discuss how to best keep her comfortable.

Nadine has fought a great fight and done so with humor, grace, and courage. Her doctor told us this week that there is simply nothing more they can do. Pray for a miracle— not to keep her alive but to give her life back in a way that allows her to go and do and remain active. With each passing day it becomes more difficult for her to do simple tasks such as walking to the bathroom. If it weren't for her darn lungs she would probably be healthier than most of us. Oxygen is a funny thing. Our bodies need it to function.

Although we don't like time frames too much, her doctor said we are looking at a 2-3 month horizon, if that. Nadine said yesterday that the time will come sooner.

As you can imagine, we are all devastated by the impending loss of our beloved rock solid wife, mom, and grandmother, NayNay. We are mindful of not letting the im-

pending dread of her absence rob us of the gift of what little time we may have left. Thus, we are going to continue to eke out a few more precious memories.

Nadine has lived a full, thoughtful, and meaningful life, touching the hearts and lives of many. She has been a great wife, mother, grandmother, sister, aunt, friend, mentor, and neighbor.

Many of you have asked us what you can do. And many of you have asked us is there anything we need. Simply, we need the rest of our days with NayNay to be as full of laughter and love as possible. And as stress-free as possible. The greatest gift you can give us is to help celebrate Nadine's life while she is alive. Our family is asking all of you who love Nadine and have been touched by her to reach out to her with funny cards (no sad or sappy shit!) and written stories about what she means to you or to share funny or happy memories you may have of her. Laughter and silliness are the absolute best medicine.

For those that will want to honor her memory with flowers or a memorial donation to the Travis County 4-H Scholarship, we ask that you do that NOW while she is alive to see the fruits of her life and to enjoy your kindness. Nadine has always said, "Send the flowers to people while they are alive and can enjoy them." Let's honor her while she is alive so she can move on with as much love and satisfaction as possible!

Many of you have contacted us about visiting Nadine or dropped in to visit. We appreciate your care, concern, and support. At this time, she is still accepting a few visitors throughout the day. However, we have a few requests for all of you who want to come see her:

A) Please keep your visits to less than 20 minutes. She tires easily.

B) Please call before you come to confirm that it is a good time.

C) *Please come with a smile on your face! This is a difficult time for all of us—especially Nadine. We want to focus on celebrating her life and the joy that she has brought to us. That is a delicate way of saying what Nadine said, "they can come for a short visit but if they can't come and be happy and up-lifting ...don't come."*

D) *And please come between 10:00 and 4:00; our evenings are selfishly reserved for Wesley and family time.*

Thank you kindly for your understanding, love, and support. We are lucky to have such a wonderful support network.

The Whiteley Family

Bibliography

Abrams, Donald. 2010. "Cannabis in Pain and Palliative Care." *The Pain Practitioner* 20 (4): 35-45.

Abrams, Donald I., and Manuel Guzman. 2009. "Cannabinoids and Cancer." In *Integrative Oncology,* by Donald Abrams and Andrew Weil, 150. Tuscon, Arizona: Oxford University Press.

Abrams, Donald I., Roslyn J. Leiser, Starley B. Shade, Tarek A. Elbeik, Francesca T. Aweeka, Neal L. Benowitz, Barry M. Bredt, et al. 2003. "Short-term effects of cannabinoids in patients with HIV-1 infection: a randomized, placebo-controlled clinical trial." *Annals of Internal Medicine* 139 (4): 258-66.

Abrams, Donald. 2011. *Project CBD Continuing Medical Education The Science of Cannabis.* Accessed April 23, 2012. *http://projectcbd.org/.*

Aggarwal, Sunil K. 2013. "Cannabinergic pain medicine a concise clinical primer and survey of randomized-controlled trial results." *Clinical Journal of Pain* 29 (2): 162-171.

Aggarwal, Sunil K. 2010. "Cannabis: A Commonwealth Medicinal Plant, Long Suppressed, Now at Risk of Monopolization." *Online Supplement to the Denver University Law Review.*

Aggarwal, Sunil K., interview by Nishi Whiteley. 2014. *Chronic Relief Book Review* (February 7).

—. 2014. "Health Scientist Blacklisting and the Meaning of Marijuana in the Oval Office in the Early 1970's." *CASP Communications Medium.com.* December 2. Accessed February 16, 2016. *https://medium.com/@ReachCASP/health-scientist-blacklisting-and-the-meaning-of-marijuana-in-the-oval-office-in-the-early-1970s-71ea41427b49#.68zrqx1d2.*

Akerman, Simon, Philip R. Holland, Michele P. Lasalandra, and Peter J. Goadsby. 2013. "Endocannabinoids in the Brainstem Modulate DuralTrigeminovascular Nociceptive Traffic via CB_1 and "Triptan" Receptors: Implications in Migraine." *The Journal of Neuroscience* 33 (37): 14869-14877.

Alhamoruni, A., A. C. Lee, K. L. Wright, M. Larvin, and S. E. O'Sullivan. Oct 2010. "Pharmacological Effects of Cannabinoids on the Caco-2 Cell." *The Journal of Pharmacology and Experimental Therapeutics* 335 (1): 92-102.

Alhouayek, Mireille, and Giulio G. Muccioli. 2012. "The endocannabinoid system in inflammatory bowel diseases: from pathophysiology to therapeutic opportunity." *Trends in Molecular Medicine* 18 (10): 615-25.

Allen, Darina, and Rosemary Kearney. 2005. *Healthy Gluten-Free Cooking: 150 Recipes for Food Lovers.* Lanham, MD: Kyle Cathie Ltd.

Alzhiemer's Association. 2014. *Alzheimer's Association Alzheimer's Disease Facts and Figures.* Accessed January 13, 2015. *http://www.alz.org/alzheimers_*

disease_facts_and_figures.asp.

American Academy of Pain Medicine. n.d. "AAPM Facts and Figures on Pain." *The American Adacemy of Pain Medicine.* Accessed September 24, 2014. *http:// www.painmed.org/patientcenter/facts_on_pain.aspx#burden.*

American Chronic Pain Association. n.d. *American Chronic Pain Association.* Accessed September 23, 2014. *http://www.theacpa.org/condition/ neuropathic-pain.*

American College of Physicians. 2008. *Supporting Research into the Therapeutic Role of Marijuana.* Philedelphia: American College of Physicians.

Americans for Civil Liberties Union. n.d. *Photo Gallery: Marijuana Arrests by the Numbers.* Accessed August 22, 2014. *https://www.aclu.org/ criminal-law-reform/marijuana-arrests-numbers.*

Armamento, Paul. 2014. "Medical Marijuana More Effective Than Big Pharma for Fibromyalgia." *High Times.* April 22. Accessed January 13, 205. *http://www.hightimes.com/read/ medical-marijuana-more-effective-big-pharma-fibromyalgia.*

Atakan, Zerrin. 2012. "Cannabis, a complex plant: different compounds and different effects on individuals." *Advances in Psychopharmacology* 2 (6): 241-254.

Backes, Michael. 2014. *Cannabis Pharmacy.* New York: Black Dog & Leventhal.

Bienenstock, David. 2015. "How to Make Weed 'Dabs' at Home With a Hair Straightener." *David Bienenstock.* August 4. Accessed January 27, 2016. *http://motherboard.vice.com/read/ how-to-make-weed-dabs-at-home-with-a-hair-straightener.*

Blázquez, C, L González-Feria, L Alvarez, Haro A, ML Casanova, and M. Guzmán. 2004. "Cannabinoids inhibit the vascular endothelial growth factor pathway in gliomas." *Cancer Research* 64 (16): 5617-23. Accessed April 23, 2012. *http:// www.ncbi.nlm.nih.gov/pubmed/15313899.*

Bone, Kerry. 2003. *A Clinical Guide to Blending Herbs, Herbal Formulations for the Individual Patient.* Missouri: Churchhill Livingston.

Borrelli, Francesca, Ester Pagano, Barbara Romano, Stefania Panzera, Francesco Maiello, Dianna Coppola, Luciano De Petrocellis, Lorena Buono, Pierangelo Orlando, and Angelo A. Izzo. 2014. "Colon carcinogenesis is inhibited by the TRPM8 antagonist cannabigerol, a Cannabis-derived non-psychotropic cannabinoid." *Carcinogenisis* 35 (12): 2787-2797.

Braverman, Eric. 2004. *The Edge Effect.* New York, NY: Sterling Publishing Co., Inc.

Byer, Stephen, and Barbara Byer. 2013. *Medical Marijuana.* Madison, Wisconsin: ALS World Wide.

California NORML. 2013. "Warnings on Butane Extractions and Dabbing." *California NORML.* October 10. Accessed October 18, 2014. *http://www. canorml.org/news/warnings_on_cannabis_butane_extractions_and_dabbing.*

Campos, Alline C., Zaira Ortega, Javier Palazuelos, Manoela V. Fogaca, Daniele C. Aguiar, Javier Diaz-Alonso, Silvia Ortega-Gutierrez, et al. 2013. "The anxiolytic effect of cannabidiol on chronically stressed mice depends on hippocampal neurogenesis: involvement of the endocannabinoid system." *International Journal of Neuropsychopharmacology* 16 (6): 1407-1419.

Cannabis Digest. 2014. "Backdoor Medicine: How Cannabis Suppositories Can Save Lives." *Cannabis Digest*. September 23. Accessed October 20, 2014. *http://cannabisdigest.ca/cannatory/*.

Carskadon, Mary A., and William C. Dement. 2011. "Normal Human Sleep: An Overview." Chap. 2 in *Principles and Practice of Sleep Medicine*, by Meir H. Kryger, Thomas Roth and William C. Dement, 16-26. St. Louis: Elsivier Saunders.

Carter, Gregory T. 2014. "Cannabis in the Management of Neuromuscular Disorders." *Endocannabinoid System and Age Related Illnesses Conference Binder*. Portland: Patients Out of Time.

Carter, Gregory T., and Bill S. Rosen. 2001. "Marijuana in the management of amyotrophic lateral sclerosis." *American Journal of Hospice & Palliative Care* 18 (4): 264-270.

Carter, Gregory T., Patrick Weydt, Muraco Kyashna-Tocha, and Donald Abrams. 2004. *Medical cannabis: Rational guidelines for dosing*. IDrugs 2004 7 (5): 464-470.

Cascio, Maria Grazia, Erica Zamberletti, Pietro Marini, Daniela Parolaro, and Roger G. Pertwee. 2015. "The phytocannabinoid, Δ(9) -tetrahydrocannabivarin, can act through 5-HT1 A receptors to produce antipsychotic effects." *British Journal of Pharmacology* 172 (5): 1305-1318.

Centers for Disease Control. 2014. "Economic Facts About U.S. Tobacco Production and Use." *Centers for Disease Control*. Accessed June 6, 2015. *http://www.cdc.gov/tobacco/data_statistics/fact_sheets/economics/econ_facts/index.htm#costs*.

—. n.d. "Public Health Grand Rounds." *Centers for Disease Control*. Accessed 12 27, 2012. *http://www.cdc.gov/about/grand-rounds/archives/2011/01-February.htm*.

—. 2008. *Smoking-Attributable Mortality, Years of Potential Life Lost, and Productivity Losses --- United States, 2000-2004*. Nov 14. Accessed April 23, 2012. *http://www.cdc.gov/mmwr/preview/mmwrhtml/mm5745a3.htm*.

Centonze, Diego, Alessandro Finazzi-Agro, Giorgio Bernardi, and Mauro Maccarrone. 2007. "The endocannabinoid system in targeting inflammatory neurodegenerative diseases." *TRENDS in Pharmacological Science* 28 (4): 180-187.

Chicca, Andrea, Diego Caprioglio, Alberto Minassi, Vanessa Petrucci, Giovanni Appendino, Orazio Taglialatela-Scafati, and Jürg Gertsch. 2014. "Functionalization of β-caryophyllene generates novel polypharmacology in the endocannabinoid system." *ACS Chemical Biology* 9 (7): 1499–1507.

Clarke, Robert C., interview by Nishi Whiteley. 2016. *Personal Communication* (March 10).

Clarke, Robert C., and Mark D. Merlin. 2013. *Cannabis: Evolution and Ethnobotany*. Los Angeles: University of California Press.

Commission on Marihuana and Drug Abuse. 1972. *Marihuana: A Signal of Misunderstanding*. Washington D.C.: Commission on Marihuana and Drug Abuse.

Common Sense for Drug Policy. 2002. *Nixon Tapes Show Roots of Marijuana Prohibition: Misinformaiton, Culture Wars and Prejudice*. Washington D.C.:

Common Sense for Drug Policy.

Corey-Bloom, Jody, Tanya Wolfson, Anthony Gamst, Shelia Jin, Thomas D. Marcotte, Heather Bentley, and Ben Gouaux. 2012. "Smoked cannabis for spasticity in multiple sclerosis: a randomized, placebo-controlled trial." *Canadian Medical Association Journal* 184 (10): 1143-50.

Corral, Valerie, interview by Nishi Whiteley. 2014. Email August 28, 2014 *Re: Blurb from my book* (August 28).

Courtney, William, interview by The New Settler Interview. 2010. *Medical Marijuana Sagas http://www.cannabisinternational.org/interviews.php.*

Crippa, Jose Alexadre, Antonio Waldo Zuardi, Rocio Martin-Santos, Sagnik Bhattacharyya, Zerrin Atakan, Philip McGuire, and P Fusar-Poli. 2009. "Cannabis and anxiety: a critical review of the evidence." *Human Psychopharmacology* 24 (7): 515-23.

Curry, Wei-Ni Lin. 2002. "Hyperemesis Gravidarum and Clinical Cannabis: To Eat or Not to Eat." *Journal of Cannabis Therapeutics* 2 (3/4): 63-83.

Davis, Jeanie Lurche. 2003. *Cannabis May Suppress Immune System Could Lead to New Autoimmune Disorder Treatments.* April 15. Accessed August 12, 2015. *http://www.webmd.com/lupus/news/20030415/cannabis-may-suppress-immune-system.*

Dempsey, Jerome. 2002. "Functional Role for Cannabinoids in Respiratory Stability During Sleep." *SLEEP* 25 (4): 396-397.

Denson, Thomas F., and Mitch Earleywine. 2006. "Decreased depression in marijuana users." *Addictive Behaviors* 31 (4): 738-42.

Desprez, Pierre-Yves, Sean D. McAllister, Rigel T. Christian, Maxx P. Horowitz, Amaia Garcia, and Pierre-Yves Desprez. 2007. "Cannabidiol as a novel inhibitor of Id-1 gene expression in aggressive breast cancer cells." *Molecular Cancer Therapeutics* 6: 2921-7. *http://mct.aacrjournals.org/content/6/11/2921.long.*

Di Marzo, Vincenzo. 2011. "Endocannabinoid signaling in the brain: biosynthetic menchanisms in the limelight." *Nature Neuroscience* 14 (1): 9-15.

Di Marzo, Vincenzo. 1998. "'Endocannabinoids' and other fatty acid derivatives with cannabimimetic properties: biochemistry and possible physiopathological relevance." *Biochimica et Biophysica Acta (BBA) - Lipids and Lipid Metabolism* 1392 (2-3): 153-175.

Di Marzo, Vincenzo, and Luciano DePerocellis. 2012. "Why do cannabinoid receptors have more than one endogenous ligand?" *Philosophical Transactions of the The Royal Society* 367 (1607): 3216-3228.

Dreher, Emily. 2007. "Jamaican Study - Cannabis Use in Pregnancy." *Patients Out of Time.* Ruby Dunes Video.

Earlywine, Mitch. 2002. "Highlights in the history of cannabis." In *Understanding Marijuana,* by Mitch Eerlywine, 25-26. New York: Oxford Press.

ElSohly Laboratories. n.d. *ElSohly Laboratories* Inc. Accessed September 21, 2014. *http://www.elsohly.com/.*

ElSohly, Mahmoud, interview by Nishi Whiteley via email. 2013. *Research Professor of the Research Institute of Pharmaceutical Sciences and Professor of Pharmaceutics* (July 9).

Erkelens, Jacob L., and Arno Hazekamp. 2014. "That which we call Indica, by any other name would smell as sweet." *Cannabinoids* 9 (1): 9-15.

Ferlay, Jacques, Hai-Rim Shin, Freddie Bray, David Forman, Colin Mathers, and Donald Maxwell Parkin. 2010. "Estimates of worldwide burden of cancer in 2008: GLOBOCAN 2008." *International Journal of Cancer* 127 (12): 2893-2917.

Fernandez-Ruiz, Javier, Eva de Lago, Maria Gomex-Ruiz, Concepcion Garcia, Onintza Sagredo, and Moises Garcia-Arencibia. 2014. "Neurodegenerative Disorders Other Than Multiple Sclerosis." In *Handbook of Cannabis*, by Roger Pertwee, 505-517. Oxford: Oxford University Press.

Fernandez-Ruiz, Javier, Onintza Sagredo, M. Ruth Pazos, Concepcion Garcia, Roger Pertwee, Raphael Mechoulam, and Jose Martinez-Orgado. 2013. "Cannabidiol for neurodegenerative disorders: important new clinical applications for this phytocannabinoid?" *British Journal of Clinical Pharmcocology* 75 (2): 323-333.

Finley, Constance, interview by Nishi Whiteley. 2016. *Personal Correspondence* (January 25).

Gable, Robert S. 2006. "The Toxicity of Recreational Drugs." *American Scientist*, May-June: 206-208.

Gardner, Fred. Autumn 2011. "Terpenoids, 'minor' cannabinoids contribute to 'entrourage effect' of cannabis-based medicines." *O'Shaughnessy's* 20.

Gerdeman, Gregory L., and Jason B. Schechter. 2010. "The Endocannabinoid System." In *The Pot Book*, by Julie Holland, 52-62. Rochester, Vermont: Park Street Press.

Gertsch, Jurg. 2008. "Anti-inflammatory cannabinoids in diet towards a better understanding of CB_2 receptor action?" *Communicative & Integrative Biology* 1 (1): 26-28.

Gettman, John. 1999. *The Bulletin of Cannabis Reform.* June 28. Accessed January 15, 2013. *http://www.drugscience.org/Archive/bcr3/n3_Marinol.html.*

Gieringer, Dale, and Arno Hazekamp. 2011. "How Accurate is Potency Testing?" *O'Shaughnessy's: The Journal of Cannabis in Clinical Practice* 17-18.

Gieringer, Dale, Joseph St. Laurent, and Scott Goodrich. 2004. "Cannabis Vaporizer Combines Efficient Delivery of THC with Effective Suppression of Pyrolytic Compounds." *Journal of Cannabis Therapeutics* 4 (1): 7-27.

Grant, Igor, Raul Gonzalez, Catherine L. Carey, Loki Natarajan, and Tanya Wolfson. 2003. "Non-acute (residual) neurocognitive effects of cannabis use: A meta-analytic study." *Journal of the International Neuropsychological Society* 9 (5): 679-689.

Grinspoon, Lester. 2005. "History of Cannabis as a Medicine." Boston.

Guindon, Josee, and Andrea G. Hohmann. 2011. "The endocannabinoid system and cancer: therapeutic implication." *British Journal of Pharmacology* 1447-1463.

Gupta, Sanja. 2013. "WEED." *CNN Television Special Report.* August 8.

Gupta, Sanjay, interview by Pierce Morgan. 2013. Neurosurgeon, *CNN Correspondent* (August 7).

Guzman, M, M J Duarte, C Blàzquez, J Ravina, M C Rosa, I Galve-Roperh, C Sànchez, and G Velasco. 2006. "A pilot clinical study of Delta9-

tetrahydrocannabinol in patients with recurrent glioblastoma multiforme." *British Journal of Cancer* 95 (2): 197-203.

Guzman, Manuel. 2003. "Cannabinoids: Potential Anticancer Agents." *Nature* 745-756.

Hampson, A J, M. Grimaldi, J. Axelrod, and D. Wink. 1998. "Cannabidiol and (-) Δ9-tetrahydrocannabinol are neuroprotective antioxidants." *Proceedings of the National Academy of Sciences* 95 (14): 8268-8273.

Hampson, Aidan J., Juilius Axelrod, and Grimaldi Maurizio. 1999. "Cannabinoids as antioxidants and neuroprotectants." *U.S. Patent Office Full Text and Image Database.* October 28. Accessed August 2, 2014. *http://patft.uspto.gov/ netacgi/nph-Parser?Sect1=PTO1&Sect2=HITOFF&d=PALL&p=1&u=%2Fnet ahtml%2FPTO%2Fsrchnum.htm&r=1&f=G&l=50&s1=6630507.PN.&OS=PN/ 6630507&RS=PN/6630507.*

Hargenrather, Jeffrey. 2014. "Creating Cannabis Policies in Extended Care Facilities." *Patients Out of Time: The Endocannabinoid System and Age-Related Illness.* Portland: Patients out of Time.

Hazekamp, Arno, Krishna Bastola, Hassan Rashidi, Joahn Bender, and Rob Verpoorte. 2007. "Cannabis tea revisited: a systematic evaluation of the cannabinoid composition of cannabis tea." *Journal of Ethnopharmacology* 113 (1): 85-90.

Hegde, Venkatesh L., Shweta Hegde, Benjamin F. Cravatt, Lorne J. Hofseth, Mitzi Nagarkatti, and Prakash S. Nagarkatti. 2008. "Attenuation of experimental autoimmune hepatitis by exogenous and endogenous cannabinoids: involvement of regulatory T cells." *Molecular Pharmcology* 7 (1): 20-33.

Hill, Matthew N., Gregory E. Miller, Erica J. Carrier, Boris B. Gorzalka, and Cecilia J. Hillard. 2009. "Circulating endocannabinoids and N-acylethanolamines are differentially regulated in major depression and following exposure to social stress." *Psychoneuroendrocrinology* 34 (8): 1257-62.

Hillard, Cecilia. 2014. "Endocannabinoids in the circulation and psychopathology." *The Eighth National Clinical Conference on Cannabis Therapeutics Conference Binder.* Portland: Patients Out of Time.

Holland, Julie. 2010. The Pot Book: *A Complete Guide to Cannabis.* Rochester, VT: Park Street Press.

Howlett, A C, F Barth, T I Bonner, G Cabral, P Casellas, W A Devane, C C Felder, et al. 2002. "International Union of Pharmacology. XXVII. Classification of cannabinoid receptors." *Pharmacological Reviews* 54 (2): 161-202.

Huestes, Marilynn A. 2007. "Review: Human Cannabinoid Pharmacokinetics." *Chemistry & Biodiversity* 4 (8): 1770-1804.

Huffington Post UK. 2013. "Cannabis 'May Help Stroke Recovery By Improving Brain Functions After The Attack'." *The Huffington Post UK*, March 12.

Institute of Medicine. 2011. *Reforming Pain in America: A blueprint for transforming prevention, care, education and research.* Washington DC: National Academies Press.

Integr8 Health, LLC. 2012. *Maine Medical Marijuana Patient Handbook.* Flamouth, ME: Integr8 Health, LLC.

International Associaton of Cannabinoid Medicine. 2014. *IACM - Bulliten of 07 September 2014.* September 7. Accessed October 11, 2014. *http:// www.cannabis-med.org/english/bulletin/ww_en_db_cannabis_artikel. php?id=433#1.*

Irwin, Michael R., Minge Wang, Capella O. Campomayor, Alicia Collado-Hidalgo, and Steve Cole. 2006. "Sleep deprivation and activation of morning levels of cellular and genomic markers of inflammation." *Archives of Internal Medicine* 166 (16): 1756-1762.

Izzo, Angelo A., Francesca Borrelli, Raffaele Capasso, Vincenzo Di Marzo, and Raphael Mechoulam. 2009. "Non-psychotropic plant cannabinoids: new therapeutic opportunities from an ancient herb." *Trends in Pharmacological Sciences* 30 (10): 515-527.

Izzo, Angelo A., Raffaele Capasso, Gabriella Aviello, Francesca Borrelli, Barbara Romano, Fabiana Piscitelli, Laura Gallo, Francesco Capasso, Pierangelo Orlando, and Vincenzo Di Marzo. 2012. "Inhibitory effect of cannabichromene, a major non-psychotropic cannabinoid extracted from Cannabis sativa, on inflammation-induced hypermotility in mice." *British Journal of Pharmacology* 166 (4): 1444-1469.

Jackson, Mark. 2010. "'Divine Stramonium': The Rise and Fall of Smoking for Asthma." *International Journal for the History of Medicine and Related Sciences* 54 (2): 171-194.

Jager, Walter. 2010. "8 Metabolism of Terpenoids in Animal Models and Humans." In *Handbook of Essential Oils: Science, Technology, and Applications*, by K. Husnu Can Baser and Gerhard Buchbauer, 209-232. Boca Raton, FL: CRC Press.

Jensen, R. Paul, Wentai Luo, James F. Pankow, Robert M. Strongin, and David H. Peyton. 2015. "Hidden Formaldehyde in E-Cigarette Aerosols." *New England Journal of Medicine* 372: 392-294.

Johnson, J R, M Burnell-Nugent, D Lossignol, E D Ganae-Motan, R Potts, and M T Fallon. 2010. "Multicenter, double-blind, randomized, placebo-controlled, parallel-group study of the efficacy, safety, and tolerability of THC:CBD extract and THC extract in patients with intractable cancer-related pain." *Journal of Pain Symptom Management* 39 (2): 167-179.

Johnson, Renee. 2013. Hemp as an Agricultural Commodity. Congressional Report, Washington DC: Congressional Research Service.

Joy, Janet E., Stanley J. Watson, and John A. Benson, Jr. 1999. "Marijuana and Medicine: Assessing the Science Base." *National Academy of Sciences.* Washington D.C.: Institute of Medicine. 83.

Klein, Zach. 2014. "Cannabis in a Nursing Home Setting." *The Endocannbinoid System and Age-Related Illnesses.* Portland: Patients Out of Time.

Kubasak, Lisa. 2013. *Email with CDER Trade Press.* July 29. Accessed October 21, 2014. *http://www.beyondthc.com/wp-content/uploads/2013/10/CBD-sked-1. png.*

Lal, Simon, Neeraj Prasad, Manijeh Ryan, Sabrena Tangri, Mark S. Silverberg, Allan Gordon, and Hillary Steinhart. 2011. "Cannabis use amongst patients with inflammatory bowel disease." *European Journal of Gastroenterology & Hepatology* 23 (10): 891-6.

Lee, Martin A. 2011. "CBD: How It Works." *O'Shaugnessy's The Journal of Cannabis in Clinical Practice* Autumn: 14.

Lee, Martin A. 2011. "CBDiary." *O'Shaugnessy's: Journal of Cannabis in Clinical Practice* 16.

Leson, Gero. 2011. "Benefits of Hemp Seed." *O'Shaughnessey's: A Journal of Cannabis in Clinical Practice* 35.

Life Extension Foundation. 2011. "Inflammation: Chronic." *Life Extention Foundation.* Accessed June 4, 2013. *http://www.lef.org/protocols/prtcl-146. shtml?source=search&key=Inflammation%20chronic.*

Life Extension Foundation. 2003. "Inflammation: Chronic." In *Disease Prevention and Treatment Expanded Fourth Edition Scientific Protocols that Integrate Mainstream and Alternative Medicine*, 1039-1047. Hollywood, Florida: Life Extension Media.

Liou, Gregory I. 2010. "Diabetic retinopathy: Role of inflammation and potential therapies for anti-inflammation." *World Journal of Diabetes* 1 (1): 12-18.

Lopez-Rodriguez, Ana Belen, Eleni Siopi, David P. Finn, Catherine Marchand-Leroux, Luis M. Garcia-Segura, Mehrnaz Jafarian-Tehrani, and Maria-Paz Viveros. 2015. "CB_1 and CB_2 Cannabinoid Receptor Antagonists Prevent Minocycline-Induced Neuroprotection Following Traumatic Brain Injury in Mice." *Cerebral Cortex* 25 (1): 35-45.

Loria, Kevin. 2015. "Marijuana's Surprising Effects On Athletic Performance." *Business Insider.* January 21. Accessed May 5, 2015. *http://www. businessinsider.com/how-marijuana-affects-working-out-2015-1.*

Lotan, Itay, Theresa A. Treves, Yaniv Roditi, and Ruth Djaldetti. 2014. "Cannabis (medical marijuana) treatment for motor and non-motor symptoms of Parkinson disease: an open-label observational study." *Clinical Neuropharmacology* 37 (2): 41-44.

Lucas, Philippe. 2012. "Cannabis as an adjunct to or substitute for opiates in the treatment of chronic pain." *Journal of Psychoactive Drugs* 44 (2): 125-133.

Mahlbert, Paul G. 2013. "Industrial Hemp and Its Relationship to Marijuana." *North American Industrial Hemp Council.* February 3. Accessed August 2, 2013. *http://naihc.org/images/NAIHC/hempmahlberg28feb13.pdf.*

Mahlbert, Paul G., interview by Nishi Whiteley. 2013. *THC Content in Hemp Seeds* (August 2).

Marsicano, Giovanni, Carsten T. Wotjak, Shahnaz C. Azad, Tiziana Bisogno, Gerhard Rammes, Maria Grazia Cascio, Heike Hermann, et al. 2002. "The endogenous cannabinoid system controls extinction of aversive memories." *Nature* 418 (6897): 530-534.

Martin, William. 2015. *Rx for U.S. Drug Policy: A New Paradigm.* Policy Report, Houston: Baker Institute for Public Policy of Rice University.

Martín-Moreno, Ana María, Begoña Brera, Carlos Spuch, Eva Carro, Luis García-García, Mercedes Delgado, Miguel A Pozo, Nadia G. Innamorato, Antonio Cuadrado, and María L. de Ceballos. 2012. "Prolonged oral cannabinoid administration prevents neuroinflammation, lowers β-amyloid levels and improves cognitive performance in Tg APP 2576 mice." *Journal of Neuroinflammation* 9: 8.

Massa, Federico, Giovanni Marsicano, Heike Hermann, Astrid Cannich, Krisztina Monory, Benjamin F. Cravatt, Gian-Luca Ferri, Andrei Sibaev, Martin Storr, and Beat Lutz. 2004. "The endogenous cannabinoid system protects against colonic inflammation." *The Journal of Clinical Investigation* 113 (8): 1202-1209.

McPartland, John M., and Ethan B. Russo. 2001. "Cannabis and Cannabis Extracts: Greater Than the Sum of Their Parts?" *Journal of Cannabis Therapeutics* (The Hawwirtg Press, Inc.) (3): 104.

Mechoulam, Raphael, email interview by Nishi Whiteley. 2013. (September 4).

Mechoulam, Raphael, and Linda A. Parker. 2013. "The Endocannabinoid System and the Brain." *The Annual Review of Psychology* 64: 21-47.

Mechoulam, Raphael, and Lumir Hanus. 2010. "Anandamide and More." Chap. 7 in *The Pot Book: A Complete Guide to Cannabis,* by Julie Holland, 65. Rochester, Vermont: Park Street Press.

Melamede, Robert. 2005. "Cannabis and tobacco smoke are not equally carcinogenic." *Harm Reducation Journal* 2: 21.

Melamede, Robert, interview by Nishi Whiteley. 2015. *Conversation about how cannabinoids impacts anxiety, depression and mood* (February 10).

—. 2011. *YouTube.* March 11. Accessed January 22, 2013. *http://www.youtube.com/watch?v=O2AY5vuz5Zg.*

—. 2010. *YouTube* CannabisTV. April 16. Accessed January 22, 2013. *http://www.youtube.com/watch?v=xa87N2XaOp4.*

Michalski, Christoph W., Milena Maier, Mert Erkan, Danguole Sauliunaite, Frank Bergmann, Pal Pacher, Sandor Batkai, et al. 2008. "Cannabinoids Reduce Markers of Inflammation and Fibrosis in Pancreatic Stellate Cells." *PLoS One* 3 (2): Published online.

Miron, Jeffrey A., and Katherine Waldock. 2010. *The Budgetary Impact of Ending Drug Prohibition.* Special Report, Washington D.C: Cato Institute.

Morgan, Celia J A, Grainne Schafer, Tom P. Freeman, and H. Valerie Curran. 2010. "Impact of cannabidiol on the acute memory and psychotomimetic effects of smoked cannabis: a naturalistic study." *British Journal of Psychiatry* 197 (4): 285-290.

Motel, Seth. 2015. "Factank: 6 facts about marijuana." *Pew Research Foundation.* April 14. Accessed August 19, 2015. *http://www.pewresearch.org/fact-tank/2015/04/14/6-facts-about-marijuana/.*

Müller-Vahl, Kristen R. 2013. "Treatment of Tourette syndrome with cannabinoids." *Behavioural Neurology* 27 (1): 119-124.

Nagarkatti, Prakash, Rupal Pandey, Sadiye Amcaoglu Rieder, Venkatesh L. Hegde, and Mitzi Nagarkatti. 2009. "Cannabinoids as novel anti-inflammatory drugs." *Future Medicinal Chemistry* 1 (7): 1333-1349. Accessed March 25, 2012. *http://www.ncbi.nlm.nih.gov/pmc/articles/PMC2828614/.*

National Institute of Health. n.d. Anxiety Disorders. Accessed February 6, 2015. *http://www.nimh.nih.gov/health/publications/anxiety-disorders/index.shtml?rf=53414.*

National Institute on Alcohol Abuse and Alcoholism. n.d. *Alcohol's Effect On the Body. Accessed* May 4, 2013. *http://www.niaaa.nih.gov/alcohol-health/*

alcohols-effects-body.

NIH National Eye Institute. 2005. *Glaucoma and Marijuana Use.* June 25. Accessed August 12, 2015. *https://nei.nih.gov/news/statements/marij.*

NORML. 2010. *Emerging Clinical Application for Cannabis and Cannabinoids: A Review of the Recent Scientific Literature 2000-1010.* Washington, DC: NORML.

Notcutt, William, Richard Landford, Philip Davies, Stuart Ratcliffe, and Ruth Potts. 2012. "A placebo-controlled, parallel-group, randomized withdrawal study of subjects with symptoms of spasticity due to multiple sclerosis who are receiving long-term Sativex® (nabiximols)." *Multiple Sclerosis Journal* 18 (2): 219-228.

Ofek, Orr, Meliha Karsak, Nathalie Leclerc, Meirav Fogel, Baruch Frenkel, Karen Wright, Joseph Tam, et al. 2006. "Peripheral cannabinoid receptor, CB2, regulates bone mass." *Proceedings of the National Academy of Sciences* 103 (3): 696-701.

Office of National Drug Control Policy. 2011. *A Fact Sheet: A Response to the Epidimic of Perscription Drug Abuse.* Government Fact sheet, Washington DC: Office of National Drug Control Policy.

O'Shaugnessy's News Service. 2011. "Medical Hemp: The Story to Date." *O'Shaugnessy's The Journal of Cannabis in Clinical Practice* 7.

Pacher, Pal, and George Kumos. 2013. "Modulating the endocannabinoid system in human health and disease: successes and failures." *Federation of European Biochemical Societies* 208 (9): 1918-1943.

Pacher, Pal, and Raphael Mechoulam. 2011. "Is lipid signaling through cannabinoid 2 receptors part of a protective system?" *Progress Lipid Research* 50 (2): 193-211.

Pacher, Pal, Sandor Batkai, and George Kunos. 2006. *The endocannabinoid system as an emerging target of pharmacotherapy.* 389-462, Bethesda, Maryland: Pharmacological Reviews.

Packer, Lester, and Carol Colman. 2000. *The Antioxidant Miracle: Your Complete Plan for Total Health and Healing.* New York: John Wiley & Sons, Inc.

Park, Boram, John M. McPartland, and Michelle Glass. 2004. "Cannabis, cannabinoids and reproduction." *Prostaglandins Leukotrienes and Essential Fatty Acids* 70 (2): 189-197.

Parker, Jennifer, Francisco Atez, Ronald G. Rossetti, Ann Skulas, Rakesh Patel, and Robert B. Zurier. 2008. "Suppression of human macrophage interleukin-6 by a nonpsychoactive cannabinoid acid." *Rheumatology International* 28 (7): 631-635.

Patel, Sachin, Matthew N. Hill, and Cecilia J. Hillard. 2014. "Effects of Phytocannabinoids on Anxiety, Mood, and the Endocrine System." In *Handbook of Cannabis,* by Roger G. Pertwee, 189-199. Oxford: Oxford University Press.

Penner, Elizabeth A., Hannah Buettner, and Murray A. Mittleman. 2013. "The impact of marijuana use on glucose, insulin, and insulin resistance among US adults." *The American Journal of Medicine* 126 (7): 583-589.

Pertwee, Roger. 2004. "Receptors and pharmacodynamics: natural and synthetic cannabionoids and endocannabinoids." In *The Medicinal Uses of Cannabis and Cannabinoids*, by Geoffrey W. Guy, Brian A. Whittle and Philip J. Robson, 103-139. Pharmaceutical Press.

Pew Research Center. 2011. *The Generation Gap* and the 2012 Election. November 3. Accessed march 25, 2012. *http://www.people-press.org/2011/11/03/section-8-domestic-and-foreign-policy-views/*.

Physicians Committee for Responsible Medicine. n.d. *Essential Fatty Acids.* Accessed February 26, 2013. *http://www.pcrm.org/health/health-topics/essential-fatty-acids*.

Piomelli, Daniel, and Ethan B. Russo. 2016. "The Cannabis sativa Versus Cannabis indica Debate: An Interview with Ethan Russo, MD." *Cannabis and Cannabinoid Research* 1 (1): 44-46.

Pope, Harrison G., Amanda J. Gruber, James I. Hudson, Marilyn A. Huestis, and Deborah Yurgelun-Todd. 2001. "Neuropsychological Performance in Long-term Cannabis Users." *JAMA Psychiatry* 59 (10): 909-915.

Porter, Brenda E., and Catherine Jacobson. 2013. "Report of a parent survey of cannabidiol-enriched cannabis use in pediatric treatment-resistant epilepsy." *Epilepsy & Behavior* 29 (3): 574-577.

Project CBD. 2012. Project CBD. Accessed August 28, 2012. *http://www.projectcbd.org*.

Raber, Jeffrey C., interview by Nishi Whiteley. 2015. *President & CEO, The Werc Shop* (August 18).

Raber, Jeffrey C., interview by Nishi Whiteley. 2013. *President & CEO, The Werc Shop* (November 25).

Rajesh, Mohanraj, Partha Mukhopadhyay, Sá ndor Bátka, Vivek Patel, Keita Saito, S Matsumoto, Y Kashiwaya, et al. 2010. "Cannabidiol attenuates cardiac dysfunction, oxidative stress, fibrosis, and inflammatory and cell death signaling pathways in diabetic cardiomyopathy." *Journal of the American College of Cardiology* 56 (25): 2115-2125.

Reiman, Amanda. 2009. "Cannabis as a substitute for alcohol and other drugs." *Harm Reduction Journal* 6: 35.

Richards, Bethan, Samuel L. Whittle, Désirée M. van der Heijde, and Rachelle Buchbinder. 2012. "Efficacy and Safety of Neuromodulators in Inflammatory Arthritis: A Cochrane Systematic Review." *The Journal of Rheumatology* 90: 28-33.

Romano, Luigi L., and Arno Hazekamp. 2013. *Cannabis Oil: chemical evaluation of an upcoming cannabis-based medicine*. International Association for Cannabinoid Medicines.

Romero, Julian. 2014. "Cannabinoids and Alzheimer's Disease." *The Endocannaboniod System and Age-Related Illnesses*. Portland: Patients Out of Time.

Rose, Jeanne. 1992. *The Aromatherapy Book: Applications and Inhalations*. Berkeley, CA: Herbal Sudies Course & North Atlantic Books.

Roth, Michael D., Jose A. Marques-Magallanes, Michael Yuan, Weimin Sun, Donald P. Tashkin, and Oliver Hankinson. 2001. "Induction and Regulation of the Carcinogen-Metabolizing Enzyme CYP1A1 by Marijuana Smoke and Δ9-

Tetrahydrocannabinol." *American Journal of Respiratory Cell and Molecular Biology* 24 (3): 339-344.

Russo, Ethan B. 2015. "Synthetic and natural cannabinoids: the cardiovascular risks." *British Journal of Cardiology*, Jan-Mar: 7-9.

—. 2015. "Introduction to the Endocannabinoid System." *PHYTECS*. February. Accessed April 24, 2015. *http://www.phytecs.com/wp-content/uploads/2015/02/Russo-Introduction-to-the-Endocannabinoid-System-corr-January-2015.pdf.*

Russo, Ethan B., interview by Nishi Whiteley. 2015. Medical Director, *PHYTECS* (April 10).

Russo, Ethan B., interview by Nishi Whiteley. 2015. *Personal Dialogue* (April 5).

Russo, Ethan B., and A. G. Hohmann. 2013. "Role of Cannabinoids in Pain Management." In *Comprehensive Treatment of Chronic Pain by Medical, Interventional and Integrative Approaches: The American Academy of Pain Medicine Textbook on Patient Management*, by Timothy R. Deer, Michael S. Leong, Asokumar Buvanendran, Vitaly Gordin, Philip S. Kim, Sunil J. Panchal and Albert L. Ray. New York: Springer.

Russo, Ethan B., and Geoffrey W. Guy. 2006. "A tale of two cannabinoids: the therapeutic rationale for combining tetrahydrocannabinol and cannabidiol." *Medical Hypotheses* 66 (2): 234-246.

Russo, Ethan B., Geoffrey W. Guy, and Philip J. Robson. 2007. "Cannabis, pain & sleep: lessons from clinical trials of Sativex, a cannabis-based medicine." *Chemistry & Biodiversity* 4 (8): 1729-1743.

Russo, Ethan. 2002. "Cannabis Treatments in Obstetrics and Gynocology: A Historical Review." *Journal of Cannabis Therpeutics* 5-35.

Russo, Ethan. 2008. "Clinical endocannabinoid deficiency (CECD): can this concept explain therapeutic benefits of cannabis in migraine, fibromyalgia, irritable bowel syndrome and other treatment-resistant conditions?" *Neuro Endrocrinology Letters* 29 (2): 192-200.

Russo, Ethan. 2001. "Depression: Practical Considerations." In *Handbook of Psychotropic Herbs: A Scientific Analysis of Herbal Remedies for Psychiatric Conditions*, by Ethan Russo, 90-91. Binghampton: The Hawthorn Herbal Press.

Russo, Ethan. 2001. "Hemp for Headache: An In-Depth Historical and Scientific Review of Cannabis in Migraine Treatment." *Journal of Cannabis Therapeutics* 1 (2): 21-92.

Russo, Ethan. 2011. "Taming THC: potential cannabis synergy and phytocannabinoid-terpenoid entourage effects." *British Journal of Pharmacology* 163 (7): 1344-364.

Russo, Ethan, Mary Lynn Mathre, Al Byrne, Robert Velin, Raul J. Back, Juan Sanchez-Ramos, and Kristin A. Kirlin. 2002. "Chronic Cannabis Use in the Compassionate Investigational New Drug Program: An Examination of Benefits and Adverse Effect of Legal Clinical Cannabis." *Journal of Cannabis Therapeutics* 2 (1): Hawthorne Press.

Salazar, María, Arkaitz Carracedo, Íñigo J. Salanueva, Sonia Hernández-Tiedra, Mar Lorente, Ainara Egia, Patricia Vázquez, et al. 2009. "Cannabinoid action induces autophagy-mediated cell death through stimulation of ER stress in human glioma cells." *The Journal of Clinical Investigation* 119 (5): 1359-1372.

Schaffer, Cliff. n.d. *http://www.druglibrary.org/schaffer/hemp/taxact/woodward. htm. Shaffer Library of Drug Policy. Accessed* August 10, 2014. *http://www. druglibrary.org/schaffer/hemp/taxact/woodward.htm.*

Schlosburg, Joel E., Steven G. Kinsey, and Aron H. Lichtman. 2009. "Targeting Fatty Acid Amide Hydrolase (FAAH) to Treat Pain and Inflammation." *American Association of Pharmaceutical Scientists* 11 (1): 39-43.

Schreiner, Amy M., and Michael E. Dunn. 2012. "Residual Effect of Cannabis Use on Neurocognitive Performance After Prolonged Abstinence: A Meta-Analysis." *Experimental and Clinical Psychopharmacology* 20 (5): 420-9.

Silvestri, Cristoforo, Debora Paris, Andrea Martella, Domonique Melck, Irene Guadagnino, Mike Cawthorne, Andrea Motta, and Vencenzo DiMarzo. 2015. "Two non-psychoactive cannabinoids reduce intra-cellular lipid levels and inhibit hepatosteatosis." *Journal of Hepatology* 62 (6): 1382-90.

Skaper, Stephen D., and Vincenzo Di Marzo. 2012. "Endocannabinoids in nervous system health and disease: the big picture in a nutshell." *Philosophical Transactions of The Royal Society of London* 367 (1607): 3193-3200.

Skrabek, Ryan Quinlan, Lena Galimova, Karen Ethans, and Daryl Perry. 2008. "Nabilone for the Treatment of Pain in Fibromyalgia." *The Journal of Pain* 9 (2): 164-173.

Sloman, Larry. 1979. *Reefer Madness: A History of Marijuana.* New York City: St. Martin's Press.

Smith, G. C. n.d. *Eat Wild.* Colorado St. University. Accessed March 25, 2012. *http:// www.eatwild.com/cla.html.*

Stern, Ruth, and J. Herbie DiFonzo. 2009. "The End of the Red Queens Race: Medical Marijuana in the New Century." *Quinnipiac Law Review* 27 (673): 673-765.

Substance Abuse and Mental Health Administration. 2014. *National Survey of Drug Use and Health. Government Survey,* Rockville: Substance Abuse and Mental Health Administration.

Sulak, Dustin, interview by Nishi Whiteley. 2014. (March 21).

Susman, Ed. 2013. *Smoking Pot Eases Tremors in Parkinson's.* 18 June. Accessed August 12, 2015. *http://www.medpagetoday.com/meetingcoverage/mds/39933.*

Suzuki, David. 2013. *The Nature of Things: The Autism Enigma.* Television show, CBC.

Sylvestre, Diana L., Barry Clements, and Yvonne Malibu. 2006. "Cannabis use improves retention and virological outcomes in patients treated for hepatitis C." *European Journal of Gastroenterology & Hepatology* 18 (10): 1057-1063.

Szabo, Gyongy. 1997. "Alcohol's contribution to compromised immunity." *Alcohol Health & Research World,* 30-38.

Tashkin, Donald P. 2013. "Effects of Marijuana Smoking on the Lung." *Annals of the American Thoracic Society* 10 (3): 239-47.

—. 2008. "Smoked Cannabis Effect On Lungs Parts 1-3." *CannabisTherapeutics YouTube Channel.* Tuscon: Patients Out of Time.

Tashkin, Donald P., Bertrand J. Shapiro, Y. Enoch Lee, and Charles E. Harper.

1975. "Effects of Smoked Marijuana in Experimentally Induced Asthma." *American Review of Respiratory Disease* 112 (3): 337-86.

The Antique Cannabis Book. 2014. "Industrial Hemp in Virginia." *The Antique Cannabis Book.* January. Accessed August 7, 2014. *http:// antiquecannabisbook.com/chap04/Virginia/VA_IndHempP3.htm.*

Tudge, L, C Williams, P J Cowen, and C McCabe. 2014. "Neural effects of cannabinoid CB_1 neutral antagonist tetrahydrocannabivarin on food reward and aversion in healthy volunteers." *The International Journal of Neuropychopharmacology* 18 (6).

U.S. Center for Disease Control & Prevention. 2014. *Chronic Disease & Health Promotion.* May 9. Accessed February 7, 2015. *http://www.cdc.gov/ chronicdisease/overview/#ref1.*

U.S. Department of Health and Human Services. 2010. *A Report of the Surgeon General: How Tobacco Smoke Causes Disease: What It Means to You.* U.S. Department of Health and Human Services, Centers for Disease Control and Prevention, National Center for Chronic Disease Prevention and Health Promotion, Office on Smoking and Health.

U.S. Department of Justice. 2009. "Justice News." *United States Department of Justice.* October 19. Accessed November 8, 2014. *http://www.justice.gov/opa/pr attorney-general-announces-formal-medical-marijuana-guidelines*

United States Drug Enforcement Agency. 2011. *The DEA Position on Marijuana.* Washington DC: U.S. DEA.

University of Maryland Medical Center. 2011. 1 26. Accessed 3 25, 2012. *http://www. umm.edu/altmed/articles/garlic-000245.htm.*

Valdeolivas, Sarah, Carmen Narvarette, Irene Cantarero, Maria L. Belido, Eduardo Munoz, and Onintza Sagredo. 2015. "Neuroprotective Properties of Cannabigerol in Huntington's Disease: Studies in R6/2 Mice and 3-Nitropropionate-lesioned Mice." *Neurotherapeutics* 12 (1): 185-199.

Verhoeckx, Kitty C.M., Henrie A. Korthout, Karl A. Ehlert, Tonny Lagerweij, Lex Nagelkerken, Mei Wang, Jan van der Greef, Richard J.T. Rodenburg, and Renger F. Witkamp. 2006. "Unheated Cannabis sativa extracts and its major compound THC-acid have potential immuno-modulating properties not mediated by CB_1 and CB_2 receptor coupled pathways." *International Immunopharmacology* 6 (4): 656-665.

Vote Hemp. 2014. "Press Release: President Obama Signs Farm Bill with Amendment to Allow Industrial Hemp Research." Vote Hemp. February 7. Accessed September 24, 2014. *http://www.votehemp.com/PR/2014-02-07- vh_farm_bill_signed.html.*

Wallace, Melisa J., Robert E. Blair, Katherine W. Falenski, Billy R. Martin, and Robert J. DeLorenzo. 2003. "The endogenous cannabinoid system regulates seizure frequency and duration in a model of temporal lobe epilepsy." *The Journal of Pharmacology and Experimental Therapeutics* 307 (1): 129-137.

Weiss, Rick. 2006. Marijuana Aids Therapy. September 13. Accessed August 13, 2015. *http://www.washingtonpost.com/wp-dyn/content/article/2006/09/12/ AR2006091201444.html.*

Wenk, Gary. 2011. "Does it matter when you start smoking marijuana?" *Psychology*

Today. June. Accessed April 11, 2014. *http://www.psychologytoday.com/blog/your-brain-food/201106/does-it-matter-when-you-start-smoking-marijuana.*

Wenk, Gary L. 2010. Your Brain on Food: How Chemicals Control Your Thoughts and Feelings. New York: Oxford University Press.

Wenk, Gary. 2012. "Life Depends on This." *TEDxColumbus.* Columbus Ohio: TED Talks. *http://youtu.be/4SvkaK2Al0o.*

Werner, Clint. 2011. *Marijuana Gateway to Health: How Cannabis Protects Us from Cancer and Alzheimer's Disease.* San Francisco: Dachstar Press.

Winston, David, and Steve Maimes. 2007. *Adaptogens: Herbs for Strength, Stamina and Stress Relief.* Rochester, Vermont: Healing Arts Press.

Wissenborn, Ruth, and David J. Nutt. 2011. "Popular intoxicants: what lessons can be learned from the last 40 years of alcohol and cannabis regulation?" *Journal of Psychopharmacology* 1-8.

Wo/Man's Alliance for Medical Marijuana. n.d. *Wo/Man's Alliance for Medical Marijuana.* Accessed August 22, 2014. *https://wamm.org/.*

Wu, Tzu-Chin, Donald P. Tashkin, Behnam Djahed, and Jed E. Rose. 1988. "Pulmonary Hazards of Smoking Marijuana as Compared with Tobacco." *New England Journal of Medicine* 318 (6): 347-351.

Yap, Ivan Kok Seng, Manya Angley, Kirill A. Veselkov, Elaine Holmes, John C. Lindon, and Jeremy Kirk Nicholson. 2010. "Urinary metabolic phenotyping differentiates children with autism from their unaffected siblings and age-matched controls." *Journal of Proteome Research* 9 (6): 2996-3004.

316

Index

[t] indicates term is found in a table

2-arachydonoyl glycerol, 38, 39, 42–43
  and neurotransmitters, 66
  and pain, 89
  production, 68
5-fluorouracil, 58
11-hydroxy-THC, 194

A

Abood, Mary, 104
Abrams, Donald
  endocannabinoid system, 37
  opiates, 144
  pain, 95
  pioneer, 26
  research, 117
acetylcholine, 66, 66[t], 105
acetylcholinesterase activity, 105–106
AChE Inhibitor, 56[t]
ACP. See American College of Physicians
activism, 118–119
adaptogens, 36
addiction, 48, 66[t], 150–151[t]
ADHD. See attention deficit/hyperactivity
  disorder
adolescents, 160–163
adrenals, 107, 153[t]
advocacy, 234–243
AEA. See anandamide
age-related macular degeneration, 81[t]
Aggarwal, Sunil K.
  addiction, 151
  benefits of cannabis, 169–170
  pain, 90
  pioneer, 26
  psychoactivity, 211
  research volume, 30–31
  schedule classification, 29
aging, 9, 69–71, 77
agonists, 41–42
AIDS
  cannabis, 9, 95, 109[t]
  cannabis oil, 201
  Cesamet®, 28
  Marinol®, 28
  pharmaceuticals, 185

tetrahydrocannabinol, 45
ALA. See alpha-linolenic acids
alcohol, 19, 126–128, 150–151[t]
alcoholics and tinctures, 207
alcoholism, 47
Aldrich, Michael, 15
allergies, 81[t]
al-Mayusi, 16[t]
alpha-linolenic acids, 65
alpha-pinene, 89–90, 153[t]
ALS. See amyotrophic lateral sclerosis
Alzheimer's Association, 105
Alzheimer's disease, 36, 42, 104–106, 237
  acetylcholine, 66[t]
  cannabidiol, 47, 48
  cannabinoids, 78
  cannabis, 9
  central nervous system disease, 63, 64
  chronic inflammation, 81[t]
  delta 9 tetrahydrocannabinol, 46, 51
  free radicals, 75
  inflammation, 83
  neurodegeneration, 83
  pro-inflammatory cytokines, 79
  in U.S. patent, 30
AMD. See age-related macular degeneration
American Academy of Pain Medicine, 85, 95
American Cancer Society, The, 99, 129, 131
American Civil Liberties Union, 23, 118
American College of Physicians, 22–23
American Journal of Psychiatry, 19
American Medical Association, 19, 71
American Pharmacopoeia, 16[t]
American Psychological Association, The, 157
Americans for Safe Access, 26, 112[t]
  legal rights, 168
  political activism, 119, 235
  Security Culture webpage, 11
America. See also United States of America
amphetamine, 27[t], 125, 126, 151[t]
amyloid B-peptides, 106
amyotrophic lateral sclerosis, 9, 103–104
  cannabis oil, 201
  central nervous system diseases, 64
  effect on nervous system, 63
  inflammation, 83
  neurodegeneration, 83

symptom relief, 45
symptoms, 64, 104
anabolic steroids, 27[t]
analgesic, 48, 50[t], 56[t], 57, 89
Anandakanda, 16[t]
anandamide, 42–43, 44, 68
　digestive system, 68
　discovery of, 17[t]
　endocannabinoid system, 38, 39
　miscarriage, 165
　neurotransmitters, 66
　pain, 89
Anatomy of the Spirit: Seven Stages of Power and
　Healing, 140
anemia, 81[t]
Angel, Garyn, 255
angiogenesis, 100, 165
ankylosing spondolytis, and cannabis oil, 201
ANS. See autonomic nervous system
Anslinger, Harry, 16[t], 18–19, 21
antagonists, 41–42
anti-anxiety, 50[t], 56[t]
antibacterial, 52, 58
antibiotic, 50[t], 56[t]
antibiotic-resistant infections, 47
anti-clotting agent, 58
anti-convulsant, 47, 51, 58
anti-depressant, 48, 50[t], 56[t]
antidotes, 180
anti-emetic, 47, 48, 50[t]
anti-epileptic, 50[t], 56[t]
anti-excitotoxic agent, 103
anti-fungal, 50[t], 52, 56[t], 58
anti-inflammatory
　agents, 84
　a-pinene, 56[t], 58
　aspirin, 10
　beta-caryophyllene, 56[t], 57
　beta-myrcene, 56[t]
　brain health, 67–68
　cannabichromene, 50[t]
　cannabidiol, 47, 50[t], 105
　cannabidiol acid, 50[t]
　cannabigerol, 50[t]
　cannabinoid acids, 53
　cannabinoid acid tea, 53
　cannabinoids, 103, 105
　cannabinol, 51
　cannabis tea, 53
　diet, 84
　hydrocortisone, 10
　tetrahydrocannabinol, 10
　tetrahydrocannabivarin, 52
anti-insomnia, 50[t]
anti-ischemic, 50[t], 56[t]
anti-malarial, 56[t], 58

anti-mutagenic, 56[t]
antioxidant, 30, 67–68, 75–76, 77
　cannabidiol, 47, 50[t]
　cannabinoids, 103
　cannabis, 9, 64, 73, 76–77, 104
　Co-enzyme Q10, 76
　tetrahydrocannabinol, 50[t]
anti-proliferative, 50[t], 56[t], 100, 208
anti-psychotic
　beta-myrcene, 56[t]
　cannabidiol, 47, 48, 50[t]
　linalool, 56[t]
　tetrahydrocannabivarin, 52
Antique Cannabis Book, The, 15
anti-spasmodic, 50[t], 56[t]
anxiety, 16, 101–103
　cannabidiol, 48, 101
　central nervous system diseases, 64
　GABA, 66[t]
　glutamate, 66[t]
anxiolytic, 47, 58
aortic valve stenosis, 81[t]
a-pinene, 55, 56[t], 58
apoptosis, 100
appearance, 175
appetite, 9, 45, 48
appetite stimulant, 28, 50[t]
Apte, Viajanti "Jay", 262
arachadonoylethanolamide, 17[t]
arachidonlylglycerol, 17[t]
arachnoid cysts, 64
arrest, 7, 149[t], 231–234
arthritis, 78, 81[t], 109[t], 201
Ashworth scale, 45
aspirin, 10, 113, 237
Association of Commercial Cannabis
　Laboratories, 228
asthma, 16, 45, 109[t]
atherosclerosis, 14, 45, 75
athletes, 77–78
attention deficit/hyperactivity disorder, 64, 126
Aunt Zelda's, 25, 26, 200
autism
　delta 9 tetrahydrocannabinol, 46
　free radicals, 75
　gel caps, 210
　glutamate, 66[t]
　spectrum disorders, 120
　tetrahydrocannabinol, 51
autonomic nervous system, 63
awareness, 158
Axelrod, Juilius, 76
Ayurveda, 16[t], 35

B
Backes, Michael, 26, 174

bacteria, 9, 178–179
Bakalar, James B., 216
Balagia, Jamie, 11
balance difficulties, 153[t]
Banuelos, Ron, 140
barbiturates, 151[t]
basic recipes, 272–274
Beeman, Sean, 211
Ben-Shabat, Shimon, 42
benzodiazepines, 125–126, 151[t]
beta-amyloid plaques, 78
beta-amyloid proteins, 106
beta-caryophyllene, 55, 56[t], 57
    anti-inflammatory agent, 84
    pain, 89–90
beta-myrcene, 55, 56[t], 57
Bhang Chocolate, 221, 222[t]
BHO. See butane hash oil
biphasic response, 101, 151[t]
birth defects, 58
Bittner, Mary Ann, 118
black pepper, 55, 57
blindness, 21, 48
blood pressure, 189
blood testing, 79–80
body, 69–71
bone growth, 9, 50[t]
bone reabsorption, 48
bong, 186, 191–193
brain, 65–66
    aging, 69–71
    cancer, 44
    cannabinoid receptors, 68
    cells, 9, 68
    development, 161–162
    digestive system, 78
    energy consumption of, 68
    health, 67–68, 69
    health of, 67–69
    role in Central Nervous System, 63
Brain Maker, 78
Braverman, Eric, 65
breast cancer, 57
bronchitis, 130, 149[t]
bronchodilator
    a-pinene, 56[t], 58
    delta 9 tetrahydrocannabinol, 44, 45
    tetrahydrocannabinol, 50[t]
Brownie Mary, 26
bud, 170, 171[t], 177, 219
buprenorphine, 151[t]
Bureau of Narcotics, 21
Bureau of Prohibition, 18
butane, 189–190, 196
butane hash oil, 188
butter, 256–257

C

cancer, 9, 14, 26, 99–101, 237
    cannabidiol, 47, 48
    cannabinoid acids, 53
    cannabis, 10, 95
    cannabis oil, 200–201, 202–204
    cannabis research, 114–115
    Cesamet®, 28
    chronic inflammation, 78, 81[t]
    delta 9 tetrahydrocannabinol, 44, 45
    free radicals, 75
    limonene, 57–58
    Marinol®, 28
    nerolidol, 58
    oils, 182–183
    pain, 28
    pharmaceuticals, 185
    tetrahydrocannabinol, 51
    THCA, 208
    tumor necrosis factor alpha, 82
cannabichromene, 50[t], 52, 84, 89–90
cannabidiol, 9, 12, 16[t], 25, 46–51, 105–106
    agonist, 42
    anti-inflammatory agent, 84
    anxiety, 48, 101
    depression, 101
    diabetic cardiac dysfunction, 83
    hemp oil, 197
    inflammatory response, 82
    long-term memory, 66[t]
    in medical cannabis, 173
    for mood disorders, 102–103
    neurogenesis, 68, 106
    pain, 89
    post traumatic stress disorder, 47, 108
    Schedule I drug, 197
    short-term memory loss, 66[t], 72, 153[t]
    synergy with tetrahydrocannabinol, 89
    tachycardia, 149[t]
    tetrahydrocannabinol ratios, 200
    used separately from tetrahydrocannabinol,
        207–208
cannabidiol acid, 50[t]
cannabigerol, 48, 50[t], 52, 89–90
cannabinologist.org, 29
cannabinoid
    agents, 89
    hyperemesis, 151–152[t]
    integrity, 222
    medicines, 8, 87
    modulator, 57
    oil, 25
    ratios, 215
cannabinoid acid, 52–53
    in raw cannabis, 195–196
    research, 196

tea, 53, 208
testing, 228
cannabinoid receptors, 33, 38, 39–41, 39
    in the brain, 68
    creation of, 167
    digestive tract, 68
    endocannabionid system, 223
    reproductive systems, 165
cannabinoids, 8–9, 16[t], 33–35, 43–52, 66–67
    absence of industry standards in testing, 226
    additional receptors, 41
    Alzheimer's disease, 78
    angiogenesis, 100
    anti-excitotoxic agent, 103, 105
    anti-inflammatory, 103, 105
    antioxidant, 103
    apoptosis, 100
    beta-amyloid plaques, 78
    brain cells, 9, 68
    brain health, 67–68
    cancer, 9, 26, 100
    cognition, 72–73
    effect on brain, 65–66
    fibromyalgia, 90
    hepatitis, 84
    high doses, 147
    HIV neuropathy, 90
    inflammatory response, 82
    liver disease, 84
    modulator of inflammation, 83
    modulator of neurodegeneration, 83
    neural repair, 103
    neurogenesis, 83
    neuro-inflammation, 78
    neuropathic pain, 90
    oxidation, 75
    oxidative stress, 105
    pain, 87, 90
    pancreas, 84
    patent, 17[t]
    pro-inflammatory cytokines, 84
    rheumatoid arthritis, 90
    safety of, 100
    sleep, 90
    stress response, 36–37
    synergistic effects, 51, 175
    synthetic, 35
    testing, 170, 228
    therapeutic effects, 50[t]
    tincture, 25
    trials, 90
    tumor growth, 44
Cannabinoids and Multiple Sclerosis study, 45
cannabinoid wax, 188
cannabinol, 16[t], 50[t], 51
cannabis, 9–10, 109–114

access to hard drugs, 240
acute inflammation, 77
adaptogenic properties, 36–37
addiction rate, 19, 22, 24, 150–151[t]
advocacy, 231–243
AIDS, 95, 109[t]
American grown, 89–90
antioxidant property of, 9, 64, 73, 76–77, 104
anti-senility agent, 16[t]
appetite stimulant, 16[t]
biphasic properties, 36
botanical names, 12
brain development, 161–162
breeding, 89–90, 173
cancer, 9, 10, 95, 100
cardiovascular system, 76
central nervous system diseases, 64
children, 239–240
cigarettes, 21–22, 218
in clinical practice, 139
cognitive performance, 78
compared to alcohol, 126–128
compared to prescription medications,
    123–126, 145
compared to tobacco, 129–132
conception, 165
cultivation, 13
depression, 10, 64, 110[t]
difference from hemp, 12–13
drooling, 64
effect on brain cells, 68
effect on reaction time, 73
effect on sperm, 165
effects on terpenes, 57
efficacy of, 237
endocannabinoid system, 114
for epilepsy, 16[t], 111[t]
executive cognitive functions, 162
extractions, 26
fear, 71
fertilization, 165
flower, 35, 177
in food, 181–182
gateway drug, 7
gel caps, 209–210
hallucinogenic, 16[t]
healthy living, 69
high cannabidiol varieties, 49
history of, 15–17, 22
horticultural crop, 13
hybrids, 7, 172–173
hyperemesis gravidarum, 164
impact of cross-pollination with hemp, 13
industry, 27
inflammation, 82–84
IQ, 161

irritable bowel syndrome, 83
legality of, 10–11
legalization, 21, 23
longevity, 16[t]
lung protection, 133–134
lungs, 132–134
medical legalization, 17[t], 23
medical necessity, 21–22
medical use research, 19
medical uses, 15, 22–23, 139
medical value, 22, 28, 43, 77
medicine, 26, 43, 101, 185
memory recovery, 71
moldy, 175
morning sickness, 164
myths, 68
neurocognitive performance, 72–73
neuroprotective properties, 9, 64, 68, 71, 73, 76
oil, 26
opiates, 125, 144
overdose, 96
oxidative stress, 104
pain, 8–9, 85, 88
pain medication, 144
patents on, 237
performance enhancer, 78
pharmacologically active, 8–9
positive effects, 154–155
post-traumatic stress syndrome, 71
pregnancy, 163–165
prescription, 16
preventative, 10, 37
prohibition, 17–23
psychotherapy, 71
ratios, 200
raw, 195–196
reclassification, 23
recreational legalization, 17[t]
recreational use, history of, 18
recreation use research, 19
relief, 8–9
research, 114–115
research-grade, 23
safety, 10, 17–18, 20–21, 73, 96, 113–114, 237
Schedule I, 21, 27[t], 29
science, 33–59
side effects, 10, 114, 166–167
smoking, 130–134
society, 240
spasticity, 64
spiritual practices, 159
symptom relief, 8–9
terpenes to enhance, 55
terpenoids, 55
testing, 170, 215, 225–229
therapeutic chemicals, 33

tincture, 26, 101
tonic, 16[t]
topicals, 26
trauma, 71
trichomes, 33
use, 2, 3, 77–78
users, 3, 7
varieties, 172–174
versatility, 237
wasting, 64
Cannabis afghanica, 172
cannabis analysis, 225–229
Cannabis Awareness Collection, 226
cannabis hemp oil. See cannabis oil
Cannabis indica, 7, 12, 172–173
Cannabis International, 196
cannabis-med.org, 87
cannabis oil, 55, 101, 177, 188, 196–204
Cannabis Pharmacy, 174
cannabis plant, 7, 34, 35
    cultivation of, 13
    female, 7, 13, 16[t]
    male, 7, 13, 16[t]
    smell, 54
    variety identification, 59
Cannabis Potency Project, 44
Cannabis ruderalis, 12
Cannabis sativa, 7, 12, 34, 172–173
Cannabis Tax Act, 16[t], 18–19
cannabis tea, 53, 208–209
Cannabis Therapeutics, 132
canna butter, 256–257
CannaDX, ™, 170
Canna Kitchen and Research LLC, 211, 213
carburetor, 192, 193
cardiac death, 14
cardiovascular diseases, 81[t]
cardiovascular system, 76
Carter, Gregory T., 104, 123, 126, 218–219
Carter, Jimmy, 234
caryophyllene oxide, 55, 56[t], 58
casual dosing, 214
Cato Institute, 23
cautions, 160–165
CB_1, 17[t]
CB_1 agonist, tetrahydrocannabivarin, 52
CB_1 receptors, 39–41, 89
    benefits, 40[t]
    and delta 9 tetrahydrocannabinol, 44
    and digestive system, 83
    role in inflammation, 82
CB_2, 17[t]
CB_2 agonist, beta-caryophyllene, 57
CB_2 receptors, 89
    benefits, 40[t], 41
    cannabinol, 51

and digestive system, 83
role in inflammation, 82
CBC. See cannabichromene
CBD. See cannabidiol
cbdfarm.org, 202
CBD-only legislation, 44–45, 51
CBG. See cannabigerol
CBN. See cannabinol
Center for the Study of Cannabis and Social Policy, 36
Centers for Disease Control and Prevention
    alcohol, 127
    autism, 120
    overdoses, 124–125
    tobacco, 129, 130, 131
central nervous system, 63–64
    benzodiazepines, 125–126
    disorders, 83
    inhalation, 181
    pain, 88
Cesamet*, 27[t], 28, 29, 185
Charlotte's Web, 47
Cheech and Chong, 128
chemical composition, 33
chemotherapy, 9
    and cannabis, 10, 110[t]
    and nausea, 9, 17[t], 22
    side effect relief for, 2, 3
    and vomiting, 9
chia seeds, 65, 151[t], 252–253
children, 160–163, 239–240
Chinese medicine, 35
cholesterol, 69
chronic, 177
chronically ill patients, 25
chronic illness, development of, 61–62
chronic inflammation, 62, 78, 79, 81[t]
chronic kidney disease, 81[t]
chronic pain, 9, 85, 87–90
    cannabidiol, 48
    cannabis, 110[t]
    effects of high dose, 224
    relaxation, 94
    stress, 94
    in the United States, 85
circulation, 9
CKD. See chronic kidney disease
Clarke,Robert C., 26
clinical practice, 139
clinical trials, 113[t]
CNN, 24
CNS. See central nervous system
CO2 extraction, 189–190, 196, 197–198, 204–205
CO2 oil, 188
cocaine, 27[t], 150–151[t]
codeine, 27[t]

Code of the West, 232
Co-enzyme Q10, 76
cognition, 72–73, 78, 153[t]
cognitive decline, and chronic inflammation, 81[t]
collectives, 25
colon cancer, 52
colon health, 69
Commission on Cannabis Drug Abuse. See Schafer Commission
Common Sense for Drug Policy, 19
communication with others, 236–237
Compassionate Use Investigational New Drug Program, 17[t], 21–22
complimentary medicine, 203
Comprehensive Drug Abuse and Control Act of 1970, The. See Controlled Substances Act
concentrated cannabis oil. See cannabis oil
conception, 165
concussions, 110[t]
congestive heart failure, 81[t]
Constance Therapeutics, 202, 203
constipation, 151[t]
constitutional rights, 11
contraindications, 160
Controlled Substances Act
    classifications, 27[t], 29
    federal law, 19
    and hemp, 12
    and history, 17[t]
    war on drugs, 21
cooking, 2–3, 171, 259
cooking. See also decarboxylation
Corral, Valerie
    cancer, 46
    dosing, 207
    healing, 166
    pioneer, 26, 200
    Wo/Men's Alliance for Medical Marijuana, 25
cost, 10
"couch-lock" sensation, 57, 153[t]
Courtney, William, 196
Craker, Lyle, 117–118
C-reactive protein, 79
creativity, 156
creeping, 181
criminalization, 21
Crohn's disease, 9, 110[t]
Curry, Wei-Ni Lin, 164
CVD. See cardiovascular diseases
cystitis, 66[t]
cytokines, 79

D

dabbing, 181, 188–191
dab rig, 188, 188
DAGL. See diacyl glycerol lipase

dank, 177
Danny's story, 10
D.A.R.E., 68, 238
DEA. *See* Drug Enforcement Administration
DeAngelo, Steve, 26
decarboxylated cannabinoid testing, 228
decarboxylation, 52–53, 171, 209, 222
decriminalization, 17[t], 19–20, 24, 27
de-felonization, 24
delta 9 tetrahydrocannabinol, 28, 43–46, 51
delta 9 tetrahydrocannabinol. *See also*
    tetrahydrocannabinol
delusions, 150[t]
dementia, 66[t]
Department of Agriculture, 13
Department of Health, Education, and Welfare, 30
Department of Justice, 24, 29
depersonalization, 150[t]
depression, 9, 16, 68, 101–103
    cannabis, 10, 64, 110[t]
    central nervous system diseases, 64
    chronic inflammation, 81[t]
    dopamine, 66[t]
    limonene, 57
    risk of, 150[t]
    serotonin, 66[t]
Deuvall, Clif, 144–145
Devane, William A., 39, 42
diabetes, 79
    cannabidiol, 47
    cannabis, 10, 110[t]
    chronic inflammation, 81[t]
diabetic cardiac dysfunction, 83
diabetic retinopathy, 48
diacyl glycerol lipase, 38
diet, 62
digestive system, 68, 69, 78, 83
DiMarzo, Vincenzo, 119
Disease Curing Plan, 147
dispensary edibles, 221–222
dizziness, 152[t]
DMF. *See* Drug Master File
DMT, 27[t]
DNA, 75
doctors, 23
do-it-yourself dabs, 190–191
dopamine, 57, 66[t]
dosing, 167, 214–223
    casual, 191–192, 214
    edibles, 194–195
    intake methods, 180–186
    tinctures, 207–208
dosing chart
    dried bud, 219[t]
    Marinol®, 216[t]
Dravet syndrome, 25, 47

Dr. Diane, 198
Dreher, Melanie C., 163–164
dronabinol, 28, 29, 185
dronabinol. See Marinol®
drooling, 64
drowsiness, 173
drug addiction, 64, 110[t]
drug arrests, 23
Drug Enforcement Administration, 24, 28, 29,
    117–118, 232
    authority to reschedule, 29
    dealing with, 11–12
    efforts against rescheduling, 29–31
    Federal Bureau of Narcotics, 18
    license to grow hemp, 12–13
    position regarding tetrahydrocannabinol
        levels, 12
    resistance to rescheduling, 17[t], 30
    role in research, 116
Drug Master File, 117
drug overdose, 124–125
Drug Policy Alliance, 27, 233, 235
drugpolicy.org/drug-war-statistic, 234
drug testing, 169
dry mouth, 152[t]
Dunn, Michael E., 72–73
duodenal ulcers, 57
Dutch Office of Medical Cannabis, The, 208
dying process, 62, 85, 148
dysmenorrhea, 16
dysphoria, 150[t]

E

Earlywine, Mitch, 15, 16
eating disorders, 66[t]
*Eating on the Wild Side: The Missing Link to
    Optimum Health*, 252, 255
ECS. See endocannabinoid system
Edge Effect, The, 65
edibles, 181–182, 194–195, 220–223
EFA. See essential fatty acids
elder care, 104–106, 160
Eli Lily, 16
ElSohly, Mahmoud A., 44, 118
encephalitis, 64
endocannabinoid deficiency, 90
endocannabinoids, 8, 33–35, 37–39, 42–43
    creation of, 67
    digestive system, 68
    discovery, 17[t]
    effect on brain, 65–66
    essential fatty acids, 65
    harm reduction system, 61–62
    homeostasis, 14
    neurotransmitters, 66–67
    overall health, 71

endocannabinoid system, 8, 37–39, 61–62, 237
  acute inflammation, 77
  addiction, 151[t]
  autism, 120
  cancer, 100
  cannabinoid receptors, 44, 223
  cannabis, 114
  dabbing, 190
  difficulty of research, 117
  inflammation, 80, 82–84
  irritable bowel syndrome, 83
  nervous system, 62–64
  pain, 88, 89
  pancreas, 82, 84
  post traumatic stress disorder, 107
  and reproductive systems, 165
  research needed, 41, 42–43, 87
  resensitizing program, 224–225
  stress, 101–102
  support for, 69
  tolerance, 223–225
end-of-life care, 1, 2–3, 4
entourage effect, 17[t], 35, 45, 55
enzymes, 38–39
epilepsy, 9, 25, 237
  cannabidiol, 47
  cannabis, 111[t]
  central nervous system diseases, 64
  oils, 182
Epstein, Jerry, 239
equipment, 169
Erh-Ya, 16[t]
essential fatty acids, 14, 65
essential oils, 53, 55
essential oils. See also individual oils
ethanol, 189–190, 196, 198
ethanolic extraction recipe, 206–207
ethanolic tinctures, 204, 205
ether, 198
Eubanks, Lisa M., 106
euphoria, 159
euphoriant, 50[t]
Europe, 15
excitoxicity, 105
executive cognitive functions, 162
extraction methods, 190–191, 197–198
extractions, 26, 204–208

F
FAAH. See fatty acid amide hydrolase
Fallon, Sally, 84, 253, 255
family communication, 236–237
Farm Bill, 12–13
fats, 69
fatty acid amide hydrolase, 38–39, 42, 89
fatty liver disease, 52

FBI. See Federal Bureau of Investigation
FDA. See Food and Drug Administration
fear, 71
Federal Bureau of Investigation, 231
Federal Bureau of Narcotics, 16[t], 18
Federal Trade Commission, 130
female plants, 33
fertilization, 165
fibromyalgia, 81[t], 90, 111[t]
fibrosis, 81[t]
Figgy, Charlotte, 25
fingerprinting, 59
Finley, Constance, 26, 200–201, 203, 207
flavonoids, 9, 33, 75
flax seeds, 252–253
flowers, 170
focus, 68
follicle-stimulating hormone, 51
Food and Drug Administration
  amyotrophic lateral sclerosis, 103
  pharmaceuticals, 29, 162
  role in research, 49, 116, 117
  safety, 123, 126, 237
  terpenes, 55
  trials, 146
  whole plant, 52
forgetfulness, 157–158
formal dosing, 214
frail users, 160
freedom from pain, rights, 94–95
free radicals, 75–76
freshness, 175–177
FSH. See follicle-stimulating hormone
fungus, 178–179

G
GABA, 56[t], 58, 66, 66[t], 125
Gaoni, Yechiel, 43
Gardner, Fred, 26
gas chromatography, 228
gastric cytoprotective, 57
gastrointestinal disorders, 66[t]
gateway drug, 7, 238–239
GC. See gas chromatography
gel caps, 209–210, 213
Genesis Pharms, 211
George Washington, 12, 15
Gettman, John, 28
ginkgo biloba, 76
glandular trichomes, 14, 33, 178, 197
  content, 218
  density, 175
  powder, 209
  terpenes, 55
glaucoma, 8, 9, 21–22, 111[t]
glioblastoma, 204

glutamate, 41–42, 58, 66, 66[t], 105
glutathione, 76
gluten-free recipes, 272–273, 295
glycerin extractions, 205
glycerol extractions, 204
Gold Star, 173
Goldstein, Bonnie, 26
Gordon, Mara, 25, 26, 200, 207
Graham, Rhea, 211–212
Grain Brain, 78
Grav Labs, 188
green plant, 171[t]
Grimaldi, Maurizio, 76
Grinspoon, Lester, 10, 15, 216
Gruber, Staci, 161
Guindon, Josée, 100
Gupta, Sanjay, 24, 25, 47, 49
gut. *See* digestive system
Guzman, Manuel, 26, 44, 100, 119
GWP. *See* GW Pharmaceuticals
GW Pharmaceuticals, 8, 28–29, 198, 204

H

hallucinations, 150[t], 152[t]
Hamm, Rebecca, 138
Hampson, Aidan J., 76
Hanuš, Lumír Ondřej, 42
Happy Apple Seed Recipe, 260
Happy Cake Ball Recipe, 294
harm reduction, 149–154[t]
hashish, 171, 178, 209
Hawaii, 13
Haze, 173
Hazekamp, Arno, 198, 199, 208
Healer.com, 225
Healing Magic of Cannabis, The, 155
health, 67–69, 71, 78, 137–141
healthcare, 137–141, 143–144
healthcare providers, 138–140
health food, 14
heart attack, 79, 81[t]
heart conditions, 160
heart disease, 30
    chronic inflammation, 78
    free radicals, 75
    risks of cannabis use, 149[t]
Heart Math Institute, The, 138
hemp, 7, 12–14, 172
    bioremediator, 49–51
    cultivation in United States, 12–15
    fiber, 7, 12, 15
    history, 15–16
    industrial, 12–14, 15
    laws, 51
    oil, 65, 197
    oil. *See also* cannabis oil

pesticides used with, 49–51
plants, 197
poor source for cannabidiol, 12, 49–51
production, 12–13
seed, 13, 15, 65, 252–253
seed oil. *See* hemp oil
hepatitis, 84, 111[t]
Hergenrather, Jeffrey, 26, 105, 106, 190, 211
heroin, 27[t], 151[t]
HEW. *See* Department of Health, Education, and
    Welfare
hexane, 196
HG. See hyperemesis gravidarum
high performance liquid chromatography, 228
high performance thin layer chromatography, 228
High Times Cannabis Cup, 189, 221–222
High Times magazine, 15
Hill, Matthew N., 102
history, 15–17, 201–202
History of Cannabis as a Medicine, A, 15
HIV, 9, 22, 45, 90, 201
Hohmann, Andrea G., 89, 100
Holder, Eric, 232
holistic medicine, 71, 138–141
home extraction methods, 198
homemade edibles, 222–223
homeostasis, 37–38, 61
honey oil, 181, 188
hops, 55, 57
hormones, 42, 69–71
Howlett, Allyn, 39
How to Regulate Cannabis: A Practical Guide, 241
HPLC. *See* high performance liquid
    chromatography
HPTLC. *See* high performance thin layer
    chromatography
humulene, 55
Huntington's disease, 52, 64
hybrids, 172–173
Hyde, Kelly, 26
Hyde, Mike, 26
hydration, 69
hydrocarbons, 189–190
hydrocortisone, 10
hyperemesis gravidarum, 164
hypertension, 45, 48, 66[t]
hysteria, 16

I

IBS. *See* irritable bowel syndrome
ID-1 gene, 200
illness recovery, 144–145
illusions, 150[t]
immune
    potentiator, 56[t]
    support, 53

system, 57
system modulation, 208
immunosuppressive, 50[t]
IND. *See* Investigational New Drug Program
indica, 172–173
industrial hemp, 13
inflammation, 8, 77–84
inflammatory pain, 89
ingestion, 194–195
inhalation, 177, 180–181, 218
   dosing equations, 219
   methods, 186–191
   tips, 191–193
injury recovery, 144–145
insomnia, 16, 45, 64
Institute of Medicine, 150–151[t]
Institutional Review Board, 116
intake methods, 147, 167
   cancer, 101
   cannabis based medicines, 185
   dabbing, 188–191
   edibles, 181–182
   inhalation, 186–193
   inhalation of concentrates, 181
   inhalation of dried plant material, 180–181
   lungs, 194
   oils, 182–183
   overview, 180–186
   raw juice, 184–185
   Sativex®, 185
   for sleep, 157
   smoking, 180–181, 186
   suppositories, 184
   tinctures, 182
   topical applications, 183
   vaporization, 180–181, 187–188
integrative medicine, 71, 203
Internal Revenue Service, 11–12
International Association of Cannabinoid
   Medicines, 27, 112[t], 235
International Cannabinoid Research Society,
   The, 27
international law, 115
intestinal flora, 69
intoxication, 152[t]
intraocular pressure, 45
Investigational New Drug Program, 217–218
IQ, 161
irritable bowel syndrome, 52, 83, 90
IRS. *See* Internal Revenue Service
isopropyl alcohol, 196
itching, 152[t]

J

James A. Baker III Institute for Public Policy, 239
joint, 186

Journal of Cannabis Therapeutics, 22
Journal of Psychopharmacology, 126
Joy, Dan, 155
Justice, Charleen, 226

K

K2, 173
Kali Mist, 173
Kaneh bosem, 16[t]
keef. *See* kif
keif. *See* kif
Kennedy, Edward, 118
Kerry, John, 118
ketamine, 151[t]
kidney failure, 81[t]
kif, 171[t], 178, 209
kif resin powder capsules, 183–184
kind bud, 177
kitchen equipment, 254–255
Kiva Confections, 222[t]
Klein, Zach, 41, 104–105

L

LA. *See* linolenic acids
Laboratory of Physiologic Studies, 45
lab testing, 174
La Guardia Committee Report, 16[t], 19
La Guardia, Fiorello, 19
La Guardia Report. *See* La Guardia Committee
   Report
lavender, 55, 58
law enforcement, 29
   consequences of, 21
   dealing with, 11–12, 167
   and fingerprinting, 59
   and hemp fields, 13
laws
   dealing with, 11–12
   differences in enforcement, 11
   federal, 10–11, 19, 23, 24, 232–234
   international, 115
   state, 10–11, 12–13, 19, 23, 168, 232–233
leaf, 170–171, 171[t], 178
Leafly.com, 173–174
Leaf Science, 113[t]
Leary, United States v., 19
Leary, Timothy, 166
Lee, Martin A., 26, 46, 196
Lee, Richard, 26
legality, 2, 10–12, 27–29, 149[t]
   at federal level, 10–11, 19, 27
   at state level, 10–11, 19, 27
legalization, 17[t]
   advocacy, 231–243
   benefits of, 178–179
   economic impact, 27

effect of cannabidiol use in children, 47
effect on pharmaceutical companies, 27
effect on research, 27
effects of, 125, 126
    national level, 11, 23
    public feeling, 234
    support for, 23–24, 168–169
legal representation, 11
Legionella, 160
legislation, cannabidiol-only, 44–45
lemon balm, 55, 58
Life Extension Foundation, The, 80
limonene, 55, 56[t], 57–58
linalool, 55, 56[t], 58, 89–90
linolenic acids, 65
lipoic acid, 76
liver disease, 84
locked-in syndrome, 64
long-term memory, 65–66, 68
low energy, 66[t]
LSD, 27[t]
lungs
    cannabis, 132–134
    intake method, 194
    irritation, 149[t], 150[t]
    protection, 133–134
    smoking, 194
lupus, 81[t], 111[t]
Lyme disease, 201

M

McCarthy Test, 164
McGhee, David, 190
McPartland, John M., 35, 62
Magical Butter Machine, 255
Magic Flight Launch Box, 187, 193
MAGL. See monoacylglycerol lipase
Magnolia Wellness, 222[t]
Maine, 13
Maintenance Plan, 145–147
Management Plan, 145–147
Marihuana:A Signal of Misunderstanding,
    17[t], 19–21
Marihuana:The Forbidden Medicine, 216
marijuana, 7, 20
Marijuana Gateway to Health, 39
Marijuana Policy Project, The, 26, 119, 235
Marijuana Tax Act, 71
Marinol*, 27–28, 27[t]
    approved, 17[t]
    dosing, 215, 216[t], 218
    drug testing, 52
    providing cover, 169
    synthetic, 35
Martin, William, 239
Mathre, Mary Lynn, 15, 26

Mayor's Committee on Marihuana. See La
    Guardia Committee Report
MD Anderson Cancer Center, 204
MDMA, 27[t]
Mechoulam, Raphael
    anandamide, 42
    cannabis science, 41
    endocannabinoid system, 61
    pioneer, 26
    post traumatic stress disorder, 108
    researcher, 119
    scholarly work, 15
    short-term memory, 72
    value of cannabis, 33, 62, 166
medical cannabis, 24, 173
    cards, 7
    federal government, 232–233
    high, 154
    laws, 7, 11, 27
    opiate use, 125
    plants, 197
    properties of, 7
    scientists, 8
    testing facilities, 228
    use, 25
medical cannabis. See also cannabis
Medical Cannabis Institute, The, 105
medical marijuana. See cannabis, medical
    cannabis
medical practitioners, 71
Medicina Britannica, 16[t]
medicine, alternative, 203
Melamede, Robert, 61
memory recovery, 71
meningitis, 64
menses, 16[t]
menstrual cramps, 16
metabolism, 111[t]
methadone, 27[t], 151[t]
methicillin-resistant staphylococcus aureus, 48, 58
Mexican cannabis, 167–168
microbial screen, 179
microbiome, 78
migraines, 9
    cannabis, 111[t]
    endocannabinoid deficiency, 90
    serotonin, 66[t]
    tetrahydrocannabivarin, 52
Mikuriya, Tod, 26, 137
Milagro Oil. See cannabis oil
minerals, 75
Miron, Jeffrey, 23
miscarriage, 165
mold, 175, 177, 177, 178–179
monoacylglycerol lipase, 38–39
mood, 14

adverse, 150[t]
cannabidiol, 102–103
cannabigerol, 52
disorders, 101–103
glutamate, 66[t]
limonene, 57
reactions, 150[t]
morality, 2
Morgan, Celia, 72
Morgan, Piers, 24
morning sickness, 164
motor skill loss, 153[t]
MRSA. See methicillin-resistant staphylococcus aureus
Multidisciplinary Association for Psychedelic Studies, 27, 108–109, 117
multiple sclerosis, 9, 22, 63, 237
acetylcholine, 66[t]
cannabis, 112[t]
central nervous system diseases, 64
delta 9 tetrahydrocannabinol, 45
and Sativex*, 28–29
muscle relaxant, 57
muscle spasticity, 9, 45
myrcene, 57, 84, 89–90, 150[t]
myrcene. See also beta-myrcene
Myss, Caroline, 140
myths, 238–240

N

nabilone. See Cesamet*
nabiximols. See Sativex*
naptha, 196, 198
National Center for National Products Research, 44
National Commission on Marihuana, 17[t]
National Conference of State Legislators, 13
national drug policy, 11, 233
National Epilepsy Foundation, 48
National Institute of Mental Health, 21, 107
National Institute on Alcohol Abuse and Alcoholism, 45
National Institute on Drug Abuse
control of United States medical research, 30, 115–119
research, 109, 115–119, 163, 164, 217
Robert Randall, 21
THC production, 28
National Institutes of Health, The, 42–43, 101, 116
National Organization for the Reform of Marijuana Laws
advocacy, 119, 235
classification, 30
Freedom Card, 12
Guide to Drug Testing, 169
law enforcement, 11

legalization, 27
pioneering, 26
National Survey of Drug Use and Health, 238–239
nausea, 9, 10, 22, 28, 64
Nelson, Willie, 143, 156
nerolidol, 55, 56[t], 58
nerves, 63, 68, 88
nervous system, 57, 62–64
nervous system. See also central nervous system and individual parts of the nervous system
neural repair, 103
neurocognitive performance, 72–73
neurodegeneration, 83, 104
neurodegenerative diseases, 47, 76
neurodegenerative disorders, 103
neurogenesis, 68, 83, 106
neuro-inflammation, 78
neurological disorders, 47
neuromodulation, 66–67
neurons, 66
neuropathic pain, 88, 95
cannabidiol, 48
cannabinoid agents, 89
cannabinoids, 89, 90
delta 9 tetrahydrocannabinol, 45
neuropathy, 9
neuroprotectant, 30
cannabidiol, 48, 50[t]
cannabigerol, 52
cannabis, 9, 64, 68, 71
neurotoxins, 190
neurotransmitters, 42, 66–67
in the brain, 68
in the digestive system, 68
levels, 69–71
modulation, 89
overall health, 71
system, 62
nicotine, 150–151[t]
Nixon, Richard M., 19–21
NORML. See National Organization for the Reform of Marijuana Laws
NORML Guide to Drug Testing, 169
North American Industrial Hemp Council, 14
North Dakota, 13
Northern Lights, 173
Nourished Kitchen, 253
Nourishing Traditions, 253, 255
nugs, 176, 177
nutrition, 249–254

O

Obama, Barack, 24
obesity, 52
obsessive compulsive disorder, 112[t]
ocimene, 55

O'Leary Randall, Alice, 21–22, 26
olive oil, 196, 198, 199
omega-3, 14, 65
omega-6, 14, 65
opiates, 125, 144, 150–151[t]
opioids, 89, 125
Opium, 27[t]
oral mucosal sprays, 204
oranges, 55, 58
Organic Center, The, 252
organic standards, 179
O'Shaughnessy's News Service, 47
O'Shaughnessy's The Journal of Cannabis in
    Clinical Practice, 26, 49, 113[t], 227
O'Shaughnessy, W. B., 15, 16
osteoporosis, 81[t]
overdoses, 95–96
oxidation, 75–77
oxidative damage, 76, 105
oxidative stress, 75–77, 104, 105
Oz, Mehmet, 78

P

Packer, Lester, 76
pain, 16, 84–85, 88, 89–90
    cannabinoids, 87, 89, 90
    dangers of, 124–125, 237
    delta 9 tetrahydrocannabinol, 43, 45
    medication, 144
    musculoskeletal, 22
    myrcene, 57
    perception, 48
    relaxation, 94
    relief from cannabis, 9
palliative care, 101
Palliative Care Plan, 148
pancreas, 84
pancreatitis, 81[t]
panic, 150[t]
parasympathetic nervous system, 63
Parke Davis, 16
Parker, Lewis F., 17[t], 30
Parker, Linda A., 72
Parkinson's disease, 9, 30, 237
    cannabidiol, 47
    cannabis, 112[t]
    central nervous system diseases, 64
    dopamine, 66[t]
    free radicals, 75
    inflammation, 83
    neurodegeneration, 83
patient control, 10
Patients Out of Time, 26, 112[t], 119, 235
PCP, 27[t]
PD. See Parkinson's disease
peripheral nervous system, 63

Perlmutter, David, 78, 84
Peron, Dennis, 26
Peskuski, Kristen, 195–196
pesticides, 178–179
petroleum ether, 198
Pew Research Foundation, 234
phantom limb pain, 9
pharmaceutical companies
    effect of legalization on, 27
    profiting from cannabis, 28–29
    role in prohibition, 18
    synthetic cannabinoids, 28
    use of fingerprinting, 59
pharmaceutical drugs, 10, 35, 162–163, 185
Phoenix Tears. See cannabis oil
Phytalab, 36
PHYTECS, 8
phytocannabinoids, 35, 43–52, 62, 67
    effect on brain, 65–66
    entourage effect, 55
    and pain, 89–90
    synergy with terpenes, 54
phytol, 55, 56[t], 58
phytosterol, 33
pine, 55
pioneers, 25–27
pipe, 186, 191–193
plant cannabinoids, 39–41, 67
PMS. See premenstrual syndrome
PNS. See peripheral nervous system
police. See law enforcement
politics, 117–119
polypharmaceutical herbs, 35
possession, 24
    arrests, 21, 23
    decriminalization, 27
    felony, 10
    legal consequences of, 11, 231–234
    race, 233
    social stigma of, 11
post traumatic stress disorder, 9, 47, 71,
    107–109, 117
potency, 171, 174–176, 178
Potter, Beverly, 155
pregnancy, 163–165
premenstrual syndrome, 9, 66[t]
Prescribed Grass, 104–105
prescription medications, 123–126, 145
Prevention Plan, 143–144
Price, Weston A., 84
pricing, 178
pro-apoptotic, 208
pro-cannabis legislation, 235–236
product quality, 51
pro-inflammatory cytokines, 79, 84
Project CBD, 27, 46, 49, 196

propaganda, 238–240
prostate cancer, 52
protozoan parasites, 58
psoriasis, 81[t]
psychiatric disorders, 66[t]
psychoactivity, 152[t]
psychosis, 160
psychotherapy, 71
PTSD. *See* post traumatic stress disorder
Public Health Service, 116
PubMed, 113[t], 138
pulmonary function, 22
purity, 51

Q
quality, 170–171, 174–177, 197
quality of life, 9
Queen Victoria, 16

R
Raber, Jeffrey C., 171, 210, 225
race, 233
Randall, Robert, 17[t], 21–22, 26
Rather, Rebecca, 278
raw cannabis, 195–196
raw food, 69
raw juice, 184–185
reaction time, 73
Realm of Caring, 25, 47
recipes, 256–295
    cannabis oil, 199
    cannabis tea, 208–209
    ethanolic extraction, 206–207
reclassification, 30, 31
Recovery Plan, 144–145
recreational use, 27, 154
Reefer Madness, 16[t], 18
Reefer Madness: A History of Marijuana, 15
Reiman, Amanda, 26
relaxation, 94, 156
relief, 187, 194–195
reproductive systems, 165
research, 114–120
    cannabinoid acid, 196
    effect of legalization on, 27
    endocannabinoids, 38
    United States, 19, 23, 115–119
    volume of, 31
resensitizing program, 224–225
resin, 188
resin powder, 178, 209
rest, 68
retail markets, 24
retinol conversion, 58
rheumatic diseases, 9
rheumatoid arthritis, 14, 47, 90

Rick Simpson Oil. *See* cannabis oil
Rick Simpson's story, 201–202
right to freedom from pain, 94–95
ring test, 227, 228
risks, 114, 149–154[t]
Robinson, Jo, 252, 255
Romano, Luigi L., 198, 199
RSO. *See* cannabis oil
Run 2 the Cure, 201
Run from the Cure, 201
Russo, Ethan B., 8
    digestive system, 68
    endocannabinoid system, 43
    entourage effect, 55
    history of cannabis, 15
    myrcene, 57
    pain, 89, 90
    pioneer, 26
    research, 117
    Sativex®, 157
    value of cannabis, 99
    women's health, 211

S
safety
    aspirin, 10
    cannabinoids, 100
    cannabis, 8, 10, 20–21, 73, 96, 113–114
    pharmaceutical drugs, 162–163
SAMHSA. *See* Substance Abuse and Mental
    Health Service Administration
Sanchez, Christina, 26, 119
SatiMed, Inc., 51
sativa, 172–173
SatiVera, 51
Sativex®, 45, 185
    classification, 28–29
    dosage, 207, 215
    manufacture, 197–198
    and sleep, 157
    sublingual, 204–205
scarring, 58
Schafer Commission, 17[t], 19–21
Schafer, Raymond P., 19
Schedule I, 27[t]
    appropriateness, 24
    cannabidiol, 197
    history, 17[t], 21, 23
    research, 116
    validity of classification, 115
Schedule II, 17[t], 27[t], 28
Schedule III, 27[t], 28
schizophrenia, 64
Schreiner, Amy M., 72–73
schwag, 177
search warrants, 11

sedative, 50[t], 56[t], 57, 58, 150[t]
seizures, 9, 53, 68, 201
seniors, 160
senses, 156
Sensi Star, 173
sensory neurons, 63
serotonin, 48, 57, 66, 66[t], 83
Sexton, Michelle, 36–37, 207
sexual dysfunction, 66[t]
sexual enhancement, 155–156
shake, 170–171, 177
shame, 153–154[t]
shatter, 188
Shen Neng, 15
Shen Nong Ben Cao Jing, 16[t]
Sherer, Steph, 26
short-term memory, 58, 65–66, 72, 153[t]
Siddhi Tonics, 221
side dish recipes, 286–290
side effects, 10, 100, 114
Simpson, Rick, 198, 201–202
sinsemilla, 170, 172, 177
Sisley, Sue, 109
SLE. See lupus
sleep, 156–157
    and cannabinoids, 90
    disorders, 66[t]
    and inflammation, 82
    myrcene, 57
Sloman, Larry, 12, 15, 18
smell, 174–175, 176
smoke shops, 169
smoking, 150[t], 186, 194
    cherry, 193
SNS. *See* somatic nervous system
social stigma, 3, 11
society, 240
Society of Cannabis Clinicians, The, 27, 104, 105, 113[t], 190
somatic nervous system, 63
sources, 167
spasticity, 64
spent plant material, 171[t]
sperm, 165
spinal cord, 63
spiritual enhancement, 158–159
spiritual practices, 159
sports recovery, 77–78
Squibb, 16
Stanley family, 25, 26
State Industrial Hemp Statutes webpage, 13
Steenstra, Eric, 13
Steep Hill Halent Laboratories of California, 43–44
stimulation, 173
stomach problems, 16

storage, 179–180
strain drain, 174
stress, 85, 94, 101–102
stroke
    cannabis, 112[t]
    central nervous system diseases, 64
    chronic inflammation, 81[t]
    free radicals, 75
    pro-inflammatory cytokines, 79
Stroup, Keith, 26
sublingual applications, 204–205
Substance Abuse and Mental Health Service Administration, 127
Sugiura, T., 42
Sulak, Dustin
    adrenals, 153[t]
    dosing, 207
    endocannabinoid system, 43, 223–225
    first time use, 167
    pioneer, 26
suppliers, 173
Supporting Research into the Therapeutic Role of Marijuana, 22–23
suppositories, 184, 210–214
surgery, 81[t], 144–145
sympathetic nervous system, 63
symptom relief, 3–4
synapses, 66
synergistic effect
    anti-inflammatory agents, 84
    cannabinoids, 51, 175
    myrcene, 57
    terpenoids, 51, 175
synthetic cannabinoids, 28, 62, 65–66

T

tachycardia, 149[t]
talking points, 236–237
Tamisium Extractors, 190
Tashkin, Donald, 132, 133–134
taste, 175–176
tea, 182, 208–209
tea tree, 55
teens, 160–163
terminally ill patients, 25
terpenes, 47, 53–59
    anti-inflammatory agents, 84
    brain health, 67–68
    inflammatory response, 82
    pain, 88
    ratios, 215
    smell, 175
    storage, 179
    synergistic effects, 54, 175
    synergy of, 51
    testing, 228

testing protocols, 226
therapeutic effects, 56[t]
See also terpenoids
terpenoids, 9, 33, 55
content, 170
in medical cannabis, 173
pain, 89–90
terpinolene, 55
testing, 215, 225–229
for cannabinoid content, 170, 226
cannabis, 170
importance of, 174
labs, 178–179, 225–229
microbial screen, 179
for purity, 51
for terpenoid content, 170, 226
testosterone production, 51
tetrahydrocannabinol, 10, 16[t], 25, 37
acetylcholinesterase activity, 105–106
affinity for CB$_1$ receptors, 39
agonist, 42
amyloid B-peptides, 106
analgesic, 50[t]
anti-emetic, 50[t]
anti-inflammatory agent, 84
anti-inflammatory, 10, 50[t]
antioxidant, 50[t]
anti-proliferative, 100
anti-spasmodic, 50[t]
anxiety, 101
appetite stimulant, 50[t]
autism, 51
benefits of, 51
biphasic response, 101, 151[t]
bronchodilator, 50[t]
cancer, 51
cannabidiol ratios, 200
in cannabis, 12–13
cognition, 72–73
depression, 101
effect on brain, 65–66
euphoriant, 50[t]
inflammatory response, 82
lack of in seeds, 14
liver disease, 84
long-term memory, 65–66
in medical cannabis, 173
myrcene, 57
neurodegeneration, 104
pain, 89
post traumatic stress disorder, 108
potency of, 44
short-term memory, 65–66
smell, 175
synergy with cannabidiol, 89
synthetic, 17[t]

tachycardia, 149[t]
tolerance, 191
used separately from cannabidiol, 207–208
See also delta 9 tetrahydrocannabinol
tetrahydrocannabinol acid, 50[t], 208
tetrahydrocannabivarin, 50[t], 52, 84, 89–90
Th1 immune response, 160
THC. *See* tetrahydrocannabinol
THCV. *See* tetrahydrocannabivarin
theanswerpage.com, 139
therapeutic dose range, 216–217
Thomas Jefferson, 12, 15
threshold dosage, 224–225
throat irritation, 150[t]
time, 153[t]
tinctures, 26, 171[t], 182, 204–208
tingling, 152[t]
tinnitus, 66[t]
titration, 191–192, 194–195, 199, 214–223
TNFα. *See* tumor necrosis factor alpha
tobacco, 19, 129–135
tolerance, 189, 191, 223–225
topical applications, 26, 183
Tourette's syndrome, 64, 112[t]
Trainwreck, 173
transdermal applications, 185–186
trauma, 71
traumatic brain injury, 66[t]
treatment program, 203
trichome. See glandular trichome
tuberculosis, 201
tumor necrosis factor alpha, 82

U

ulcerative colitis, 9, 110[t]
Understanding Marijuana: A New Look at the Scientific Evidence, 15
United States
medical cannabis research, 115
usage in, 16[t], 20
United States Government, 115, 217
advocating legalization, 235–236
Attorney General, 29
Congress, 127
denial of medical value, 30
Department of Health and Human Services, 17[t], 30–31, 117
drug policy benefits, 234
hemp oil, 197
nabiximols, 29
National Institute of Health, 119
Office of National Drug Control Policy, 95–96
patents on cannabis, 9, 30, 237
See also United States Patent
position on medical value, 22, 76
prohibition, 21–23

state laws, 232–233
Treasury Department, 16[t], 18
United States Patent, 52, 64, 76
United States Patent and Trademark Office, 29
United States Pharmacopoeia, 15–16, 19
United States v. Leary, 19
University of Mississippi, 117–118
usage tips, 166–169
USP. *See* United States Pharmacopoeia
Utah, 13

V

vaginal suppositories, 211
Van Rixel, Scott, 221
vape pen, 188
vaporizers, 134, 150[t], 187–188, 191–193
Vegetable Glycerin Tincture Recipe, 258
Venice Cookie Co., The, 222[t]
Veterans for Medical Marijuana, 108
viruses, 9
vitamin A-related birth defects, 58
vitamin C, 76
vitamin E, 76
vitamins, 75
Volcano, 187, 187, 193
vomiting, 9, 10, 28, 64
Vote Hemp, 13

W

Waldock, Katherine, 23
WAMM. *See* Wo/Men's Alliance for Medical
Marijuana
Ware, Marc, 119
war on drugs, 19, 21, 23, 231, 239
Washington D.C., 24
wasting
cannabis, 64
Cesamet®, 28
delta 9 tetrahydrocannabinol, 45
HIV, 22
Marinol®, 28
relieved by cannabis, 9
water pipe, 150[t], 191–193
WEED, 24, 25, 47
weight, 178
weight loss, 52
Weil, Andrew, 78
Wenk, Gary, 68, 143, 161–162
Werc Shop, The, 55, 179, 198, 225
Werner, Clint, 39
West Virginia, 13
What Plants Talk About, 54
Wheat Belly, 78
White Berry, 173
White Russian, 173
WHO. *See* World Health Organization

whole plant, 170–172
antioxidants, 76
benefits, 9, 35, 45, 54, 217
cannabis extract, 28
future of, 47
marker for consumption, 52
medicine, 35, 49, 215
therapeutic benefits, 29
Williams, Chris, 232–233
William's story, 91–94
Wilson, Hollis, 153[t]
Wo/Men's Alliance for Medical Marijuana, 25, 46, 166
Woodward, Willliam C., 71
World Health Organization, 29
World War II, 12

Y

Young, Francis L., 17[t], 30

Z

Zelda Therapeutics, 26, 200

Made in the USA
San Bernardino, CA
27 July 2017